Death and Dying
A Reader

Edited by
Sarah Earle, Carol Komaromy and Caroline Bartholomew

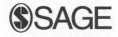

Los Angeles • London • New Delhi • Singapore • Washington DC

The Open University

First published 2009

SAGE Publications Ltd
1 Oliver's Yard
55 City Road
London EC1Y 1SP

SAGE Publications Inc.
2455 Teller Road
Thousand Oaks, California 91320

SAGE Publications India Pvt Ltd
B 1/I 1 Mohan Cooperative Industrial Area
Mathura Road
New Delhi 110 044

SAGE Publications Asia-Pacific Pte Ltd
33 Pekin Street #02-01
Far East Square
Singapore 048763

Library of Congress Control Number: 2008924627

British Library Cataloguing in Publication data

A catalogue record for this book is available from
the British Library

ISBN 978-1-84787-509-9
ISBN 978-1-84787-510-5 (pbk)

Typeset by C&M Digitals (P) Ltd., Chennai, India
Printed and bound in Great Britain by TJ International Ltd, Padstow, Cornwall
Printed on paper from sustainable resources

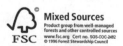

Mixed Sources
Product group from well-managed
forests and other controlled sources
www.fsc.org Cert no. SGS-COC-2482
© 1996 Forest Stewardship Council

Contents

Acknowledgements

Every effort has been made to trace all the copyright holders, but if any have been inadvertently overlooked the publishers will be pleased to make the necessary arrangement at the first opportunity.

Reading 1
From S. Fisher (1973) *Body Consciousness*. London: Calder and Boyars, pp. 147–64 (abridged).

Reading 2
Excerpts from 'The sight and sound of death: The management of dead bodies in residential and nursing homes for older people', Carol Komaromy, *Mortality*, 5(3): 299–315, 2000, Taylor & Francis Ltd. Reprinted by kind permission of the publisher (www.informaworld.com).

Reading 3
Excerpts from 'Foucault and the medicalisation critique' by Deborah Lupton in A. Petersen and R. Bunton (eds), *Foucault, Health and Medicine*, Routledge. Copyright © 1997 Deborah Lupton. Reproduced by permission of Taylor & Francis Books UK.

Reading 4
'Death and the maiden: end-of-life policy in the USA' presented at Making sense of death and dying, 4th Global Conference, 12–14 July 2006, Mansfield College, pp. 2–7. Reproduced by kind permission of the author.

Reading 5
Excerpts from 'The dying soul: Spiritual care at the end of life' by Mark Cobb, Open University Press Copyright © Mark Cobb, 2001, reproduced by kind permission of the author and the Open University Press Publishing Company.

Reading 8
Excerpts from *A Social History of Dying* by Allan Kellehear, copyright © Allan Kellehear 2007, published by Cambridge University Press, reproduced with permission.

Reading 9
Excerpts from 'Quality end-of-life care: A global perspective' by Peter A. Singer and Kerry W. Bowman, *BMC Palliative Care*, 1(4): 3–10.

Reading 11
Excerpts from 'The need to revise assumptions about the end of life: implications for social work practice' by Mercedes Bern-Klug, Charles Gessert and Sarah Forbes, *Health and Social Work*, 26(1): 38–47, incl. Table 3, Copyright © 2001, National Association of Social Workers, Inc., Health & Social Work. Reprinted with permission

Reading 12
Originally published in *The Practising Midwife*, 8(10).

Reading 13
'What is the best way to help caregivers in cancer and palliative care?' by Richard Harding and Irene J. Higginson, *Palliative Medicine*, 17, excerpts from pp. 63–74. Reprinted by kind permission of the publisher and authors.

Reading 16
'The role of the family in patient care' by A.-M. Slowther, *Clinical Ethics*, 2006; 1(4): 191–3. Reproduced by permission of The Royal Society of Medicine Press, London.

Reading 17
Originally published in *Journal of Medical Ethics* (2006), 32: 21–3.

Reading 18
Excerpts from *Critical Moments: Death and Dying in Intensive Care* by Jane E. Seymour, Open University Press, Copyright © Jayne E. Seymour, 2001 reproduced by kind permission of the author and the Open University Press Publishing Company.

Reading 20
'Palliative care and the doctrine of double effect' by Stephen Wilkinson in Dickenson, Johnson, Samson, Katz (eds), *Death, Dying and Bereavement*, 2nd edn. SAGE, 2000, pp. 299–302. Reprinted by kind permission of the publisher and author.

Reading 21
Excerpts from 'Theories of grief: A critical review', by Neil Small in J. Hockey, J. Katz and N. Small (eds), *Grief, Mourning and Death Ritual*, Open University Press, Copyright © Neil Small, 2001. Reproduced by kind permission of the Open University Press Publishing Company.

Reading 22
'In the shadow of the traditional grave' by Leonie Kellaher, David Prendergast and Jenny Hockey, *Mortality*, 10(4), 2005, Taylor & Francis Ltd. Reprinted by kind permission of the publisher and Leonie Kellaher (www.informaworld.com).

Reading 23
Excerpts from 'A voice unheard: Grandparents' grief over children who died of cancer' by Miri Nehari, Dorit Grebler and Amos Toren, *Mortality*, 12(1): 66–78, 2007, Taylor & Francis Ltd, reprinted by kind permission of the publisher and Miri Nehari (Taylor & Francis Ltd., www.informaworld.com).

Reading 26
Excerpts from 'The making of roadside memorials' by Jennifer Clark and Majella Franzman, *Death Studies*, 30: 584–99, 2006, Taylor & Francis, reprinted by kind permission of the publisher and Jennifer Clark (Taylor & Francis, www.informaworld.com).

Reading 27
'Online memorialisation' by Kylie Veale, *Fibreculture*, Issue 3 [extract]. Reprinted by kind permission of the author and journal.

Reading 30
Excerpts from 'Being in, being out, being with: affect and the role of the qualitative researcher in loss and grief research' by Louise Rowling, *Mortality*, 4(2): 167–81, 1999, Taylor & Francis Ltd, reprinted by kind permission of the publisher and author (Taylor & Francis Ltd., www.informaworld.com).

Reading 32
From 'Death does not become us: The absence of death and dying in intellectual disability research' by Stuart Todd, *Gerontological Social Work*, 38: 225–40, 2002, Taylor & Francis, reprinted by kind permission of the publisher and author (Taylor & Francis, www.informaworld.com).

Reading 34
Excerpts from 'Bridging the gap between research and practice in bereavement' by Bridging Work Group, *Death Studies*, 29: 93–122, 2005, Taylor & Francis, reprinted by kind permission of the publisher and Irwin Sandler (Taylor & Francis, www.informaworld.com).

An Introduction to Death and Dying

Sarah Earle, Carol Komaromy and Caroline Batholomew

This book, which brings together a collection of classic and contemporary writing in the field of death and dying, draws on a wide range of disciplines and perspectives. The book is organised into five discrete sections exploring: the meaning of death, caring at the end of life, moral and ethical dilemmas, grief and bereavement, and researching death, dying and bereavement. However, each part of the book, and the contributions within them, also explore overlapping themes and issues.

Part I focuses on the ways in which death can be conceptualised and understood. The readings draw on a range of disciplines to examine the meaning of death, for example, the first reading takes a psychological approach to explore the way in which children make sense of death. Other readings in Part I use sociological perspectives to examine how the dead body can become a source of meaning and what that meaning might be. For example, one reading examines the role of the body in the management of the boundary between life and death while another reflects on the body as a site of power and resistance. Other readings explore the meaning of death from a spiritual perspective or from the perspective of diverse religious traditions. The final reading in Part I uses a combined epidemiological and demographic approach to explore changes in death over time and reflects on how a global perspective can enrich understandings of the meaning of death.

In Part II attention turns to the issue of caring at the end of life and focuses on the roles of individuals, organisations and systems – and the relationships between them. The first pair of readings examine care at the end of life within a global context, exploring issues of social deprivation and public health. The next contribution – drawing on an ethnographic study of dying and death in care homes for older people – considers how the period of dying is defined and the impact of this diagnosis on end-of-life care. The remaining readings in this part of the book discuss the role of professional caregivers, such as social workers and, focusing specifically on the management of emotions, on the role of midwives at the end of life. These readings also consider the role of families and other informal caregivers and the relationships between these and formal caregivers.

Making sense of moral and ethical dilemmas is also vital to developing an understanding of death and dying in practice. Part III begins by exploring moral theory and considers the question: 'what is ethics?' The remaining selection of readings examine a range of moral and ethical issues such as the role of the family in patient care and – focusing specifically on children – the principle of respect for autonomy. Consideration is also given to sociological approaches to moral and ethical decision making in two readings which focus on withdrawal of treatment in intensive care, and brain death. The final contribution to Part III examines the doctrine of double effect, and concludes with a discussion on euthanasia.

In Part IV the focus is on grief, bereavement and post-death ritual. This part begins with a brief critical overview of theories of grief, before moving on to explore the subject of disposal and the modern practice of cremation. The next selection of readings focus specifically on bereavement. Here, attention is given to the experiences of grandparents and children and one reading focuses specifically on the facilitation of bereavement for survivors of genocide. Moving on from the subject of bereavement, the final contributions in Part IV explore the issue of memorialisation. The growing global phenomenon of road-side memorialisation and the increasingly popular practice of online memorialisation are explored.

There is a growing body of research on and about death, dying and bereavement. The final part of this book explores some of the issues which arise when carrying out research in this field and contributions challenge some of the assumptions that underpin the possible dangers inherent in conducting research at the end of life and with bereaved people. The readings explore whether death, dying and bereavement are taboo and the implications for research with dying people perceived as vulnerable. Some readings examine the role and emotional needs of the researcher, as well as those who are the subjects of research. Drawing on empirical research, other contributions explore the experiences of young people living with HIV, researching people with intellectual disabilities and the subject of reproductive loss. The final reading in this part of the book focuses on the relevance of practice for research and the role of research in practice at the end of life.

The collection of readings in this book – some of which have been especially commissioned for this volume – is not exhaustive and, of course, there are many other interesting and relevant readings which we, as editors, would have liked to include had there been more space. Although the purpose of this book is not to provide a comprehensive digest of the literature in the field, it is intended to be thought-provoking, encouraging critical thinking on the subject of death and dying; we hope you enjoy reading it.

Part I

Understanding Death

Introduction

Carol Komaromy

The focus of this first part of the book is on the meaning of death. The opening reading by Seymour Fisher takes a psychological approach to the way that children make sense of death through what he calls, 'the motionless body'. The author argues that the body is read for signs of life and it is this stillness that marks an absence of life for young children. Furthermore, the essence of comprehension lies in the body that does not move and is entirely passive. It is this passive body that is later confined in a coffin and put into the ground that transforms the dead body into a symbol of death and something to be feared. While he argues that older children are able to grasp aspects of the inevitability and permanence of death, he explores how the interplay between reality and the irrational part of the psyche remains an enduring tension into adulthood. He argues further that it is this latter irrationality that provides a coping mechanism beyond childhood into adulthood (Readings 17, 24 and 31 also focus on children and young people).

In the second reading, the focus shifts from a psychological to a sociological approach to ways in which death is understood. Carol Komaromy uses empirical data collected through participant observations of death and dying in care homes for older people, to explore how the sight of the dead body is concealed within such institutional settings. Her observations revealed that the sight of death, even when temporally close to residents who were themselves approaching the end of life, was something that the staff tried to conceal. By contrast, the sounds of death were not concealed, although they appeared to be ignored or not acknowledged by care staff and residents. She concludes that this apparent contradiction in the denial of death in settings where death is a regular occurrence is a performance of visual conceal-ment that serves as one of several strategies deployed to manage the dead body at the boundary between life and death. Furthermore, it is at this boundary where the need for rituals is most likely to be played out and consequently, the dead body becomes invested with meanings that translate it into degrees of taboo and unsight-liness (also see Reading 10).

In Reading 3, Deborah Lupton continues with the theme of the body as the site in which of the meaning of death is translated. The focus is not on death but on the role of medical power, and she uses Foucault and a critique of the medicali-sation of the body to offer competing explanations for the way that power is played out in the sick (and dying) body. She argues that Foucault's move away from the simplistic interpretation of the dominance of doctors' medical power over the bod-ies of their patients offers a more persuasive interpretation of power. However, even allowing for Foucault's notion of resistance, her own research suggests that rather than being passively produced as medicalised bodies, patients occupy a more active role within a relationship with their doctors. Furthermore, this rela-tionship with its emotional and psychodynamic dimensions is one of mutual dependence. These ideas echo those of the collaborative enterprise of conceal-ment of death discussed in the second reading.

In the next reading, the focus remains on the body as Regis A. DeSilva explores end-of-life decision making in the US. He uses the example of three young white women with diagnoses of persistent vegetative state or brain death to show how technological changes have produced the possibility of different forms of existence (for further discussion of brain death see Reading 19). These bodies became the site of medical, legal and media scrutiny and this public attention was central to legal and clinical end-of-life decisions in the US. The media attention that was drawn to the fate of these women highlighted how different forms of interpretation were articulated. DeSilva argues that occupying the space between life and death and in which life and death can be simultaneously observed, the female body is open to many myth-ical interpretations. The author uses the ideas of Baudrillard to interpret this *other* state of life that has been technologically created and which then creates a fertile base for fear and fantasy. He argues, for example, that the mythical representation of these 'sleeping beauties' plays into the iconography of the female body in Western and Eastern cultures and provides examples of such mythical stories.

In the next two readings the emphasis shifts from the theme of the dead and dying body as a site of interpretation of the meaning of death to consider beliefs about what happens after death. The reading by Mark Cobb provides a thorough exploration of the need for spiritual care at the end of life. Much of this reading focuses on spiritual care as an essential part of end-of-life care and the author provides a strong rationale for the need for spiritual care. Not least because it is at the moment of death that people attempt to make sense of life by questioning the meaning of their own life and whether or not they will cease to exist. Cobb argues that one of the ways in which this spiritual dimension is expressed is through ritual and he draws on anthropological arguments and some examples to support this point. Underpinning these ideas is the question that philosophers have asked for centuries about the possibility of an existence that is not an embodied one. This reading leads well into the clearly defined beliefs about an afterlife, which is the focus of the next contribution.

David Webster questions what life after death means in religious traditions and how this might impact upon an understanding of the process of dying. The author describes the different faiths of Judaism, Christianity, Islam, Hinduism and Buddhism as representative of major religious traditions and suggests that while they offer a diverse range of beliefs about life after death, what they share is the belief in death as a transition. He concludes that a belief in an afterlife, while not eradicating fear, offers religious people the possibility of standing on the threshold of death with a degree of hope.

In the final reading, Cathy E. Lloyd uses an epidemiological and demographic approach to illustrate changes in death over time, as well as highlighting the way that divisions in society are continually reflected in mortality statistics. She covers distinctions between and within developing and developed countries, changes in the cause of death over time and how mortality statistics continue to show a direct correlation between poverty and deprivation and reduced life expectancy. However, this reading cautions against simplistic data interpretation and teases out some of the problems with data collection and its impact on the quality of findings. Despite problems such as restrictions on being able to compare like with like and the absence of meaningful data for some developing countries, this global view of death provides a different interpretation of the meaning of death and one in which social inequality and injustice are impossible to ignore.

1

Motionless Body

Seymour Fisher

It may not be a coincidence that the two things we keep most secret from our children are birth and death. Somehow, we do not want them to be directly confronted with how they were created or how they will be extinguished. Perhaps the beginning and the end are linked in their common reference to the fact that there are boundaries to the state of being alive. There is a time of body existence and a time of body non-existence. To master the fear generated by this bare statement has strained the ingenuity of every known society. To witness death is to know that your own body is vulnerable to death. If someone else's body can become nothing, so can your own. An amazing repertory of strategies has been developed across the world to buffer this recognition. Elaborate myths have been invented that portray death as only temporary and leading to rebirth in a new and marvelous place. [...] The illusion that death does not exist is enhanced by the declining death rate and the consequent decrease in the frequency with which unpredictable casualties occur in any individual family. Another way of hiding death is to segregate the elderly into institutions and hospitals where their dying will be out of sight. Those most potentially ripe for dying are assigned cubicles in places where only specialized nursing personnel are likely to have much contact with them, and there are smooth, well worked-out procedures for disposing of their remains as unobtrusively as possible. The banishment of death is also reinforced by the siren-like promises of science that it will soon be able to master the major diseases and ailments. There is a half-belief, widely accepted, that soon all serious defects of the body will be repairable. If so, death can be put off – for a long, long-time. There is the implication that death will no longer be obligatory. It will be quasi-accidental. Or it will be due to carelessness and neglect. Presumably, people do not have to die if they avoid cholesterol, refrain from smoking, see their physicians regularly, fill up on the right vitamins, and so forth. When all else fails, you can always get a heart transplant or a renal dialysis. If death can be conceptualized as avoidable and subject to the control of omnipotent science, it becomes psychologically more distant. It is less a fact of personal inevitability and more the concern of a vast intellectual apparatus. Of course, in that sense the defense pattern is not so different from religious strategies that instruct the individual that his death is programmed by God and when it occurs will be a meaningful part of a vast game plan.

Motionless Body, Body Consciousness by Seymour Fisher, Calder & Boyars, 1973, excerpts fom pp. 147–64 plus references. Reproduced by kind permission of Eve Fisher Whitmore.

It should be noted that while there is less *direct* contact with death in our society than there used to be, indirect confrontation has been many times multiplied. An evening of television viewing brings more messages about death in a few hours than most people previously had to absorb in a month. After the news broadcast that gives the box score, for the entire world, of the more spectacular deaths of the day (due to floods, crashes, wars, concentration camps, and self-immolation), there usually follow a succession of dramatic programs that average several deaths each. The evening closes with another news summary of the latest mayhem. This process is duplicated in various ways in radio broadcasts, newspapers, and popular magazines. Each of us is bombarded almost hour by hour by images of death. Sometimes, as on television, the images are vivid, bloody pictures. But these encounters differ from those of a past time because they are largely impersonal. They involve people we have never met. They are quantitatively great but personally distant. Perhaps we learn to defend against them so well that they have little influence on our fantasies and behavior. But I doubt this. I read an anecdote in which a teacher talked about the reactions of a group of young children to the news that John Kennedy had been assassinated. She poignantly described one child who lay down on the floor, closed his eyes, and pretended to be dead (refusing to speak) for a long period of time. This child was obviously captured and moved by the image of death he had received in the day's news. It is likely that many others are equally moved, although they do not show their feelings so openly and dramatically. But even as I make this point, I would not argue that the impersonal death messages from television compare in intensity with those you get from actually being in the presence of the corpse. This is often brought home to the medical student when he begins to become acquainted with the cadaver assigned to him. He discovers that this brand of closeness to death is powerful stuff. He not infrequently goes through a period of being upset, has bad dreams, and experiences strange and puzzling sensations. If you will introspect about your own feelings the last time you attended a funeral you will be able to empathize with the adaptation required of the medical student.

[…]

How do children become aware of death? How do they incorporate it into their concept of their own bodies and of the world in general? Empirical studies demonstrate (Anthony, 1940; Piaget, 1929) that up to the age of five the average child has only hazy notions about it. He has difficulty at first in even distinguishing the animate from the inanimate. Anything that moves seems alive to him. He has trouble in deciding whether or not a candle flame is alive because of its dancing movements. When something is motionless it can be classified as not living or dead. Gradually, the child witnesses phenomena that educate him about life versus death, but it is difficult for him to comprehend the idea that death is a natural or final thing. He thinks of death as primarily due to accident or disease or violence. It is not inevitable and it is reversible. He assumes that things that die can, by suitable manipulation, be brought back to life. To die is somewhat like going to sleep. You can be re-awakened. This, of course, is the basic concept that most cultures have tried to maintain in their myths and religious systems. The idea that the dead can be revived in some form is a return to the child's original view of it all. Up to the age of nine interpretatious of death remain magical and unreal. Dying is attributed to arbitrary actions by evil things or people. According to some, it is also especially likely to be tied in with matters of anger and fantasies of desertion. That is, people die because they want to go away or get rid of you. It is only around the age of nine that the child seems to crystallize the adult concept that death is part of a natural impersonal cycle.

[…]

While it may be true that the child arrives at a fairly adult concept of death by the age of nine, there is also good evidence that he retains many irrational and half-baked ideas about it throughout his life-time. All sorts of irrational feelings may feed into his attitudes toward it. One that should be spelled out relates to separation anxiety. People differ in how disturbed they become when separated from the people important to them. […] With this perspective, it has been proposed that fear of death is maximized in those who are most alarmed about being alone and the possibility of losing relationships. They are so frightened by death because it conveys the possibility of losing those important to them, either through the others' death or through their own.

[…]

In time of danger some animals mimic death. They try to convince the predator that they are not worth attacking. Children, too, imitate the dead when they are playing. They may fascinatedly try out 'dead' postures.

[…]

If someone dies whom you know well, the reality of death is brought home with a vividness that is unique. You are suddenly unable to dodge the facts and must digest their implications with regard to your own career. Soldiers on the battle-field, who are called upon to live intimately and repeatedly with death, not infrequently become highly disturbed, even when those who perish are relative strangers. They have their noses rubbed in death, and they become hyperaware of its implications for their own existence.

Aside from the idea of dissolution and non-existence, what is there about the image of death that is so difficult to endure? I wonder if one of the basic elements of unpleasantness does not derive from something that has been found to be prominent in the young child's definition of death. He tends to equate death with a body that does *not move*, and when he imitates death it is the posture of being motionless that is central. If he moves a muscle, his playmates 'shoot' him again. It is the idea that your dead body will cease to have the potentiality for voluntary intention that may be most disconcerting. This idea conjures up a picture of passivity that our entire adult career has been dedicated to preventing. To be a respected personage in the world you have to show that you can do things. You have to show that you can reach out and have an effect on your environs. You must have a certain minimum capability of taking care of yourself. Not to be capable of self-care means that you are reduced to the helpless child who cannot provide his own food and who is even incapable of controlling his body sphincters. The motionless body could also be the dirty body that fouls itself with its own feces and urine. For a man, the motionless body may be one that shamefully cannot defend itself against attack. It becomes the cowardly body. For a woman, the motionless body may signify shameful exposure to sexual indignities. She may equate inability to act with a surrender to sexual looseness. The specter standing behind death may be indecent helplessness.

Death carries with it the notion of confined space. The corpse is put into a box, which in turn is tightly squeezed into the earth. The motionless body could not move even if it were magically revived. In almost every culture there are fearful tales about being accidentally buried alive. A surefire way for a horror story to arouse distress is to describe the struggles of a victim who awakens to find himself buried in a casket. Death means being put into a compartment barely big enough to hold you. The claustrophobic reactions of many when they enter an elevator or go into a small basement room may be incited in part by the death implications of putting one's body into such a small chunk of space. The metaphorical similarity to the casket may be too intense to tolerate. […]

In everyday life how do we go about reassuring ourselves that we are safe from death? What other things do we do besides avoiding contact with the dying and clinging to religious belief that assure us of immortality?

Each of us manufactures a chain of realistic and semimagical procedures for safeguarding our health and preventing potentially life-threatening illness.

[…]

It is informative and amusing to analyze the properties that we assign to our after-death selves. Probably the most typical of the post-burial forms is the ghost. The ghost lacks solidity. It is gaseous, without weight, and capable of moving freely through matter. Walls and barriers cannot stop it. But at the same time it retains recognizable human shape. It can even speak with its former live voice, although a few eerie overtones are added. The most novel thing about the ghost is the interpenetrating way in which it interacts. It lacks firmness or palpability, but all other objects also lack the firmness to keep it out. In other words, the ghost is an image of a 'body' that is not terribly different from a real one, except for the way in which it can merge with, and flow through, other objects. We are so accustomed to the ghost concept that we do not realize what a unique attribute this 'merging' and 'flowing through' represents. While at one level it may merely symbolize the idea of nonexistence, I wonder if it does not represent a widely cherished and secret body-image fantasy. In our ghost myth we are able to create a version of the body that can magically do something we ordinarily cannot but wish we could. The ghost body can become part of anything else. No object can ward it off when it wishes entry. This paradigm sounds familiar. It is the core of the concept of symbiosis. It is an abstract statement of how the very early relationship between child and mother is often pictured. Presumably, the child initially feels fused with the mother. He can tap into her body whenever he pleases (by sucking the breast), and she also taps into his in the process of caring for it. All through the early years the psychological attitude is maintained that the child's body and those of his parents are permeable to each other. Dependence and symbiosis tend to foster fantasies of interconnection that defy the usual laws of object separation. The ghost is a symbol of super symbiosis and in that sense may reveal a fundamental belief that death leads to a reinstatement of what was true in the early days of contact with one's mother. There are related ideas implicit in religious myths about the dead merging with God.

It has been pointed out that death marks off a limit to your life. No other factor so decisively declares that your existence is anchored in flesh and blood. You can't really outlast your body. I think insufficient attention has been given to the democratizing implications of this fact. No matter how glorious the fame of any person in the culture, both he and others are aware that there will be an end to it all. He will ultimately prove to be composed of the same materials as the average citizen.

[…]

References

Anthony, S. (1940). *The Child's Discovery of Death.* New York: Harcourt Brace Jovanovich, Inc.
Piaget, J. (1929). *The Child's Conception of the World.* New York: Harcourt Brace Jovanovich, Inc.

2

The Sight and Sound of Death: The Management of Dead Bodies in Residential and Nursing Homes for Older People

Carol Komaromy

[…]

In residential and nursing homes for older people death and dying is a regular event. Between one-sixth and a third of the population of homes will die each year (Sidell *et al.,* 1997). […] Several studies have highlighted the tension between 'living' and dying in residential care. Hockey (1990) talked about the creation of drying spaces in an attempt to separate 'living' residents from those who were dying, and a small study by Shemmings (1996) points out the need for staff of residential homes to recognize the reality of death and dying as the first step in being able to give better care to dying residents.

[…] Like Ariès (1981), I would argue that contemporary society places dying people in institutional settings away from the public gaze, but the question remains as to why death is hidden *within* institutions. Synott (1993) claims that, 'In every culture the dead body is treated with respect and with ceremony; and the body remains the symbol of the self' (p. 33). Yet, as Hallam *et al.* (1999) argue, the corpse is also a taboo object, 'it is the antithesis of the living body within a society where "life" and "death" are understood to stand in dichotomous relationship to one another' (p. 126). Thus, if the living body stands for attractiveness and well-being, its opposite number, the corpse, stands for disorder and decay. The process is also reiterative in that the management of bodies affects the meanings given to them. Further, the meanings attributed to the corpse are derived from a variety of social, personal, cultural and existential sources. As a result dead bodies not only represent death but also continue to represent the living person. Particularly in institutions, the way the dead are treated also reflects the treatment of living inmates. However, the body after death is much more than the

Excerpts from 'The sight and sound of death: The management of dead bodies in residential and nursing homes for older people', Carol Komaromy, *Mortality*, 5(3): 299–315, 2000, Taylor & Francis Ltd. Reprinted by kind permission of the publisher (www.informaworld.com).

representation of the living person. Occupying the space between life and death it is a powerful symbol of the particular beliefs which surround death.

What is clear from this brief introduction is that the dead body has the potential to represent a multiplicity of phenomena, all of which have to be managed by people who come into contact with death.

The data for this paper were collected as part of a large study into the management of death and dying in residential and nursing homes in England, commissioned by the Department of Health.

[…]

The following account conveys not just the events of death at that time, but also some of the emotions carried forward from that experience. It was at this time, before I was socialized into a professional role, that I first noticed and questioned why the sight but not the sound of death was concealed even though the sounds were extremely audible.

Professional experience of concealment of death in a hospital

In the early 1960s death in hospital seemed to be a taboo. Although a regular event, even in my experience at that time, the discussion of death was limited to staff mealtimes in the hospital canteen or in the ward sluice, where all body fluids were disposed of, including staff tears.

The first death I witnessed was that of a woman of 80, when I was a 16-year-old cadet nurse working on a medical ward for the first time. Although she was expected to die, her death was still a shock to all the ward staff, because it was sudden: one minute she was talking and the next she was dead. When the hospital porters collected her body to take it to the morgue, they were performing one of their least favourite tasks, which they called 'snatching a body'. My ears still resound with the thud of her body hitting the hospital's metal mortuary trolley. A hinged metal lid enclosing the corpse rang out the fullness of the coffin as it was closed. Even porters who tried hard to *place* bodies inside the metal trolley could not disguise the thud as the unresisting body collapsed noisily into it.

When a patient died, surviving ward patients were not told what was happening and questions were not invited. The screens were pulled around the beds of living patients, side room doors were closed and all ambulant non-medical people were stopped and placed out of sight of the departing corpse. In order that the body could be moved, living people were stopped in their tracks. Silence descended on the ward. The busy and obvious concealment of the dead body left patients and visitors listening acutely for clues. The porters waited outside the ward until a nurse signalled that it was 'safe' to enter, that is, no-one had visual access to what was about to take place. The patients heard a noisy trolley whose metal substance was announced by its rattling crescendo. The dull sound of heavy body hitting metal left no-one in doubt about what had transpired. The creaking, closing lid confirmed the death. The sound of the 'chariot of death', as it was known, rattling down the ward severed as an unmusical requiem.

After the removal of the body, the 'theatrical' opening of the screens revealed what I experienced as the spectacle of an empty, hideous bright orange mattress, signifying not a successful home discharge, but a warning of the reality that not everyone is saved and that perhaps no-one is safe. Patients and nurses colluded in the silence as the bed was made up ready for the next patient, someone who would be kept in ignorance of the fate of its last occupant.

These events therefore seemed to involve a collusion which required the key actors to resist asking questions which could produce answers that were difficult to deal with. It is as if the formal knowledge acquired through verbal or visual evidence makes the event real and therefore undeniable. Privately we may suspect the 'truth', but only when it is confirmed socially are we no longer able to deny it. This is reflected in the concealment of the sight of death. Despite all the aural information, those who had not actually seen the corpse had not faced death – and everyone involved could act as if death had not happened. From this experience there appeared to be two levels of silence; one produced by not talking about the event of death and one resulting from an unwillingness to acknowledge the sounds being made.

[…]

Theoretical context

Douglas (1966) describes how the body is dangerous, not only because the boundaries of the body are at risk of being breached by corporeal dirt, but also because the body is a container of death. The danger of spilling its contents is more intense, says Douglas, because the body has breached the metaphorical boundary between life and death. This further increases the need for containment and concealment of the body. Douglas' notion of the body as a container of death (1996) is echoed by Leder (1990), who describes the corpse as implicitly residing inside the living body. Death is a constantly approaching future, but one at which we as living bodies cannot arrive since, as he claims, we can never be conscious of our own death. But the body immediately after death is more than death embodied, it has an ambiguity that is also temporal, in that yesterday it was alive and today it is dead. This was shown in responses to the 80-year-old female patient who was talking one minute and dead the next, described in the account of my experience as a nurse. This simultaneous representation of both dead and living persons is contingent upon time. Bodies are translated into representations and the transformation that takes place confers a taboo status upon the dead. Heads of homes argue that to confront residents with a dead body confirms the fact that the reality of death is close to them in time. It seems that a spatial presentation of the physical reality would make the temporal closeness too real and painful.

[…]

My observations in homes revealed that when a death occurred there was a hierarchy of unsightliness.

In descending order of preferred visibility, the body contained in the coffin is at its most dignified and eminently viewable. Seeing a deceased person's body immediately after death is the next most acceptable form of visible death, and relatives and a few residents were invited by the person in charge of the home to view the body. Regardless of whether or not bodies were viewed, most staff talked about the need to make the body presentable, as the following quote from the written procedure in Oak Trees voluntary residential home illustrates:

> The resident should be washed and dressed in his or her own night-clothes. Dentures should be left in and hair combed.

The head of Beeches home described the transformation of the body of a particular resident who had died using terms which suggest the importance of the resident looking good after death:

> I made sure her teeth were in and put her wig on and made her look nice – a little cushion under her chin, the covers up over the cushion, not over the face, and she looked so peaceful, she really looked so much younger, yes – it was really lovely.

The following example from a code of practice in Rose Tree home further illustrates the point:

- Remove the pillows from the bed.
- Straighten the body and lay it gently flat.
- Leave the body for at least an hour (the hour of repose).
- Make sure the body is clean, nails clean and hair combed.

These are formal procedures but they are complemented by more implicitly understood sets of practices which are nonetheless crucial for successful management of the 'resource' of the dead body. In *The Civilising Process* Elias (1994) traces what he calls the 'layered patterning of behaviour in society that both shapes and creates taboos around pleasures and prohibitions' (p. 519). This creation, he claims, is in response to fear and anxieties that exist in different societies and historical periods. We have constructed rituals not only around what we can be permitted to see and hear but also around what we can *admit* to having seen.

Although the unsightliness of the corpse can therefore, in part, be overcome through washing and positioning the body, it still remains difficult visual evidence of the event of a death.

[…]

From both the interview and the observational data it would seem that the body is in its most taboo state when it is a corpse *and* during the period surrounding its removal from the home. Data suggest that the movement of the body makes real the liminality of its status. In some homes the body's exit was concealed from other residents even though it was taken out of the front door. In the remaining homes, which constitute the majority, the body was taken out of the nearest exit to reduce the chances of the removal being witnessed. In homes where the body had to be taken out through a public area because of the layout, staff did their best to conceal its removal, as this head of Eventide home said:

> We try to arrange to do it at a time when there aren't many residents around. I think it can be a little bit distressing for them.

The head of Bracken home told me: 'Usually, we have a back entrance, usually that way, quite private.'

[...]

In sum, the reality of death appears to have most impact when it is represented by the sight of a dead body leaving the home but less impact in the sight of a resident after death for [...] in some of these homes residents did say good-bye to their housemates after death. The protection of the residents who live in the home from the sight of a departing corpse appears to contradict a frequently expressed belief by most home staff that residents who are very old are more accepting of death (Komaromy and Hockey, 2001). Home staff frequently stated that residents accepted death because they had seen so much death during their long lives. Also they were at an age where they expected to die, and others expected them to do so. The evidence suggests that there are several problems with these explanations.

First, staff represent residents as institutionalized into a homogeneous group who all share the same life experiences, responses and expectations. Communal life, however, does not construct a communal identity. Taking into account the fact that interviews invite people to give generalized responses, during the observation in the homes and informal conversations, I found that staff constructed two main categories of residents: the collective resident group who followed general behaviour rules, and those who could be called individual exceptions to the general behaviour rules. As a result, therefore, a resident called James who died during a period of observation in one of the case study homes was described as someone who was 'afraid of death', unlike the other residents in the home who were 'used to death'.

Second, the staff's perception of the dead body as unsightly and something to protect their charges from, places residents in the position of passive beings in need of protection and contradicts their competing assertions that residents are strong enough to face and accept their own imminent mortality. The way in which the majority of staff told me that they protected their residents from the sight of the body leaving the home therefore suggests that they invest the corpse with an intrinsically distressing or frightening quality. One head of home explained the need to protect residents from the sight of the corpse leaving the home: 'We don't want to stuff it [death] under their noses.'

In contrast with staff's constructions of 'their' residents' need for protection, residents themselves sometimes made determined efforts to gain visual access to 'the reality of death' as embodied in the corpse in transit. Thus, the secrecy with which bodies are taken out of the homes could require a lot of devious cunning on the part of the staff to outwit the gaze of some residents. In Raffles home, during a colleague's observations, residents struggled to see what it was they were being protected from by attempting to look behind staff who were shielding the glass door while a corpse was being removed.

From this evidence it seems that the sight of the departing body is taboo in hospitals and homes alike. Death as the failure of biomedical supremacy and death as a natural event, occurring at the end of a long life and produced by home staff as a good death, are both equally unseeable in their embodied forms.

[...]

In most homes the staff conferred the status of something unbearable and unseeable on to the corpse, even though unmistakable sounds indicated that the body was being borne away. Staff and funeral directors collude in conferring a dangerous status onto the body by covering the corpse with sheets or placing them into thick, black plastic bags. These covered up, enclosed bodies represent death in the form of a tightly wrapped corpse. The person who has died becomes a concealed shape, no longer recognizable as a person, but transformed into a corpse. The object-like status conferred on the ageing body finds its most complete expression in this form.

[…]

The sounds of death

Closing doors, moving lifts, squeaking trolley wheels, approaching and departing hearses, all announce the departure of the corpse. Sounds do not have physical boundaries and sounds escape even soundproof rooms. It is only possible to conceal sounds with other sounds, but home staff made no attempt to do this. Instead the staff managed the sounds with verbal silence about death. The sounds of the removal of the bodies from homes, even through public spaces, were ignored and this lack of acknowledgement served to deny the sounds and became part of the silence about the departing corpse. By denying the sight of death it was assumed that residents could not legitimately discuss the sound. In everyday life, conversations behind closed doors are signalled as private conversations, unlike those heard in public spaces. To discuss an overheard conversation openly would be taboo. Likewise, the noises of departure of the corpse, with exposes the cover-up, have been constructed as non-hearable sounds. In this process death is being more than privatized, it is being ritualistically ignored in that what residents and patients are not permitted to see, they have to pretend not to have heard.

[…]

It would appear that, rather than attempting completely to conceal the fact of death, professionals who dispose of the dead are more concerned with their *performance* of concealment. This performance demonstrates that the staff feel compassion for what they perceive to be the residents' fears of the reality of death. Just as Howarth (1996) describes funeral directors' concerns with the 'visual effect', so the staff of homes enact a compassionate performance which spares the residents the harsh reality of facing death. After all, no-one is fooled, and many residents do take part in the collusion of silence surrounding the removal of dead residents from their homes. If death is not talked about or is done so in hushed tones, residents pick up a strong signal that they are not permitted to discuss the death.

[…]

I found that the residents I talked to were very much affected by deaths in the home. Flora, a resident of Orange House, a large residential home, told me tearfully about the death of a resident with whom she had become a friend:

When they told me I was upset and cried. It was silly of me, but I felt so sad. They thought they'd upset me and didn't mention it again, so I didn't know when the funeral was. Not only was I unable to go, but I couldn't, I couldn't send flowers. And I still miss her. I still feel sad.

[...]

Not making any effort to conceal the sound of death suggests that it is not the fact of death that is being denied, but more its visibility and everything which that represents and is made to represent. It is a performance of care and concern for residents' feeling which is both incomplete and also in contradiction with staff's expressed belief that residents are reconciled to the imminence of death.

Conclusion

[I have] posed the question of why the sight and not the sound of death is concealed from the residents of residential and nursing homes. My explanation is threefold. First, the performance of the concealment of the sight of death is of paramount importance as a formal and informal aspect of procedures at the time of death. I have therefore argued that a ritualized performance takes place in residential and nursing homes when a resident dies and that this is focused on the dead body, itself invested with many attributes. [...] Not just the management of the death itself but also the transformation of the body into a corpse and the removal of that corpse from the home require a performance in which there is a hierarchy of unsightliness which requires degrees of concealment. Whether it is at its least or most viewable, the non-performing dead body is ascribed with the power to produce a highly ritualized set of performances in others, mostly the home staff, supported by a cast of relatives, residents and ancillary and visiting staff who participate with varying degrees of collusion. [...]

Second, the primacy of vision over sound means that staff prevent the residents from 'facing' death in the literal sense but cannot deny the event itself. The lack of concealment of the sound of death reinforces the idea that it is less important to conceal the actual event of a death from living residents than for staff to perform the act of concealment. The privileging of sight over sound scripts this performance and this is where the preoccupation with visual concealment lies. This privilege has a traceable history to the Enlightenment and the latter's influence over the management of death remains powerful.

Finally, home staff draw upon institutional hierarchies to distance themselves from the difficult boundary between life and death and in this drama their ears have been stopped by a ritual which conceals the gap between reality and the meanings invested in death. The performance is a professional strategy which enables staff to manage the boundary between life and death and, as a performance, is a charade in which words are either not spoken or are delivered quietly.

References

Ariès, P. (1981). *The hour of death*. London: Allen Lane.

Douglas, M. (1966). *Purity and danger: an analysis of concepts of pollution and taboo*. London: Routledge.

Elias, N. (1994). *The civilising process*. Oxford: Blackwell.

Hallam, E., Hockey, J. and Howarth, G. (1999). *Beyond the body: death and social identity*. London: Routledge.

Hockey, J. (1990). *Experiences of death*. Edinburgh: Edinburgh University Press.

Howarth, G. (1996). *Last rites: The work of the modern funeral director*. Amityville: Baywood Publishing.

Komaromy, C. and Hockey, J. (2001). Naturalising death among older adults in residential care. In J. Hockey, J. Katz and N. Small (Eds) *Grief, mourning and death ritual*. Buckingham: Open University.

Leder, D. (1990). *The absent body*. Chicago, IL: University of Chicago Press.

Shemmings, Y. (1996). *Death, dying and residential care*. Aldershot: Avebury.

Sidell, M., Katz, J. and Komaromy, C. (1997). Death and dying in residential and nursing homes for older people: examining the case for palliative care. Unpublished report, Department of Health, London, UK.

Synott, A. (1993). *The body social: symbolism, self and society*. London: Routledge.

3

Foucault and the Medicalisation Critique

Deborah Lupton

[...]

The medicalisation critique was one of the most dominant perspectives in the sociology of health and illness in the 1970s and into the 1980s. It remain[ed] a dominant approach in the 1990s, particularly for feminist writers, those critics who still adhere to a Marxist perspective on health and illness and proponents of the consumerist approach to medicine. There is no doubt that the medicalisation critique represented an important shift in thinking among medical sociologists in calling attention to the possibility for inequity in medical encounters and the delivery of health care. Nonetheless, the critique may itself be criticised on a number of grounds. One major difficulty with the orthodox medicalisation critique is its rather black-and-white portrayal of Western medicine as largely detracting from rather than improving people's health status, of doctors as intent on increasing their power over their patients rather than seeking to help them, and of patients as largely helpless, passive and disempowered, their agency crushed beneath the might of the medical profession. Indeed, in much of this literature, 'The asymmetry of the relationship is exaggerated to the point that the lay client becomes not the beneficiary but the *victim* of the consultation' (Atkinson 1995: 33, original emphasis).

In their efforts to denounce medicine and to represent doctors as oppressive forces, orthodox critics tend to display little recognition of the ways that it may contribute to good health, the relief of pain and the recovery from illness, or the value that many people understandably place on these outcomes. They also fail to acknowledge the ambivalent nature of the feelings and opinions that many people have in relation to medicine, or the ways that patients willingly participate in medical dominance and may indeed seek 'medicalisation'. As de Swaan has pointed out, the power of the professions to make judgements about normality must involve complicity on the part of their clients, students, charges or patients. This complicity inevitably incorporates latent conflict and resistances, 'a shifting balance between manifest collaboration and tacit opposition in the relations between those who come for help and those who profess to provide it' (de Swaan 1990: 1). Rather than there being a struggle for power between the dominant party (doctors) and the less powerful party (patients), there is collusion between the two to reproduce medical dominance.

Excerpts from 'Foucault and the medicalisation critique' by Deborah Lupton in A. Petersen and R. Bunton (eds), *Foucault, Health and Medicine,* Routledge. Copyright © 1997 Deborah Lupton. Reproduced by permission of Taylor & Francis Books UK

Foucault and medicalisation

The gradual entry of Foucault's writings into Anglophone medical sociology over the past fifteen years or so (albeit more so in Australia and Britain than in North America) has also challenged some of the central assumptions of the orthodox medicalisation critique, particularly in relation to its conceptulisation of power and medical knowledge. Foucault's writings emphasise the positive and productive rather than the repressive nature of power. Indeed, Foucault argued, the very seductiveness of power in modern societies is that it is productive rather than simply confining:

> what makes power hold good, what makes it accepted, it simply the fact that it doesn't only weigh on us a force that says no, but that it traverses and produces things, it induces pleasure, forms knowledge, produces discourse. It needs to be considered as a productive network which runs through the whole social body, much more than as a negative instance whose function is repression.
>
> (Foucault 1984a: 61)

[...]

From the Foucauldian perspective, power as it operates in the medical encounter is a disciplinary power that provides guidelines about how patients should understand, regulate and experience their bodies. The central strategies of disciplinary power are observation, examination, measurement and the comparison of individuals against an established norm, bringing them into a field of visibility. It is exercised not primarily through direct coercion or violence (although it must be emphasised that these strategies are still used from time to time), but rather through persuading its subjects that certain ways of behaving and thinking are appropriate for them. The power that doctors have in relation to patients, therefore, might be thought of as a facilitating capacity or resource, a means of bringing into being the subjects 'doctor' and 'patients' and the phenomenon of the patient's 'illness'. From this perspective, doctors are not considered to be 'figures of domination', but rather 'links in a set of power relations', 'people through whom power passe[s] or who are important in the field of power relations' (Foucault 1984b: 247). Unlike those who assert the orthodox medicalisation critique, a Foucauldian perspective argues, therefore, that it is impossible to remove power from members of the medical profession and hand it over to patients. Power is not a possession of particular social groups, but is relational, a strategy which is invested in and transmitted through all social groups. This more complex view of power goes some way to recognising the collusive nature of power relations in relation to medicine.

Another important dimension of the Foucauldian understanding of power in the medical context is an emphasis on the dispersed nature of power, its lack of a central political rationale. Proponents of the orthodox medicalisation thesis tend to view members of the medical profession as consciously seeking to gain power and status and limit other groups' power, largely by eliciting the state's support. In contrast, Foucauldian scholars tend to argue that the clinical gaze is not intentional in terms of originating from a particular type of group seeking domination over others. There is not a single medicine but a series of loosely linked assemblages, each with different rationalities (Osborne 1994: 42). Foucault and his followers have emphasised that the fields and concerns of medicine are diverse and heterogeneous, taking place at sites such as workplaces, schools, supermarkets and homes as well as the clinic, hospital or surgery. The state is, of course, involved in the reproduction of medical dominance, including regulating the conditions for the licensing of medical practitioners, but there are also other agencies and institutions involved beyond the state, and indeed the interests of the medical profession and those of the state often clash. (This can be seen in the continual battles between doctors' lobby groups such as the Australian Medical Association and the government ministers who hold the responsibility for the administration of health portfolios.)

[...]

Medicalisation is evident in the ways in which warnings about health risks have become common events. People are constantly urged to conduct their everyday lives in order to avoid potential disease or early death. As a result, 'Sociologically speaking, everyone lives under the medical regime, a light regime for those who are not yet patients, stricter according to how dependent on doctors one becomes' (de Swaan 1990: 57). This is particularly the case for older people and the chronically ill, in relation to improvements in longevity and medical treatment for acute illnesses. Where once, for instance, physical activity might have been undertaken for the purposes of 'character formation', 'experiencing nature' or 'the pleasure of functioning', it is now often understood as a medical activity, undertaken for the purposes of good health (de Swaan 1990: 59).

[...]

Foucault himself was careful of emphasise frequently that where there is power there are always resistances, for power inevitably creates and works through resistance. He acknowledged that the existence of strategies of power does not necessarily correspond with the successful exertion of power, and that intended outcomes often fail to materialise because disciplinary strategies break down or fail. This is as true of the practice of medicine as of any other field of power. As May has stated in relation to the medical context, there is 'a massive array of practical problems which actors operating in medical (and other) settings encounter as they attempt to monitor subjects' (1992: 486; see also Porter 1996). Rather than being interested in power as an ideology, as is the concern of Marxist critiques, Foucault commented in an interview that he was interested in 'the question of the body and the effects of power on it' (Foucault 1980: 58). Frustratingly enough, however, Foucault's concept of resistance was never really explained in detail. Instead, he made various somewhat elliptical comments about the interrelationship of power, embodiment and resistance, such as the statement: 'Power, after investing itself in the body, finds itself exposed to counter-attack in the same body' (Foucault 1980: 56).

[...]

In Foucault's later work, such as volume three of *The History of Sexuality* (1986), he began to move away form the notion of power as operating on individuals via dominating institutions to speculate on the modes of the formation of personhood, or, as he termed it, the technology or practices of the self. As he commented in an interview,

> Perhaps I've insisted too much on the technology of domination and power. I am more and more interested in the interaction between oneself and others and in the

technologies of individual domination, the history of how an individual acts upon himself [sic], in the technology of self. (1988: 146)

[...]

Sociological accounts often fail to acknowledge the interpersonal aspects of the medical encounter, the mutual dependencies that doctors and patients have upon each other and the emotions and desires that motivate behaviour. In my own recent empirical research using interviews with both lay people and medical practitioners in Sydney (see Lupton 1997), the data suggested that the medical encounter involves a continual negotiation of power that is contingent upon the context in which the patient interacts with the doctor. Such factors as the type of medical complaint, the age, ethnicity and gender of the patient and doctor, emotional dimensions and the patient's accumulated embodied experiences all shaped the encounter in diverse ways. In their interviews, patients said that at times they sought to dominate their doctor, to adopt explicitly consumerist positions, sometimes directly expressing hostility and anger. At other times, they were apparently quite happy to give themselves over to the doctor without question. Indeed, this study found that the majority of lay people interviewed continued to want to invest their trust and faith in their doctor, and welcomed the doctor showing an interest in their lives, including their personal lives. For those people who had experienced serious illness or hospitalisation, it was vital that they felt they could rely upon their doctors. This investment of trust and faith, however, is also problematic for many people, because it means relinquishing some degree of autonomy, allowing oneself to become dependent upon another and exposing one's body, feelings and innermost thoughts to another. In the relationship between carer and cared-for, there is a continual tension on the part of the cared-for between wanting and appreciating care and resenting it (Fox 1995; Lupton 1997).

Foucault's notion of the practices of the self can be brought into play to analyse the ways that people respond to the medical encounter. The doctor–patient relationship is a central site at which subjugated knowledges and the practices of the self play a major role in the interrelation of institutional and localised power. When consulting a doctor, individuals may, on at least some occasions, and if they so choose, attempt to struggle against, challenge or subvert those disciplinary techniques they experience as restricting of their autonomy. That patients often fail to take 'doctors' orders' is evident in the extensive medical literature on the problem of patient compliance with medical regimens. On the other hand, those individuals who 'go along' with medical advice need not necessarily be viewed as passively accepting the orders of the doctor or the medical gaze, but rather could be seen as engaging in practices of the self that they consider are vital to their own well-being and freedom from discomfort or pain. As the above research suggests, individuals may constitute themselves as ideal-type 'consumers' as part of the presentation of the self as an autonomous, reflexive individual who refuses to take a passive, orthodox patient role. Alternatively they may present themselves as someone who 'follows doctor's orders', who is a 'good patient', working actively in the medical encounter to achieve this. Sometimes they may pursue both types of subject position simultaneously or variously. In each case, the individual has a personal, emotional investment in presenting her- or himself in a certain manner, as a certain 'type of person' engaged in 'rational' and 'civilized' behaviour consonant with her or his social or embodied position at the time.

[...]

Conclusion

Given the complexities that have been raised by the Foucauldian critique, it may seem difficult to take a position on the issue of 'medicalisation'. I would argue, however, that the awareness of these difficulties is itself an important outcome that has emerged from the entrée of Foucauldian perspectives into the debate. One possibility I have identified in furthering the insights offered by Foucauldian perspectives is taking up Foucault's later interest in the practices of the self and engaging in a phenomenological analysis of the experiences people have in the context of medical care. Neither the orthodox medicalisation critique nor the Foucauldian perspective has adequately taken account of the mutual dependencies and the emotional and psychodynamic dimensions of the medical encounter, preferring to rely upon a notion of the rational actor. Yet, as I argued, a recognition of the 'irrational' and contradictory aspects of the relationship that lay people have with members of the medical profession goes some way to explaining why it is that 'power, after investing itself in the body, finds itself exposed to a counter-attack in the same body'. It remains for scholars and researchers to devote more attention to the ways that the discourses on the human body, medicine and health care that may be identified in such sites as the mass media, medical and public health literature and policy documents are recognised, ignored, contested, translated and transformed in the context of everyday experience.

Acknowledgement

This chapter was written as part of series of papers emerging from a study on patients' and medical practitioners' views on the medical profession and the coverage of the medical profession in the mass media funded by a large grant from the Australian Research Council in 1994–5.

References

Atkinson, P. (1995) *Medical Talk and Medical Work*, London: Sage.

de Swaan, A. (1990) *The Management of Normality: Critical Essays in Health and Welfare*, London: Routledge.

Foucault, M. (1980) 'Body/power', in C. Gordon (ed.) *Power/Knowledge: Selected Interviews and Other Writings, 1972–1977*, New York: Pantheon.

Foucault, M. (1984a) 'Truth and power', in P. Rabinow (ed.) *The Foucault Reader*, New York: Panthenon.

Foucault, M. (1984b) 'Space, Knowledge, and power', in P. Rabinow (ed.) *The Foucault Reader*, New York: Panthenon.

Foucault, M. (1986) *The Care of the Self: Volume 3 of the History of Sexuality*, New York: Panthenon.

Foucault, M. (1988) 'The political technology of individuals', in L. H. Martin, H. Gutman and P. H. Hutton (eds) *Technologies of the Self: A Seminar with Michel Foucault*, London: Tavistock.

Fox, N. (1995) 'Postmodern perspectives on care: the vigil and the gift', *Critical Social Policy*, 15, 44/5: 107–25.

Lupton, D. (1997) '"Your life in their hands": trust in the medical encounter', in V. James and J. Gabe (eds) *Health and the Sociology of Emotion*, Oxford: Blackwell Publishers.

May, C. (1992) 'Nursing work, nurses' knowledge, and the subjectification of the patient', *Sociology of Health & Illness*, 14, 4: 472–87.

Osborne, T. (1994) 'On anti-medicine and clinical reason', in C. Jones and R. Porter (eds) *Reassessing Foucault: Power, Medicine and the Body*, London: Routledge.

Porter, S. (1996) 'Contra-Foucault: soldiers, nurses and power', *Sociology*, 30, 1: 59–78.

4

End-of-Life Legislation in the United States and the Semiotics of the Female Body

Regis A. DeSilva

She bestows the idea. And the idea withdraws, becomes transcendent, inaccessible, seductive. It beckons from afar ... The dream of death begins. It is woman.

Jacques Derrida

Introduction

Until thirty years ago, death was largely a matter between the patient and the physician. Since then, end-of-life care has become rather more complex and clinical decision-making has undergone significant changes. End-of-life decisions now involve lengthy, and sometimes contentious, discussions with families with legal disputes, and the involvement of ethics committees, state regulators and public advocacy groups. In the United States, three end-of-life cases resulted in litigation that reached the Supreme Court, and with a major impact on how clinical care is rendered. All three cases involved young white women and in all cases there were protracted legal proceedings. There were escalating levels of public involvement, legal action and media attention with each subsequent case. These cases raise questions about the hidden role young white women play in American society and in the public imagination. In an analysis of these cases, I will draw on the possible roles symbolism, semiotics and mythology play in making public policy at the end-of-life.

The clinical challenge

The primary reason for the complex situation at the end-of-life is the development of life-sustaining technologies within the last fifty years. Before the advent of new technologies death occurred rapidly during critical illnesses.

'Death and the maiden: End-of-life legislation and the semiotics of the female body' presented at 'Making sense of death and dying, 4th Global Conference', 9–12 July 2007, Mansfield College, Oxford, United Kingdom. Reproduced by kind permission of the author.

In the United States, more than half of all people die in a hospital, often in the intensive care unit, and the trend in Western Europe is similar. Due to technological advances, the space (caesura) between life and death has been increasing, as shown in Figure 4.1.

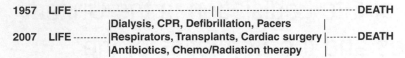

```
1957   LIFE --------------------------------------||--------------------------------------- DEATH
                     |Dialysis, CPR, Defibrillation, Pacers        |
       2007   LIFE ----------|Respirators, Transplants, Cardiac surgery|--------DEATH
                     |Antibiotics, Chemo/Radiation therapy         |
```

*A caesura is a pause denoted by the sign "| |" in Latin and Greek poetry

CPR = Cardiopulmonary resuscitation

Figure 4.1   The growing space (caesura*) between Life and Death

This space, the caesura, has been gradually expanding as new technologies and complex new drug protocols allow longer life spans. Some of these key technologies are well known, such as CPR, electrical defibrillation, artificial ventilation, pacemakers and chemotherapy for cancer and HIV. Thus, several intermediate states in the border between life and death are now recognized ranging from completely reversible coma and temporary respirator-dependent life support, to mild brain damage, to severe brain damage, to irreversible brain death. The clinical challenge is to determine the diagnostic category into which a particular patient should be placed so that the appropriate level of care can be delivered judiciously. The most difficult problem is to determine the neurological status of the person in order to make an assessment not only of the current state, but also to prognosticate the possibility of a sapient existence in the future. Unfortunately, what Derrida called the 'gift of death' (*donner la mort*) is no longer as common in Western society as it once was before, unless someone dies suddenly from an accident or a heart attack.

The clinical and legal arguments I will discuss here centre on three cases in women in their twenties and thirties who were rendered unconscious, one by a combination of alcohol and drugs, one in a motor accident and one that was of unknown cause. All three cases were litigated in the courts before a final decision regarding their disposition could be made.

Case law in the United States

The three cases that determine how we deal with irreversible brain injury leading to persistent vegetative state (PVS) will be summarized.

Case 1: Karen Ann Quinlan was the first modern icon of the right-to-die debate. The 21-year-old Quinlan collapsed at a party after swallowing alcohol and the tranquilizer diazepam (*Valium*) on 14 April 1975. Doctors saved her life, but she suffered brain damage and lapsed into a persistent vegetative state. Her family waged a much-publicized legal battle for the right to remove her life support. However, Quinlan kept breathing spontaneously for 10 years after the respirator was terminated. She remained in a coma in a New Jersey nursing home until she died in 1985.

Case 2: In 1983, 25-year-old Nancy Cruzan's car went off the road in Missouri. She was thrown from the car, sustaining severe head injury aggravated by anoxia as she did not breathe for 15 minutes. After 5 years in a persistent vegetative state, the family accepted the fact she would not recover and began a very public battle to terminate feeding and hydration. The US Supreme Court agreed to hear its first right-to-life case and Nancy Cruzan's was argued on December 6th, 1989 and decided on June 25th, 1990. In a 5–4 decision, they declined to allow termination of feeding and hydration. The Cruzan family experienced threats and underwent a public battering by activists who were enraged that they would seek to terminate her life in what was deemed an inhumane manner tantamount to murder. The Cruzan's attorney took the case back to the Missouri Supreme Court and this court reversed the original decision. The court recognized a right to refuse treatment under the common law doctrine of informed consent. It appeared that Nancy had told a roommate that she would not wish to continue her life unless she could live at least a halfway normal life. Her gravestone has 3 dates on it: Born July 20, 1957 / Departed January 11, 1983 / At Peace December 26, 1990.

Case 3: Terri Schiavo (December 3, 1962–March 31, 2005) was a Florida resident and at the age of 26 collapsed at home from cardiorespiratory arrest. She remained in a coma for 10 weeks and within 3 years was diagnosed as being in a persistent vegetative state. In 1998, her husband and guardian, Michael Schiavo, petitioned the courts to remove her feeding tube. Her parents opposed this move, but the courts found for her husband that she was in a PVS and that she should not be kept alive. Between 2003 and 2005, the case received constant and escalating media attention with 14 appeals, numerous hearings in the state courts and 5 suits in Federal District Court. The Florida Legislature intervened and a law to 'protect' Schiavo was struck down by the Florida Supreme Court. Terri Schiavo's case was similar to Cruzan's case, but evoked a far greater national outrage than Cruzan on both sides of the aisle. Moreover, there was widespread international coverage by the media on an unprecedented scale for such a case.

The Baudrillard critique

The philosopher Jean Baudrillard views technology as extensions of the human body. Thus, telescopes and microscopes are viewed as extensions of the eyes, vehicles extensions of human locomotion, and so forth. Similarly, we can view some forms of medical technology as extensions of vital internal functions of the body. The respirator is an extension of the lungs, pacemakers are extensions of the heart, and dialysis machines are extensions of the kidney. There are two differences between the kinds of technology to which Baudruillard makes reference and medical technology. First, medical instruments are intimately and physically connected to internal and life-sustaining functions of the body. Second, unlike other appliances and instruments that extend the normal external functions of the human body, these life-sustaining forms of technology create legal and ethical problems regarding discontinuation if the body becomes incapable of supporting independent existence.

A second and unrelated notion from Baudrillard is the concept of *simulation,* which is the creation of what is real through a conceptual or mythological model, or a *simulacrum.* These models, often based on images in the media and related to technology, then become the determinants of our perception of reality. In Baudrillard's critique, such idealized images provided by the media create a blurring of the boundaries between the generated image and reality. He views American society as being excessively technological and postmodern, where consciousness interacts with reality so that it fails to distinguish reality from fantasy, so creating a condition of '*hyperreality*'.

In my view, especially in the intensive care unit, the proximity of technology to living humans creates a simulation that becomes a *simulacrum* of a person in a state of life that borders on death, so that both life and death are paradoxically represented in the same person. These contrasting images of life and near-death thus accentuates the sense of 'hyperreality'. I am taking Baudrillard's discourse further in the use of technology in medicine as such technology can create two very different kinds of simulacra of a person which will be developed more fully below.

The patient in the hard drive

As described above, an unconscious person attached to both small and large pieces of technology such as oxygen masks, nasal cannulae, respirators, balloon and infusion pumps, external pacemakers, tracking computers, blood pressure monitors and oxygen sensors creates a simulacrum that provides a different kind of reality than the one we usually associate with a free-living human being. This simulacrum is a physical representation of all the invisible vital functions of a person that is now visually displayed in color on a screen. The person becomes, in effect, a *hyperreal* object that embodies both life and death.

A second kind of 'virtual' or technological simulacrum that is invisible to the casual bedside observer is created for each patient by the construction of an extensive digital database in the form of blood chemistry and hemodynamic data, X-ray, CT and MRI/MRA images, and a digitized written record of historical and demographic information in the hard drive of a computer. Such a database that can be rapidly accessed by a trained observer creates a physiological embodiment or simulacrum that represents a 'virtual' patient. What happens in reality is that this simulacrum in the computer becomes the 'patient in the hard drive'. This simulacrum, unlike the first, is accessible only to the caregivers and is hidden from other observers. A corollary of this development, for better or for worse, is that in both unconscious and conscious patients, we have arrived at a situation where the physician does not need to interact with the patient to treat him or her. Any aberration in laboratory values or the images on the screen of an organ system is subject to treatment, often without any physical contact or interaction with the living patient. The difference between the physician's simulacrum and the lay person's view of the patient is that the former model sees the patient in detached terms and as an inert substrate that is defective, needing corrective remedies.

Role of the media

What role does the media play in the creation of reality and hyperreality in end-of-life situations, and how is it relevant to these three cases? A corollary phenomenon related to excessive media attention to women merits comment. The US media – and television in particular – is obsessed with missing white women. The phenomenon has been dubbed the 'Missing White Woman Syndrome' or the 'Missing Pretty Girl Syndrome' by the media. Though the US population is roughly 50 per cent male and 35 per cent non-white, there is a preponderance of reports regarding the abduction, murder and disappearance of white women and white female children. Most of the women are below the age of 40 or young girls or teenagers, and they are often blonde and attractive. At present, this phenomenon is somewhat commoner in the US than in other Western countries.

Typically, TV coverage consists of nightly repetitions of images and videos of the victim over weeks and months, accompanied by analyses and comments by media savvy lawyers, ex-prosecutors and ex-judges, psychologists, pathologists and other 'experts', as well as family members and friends. In some cases, even suspects are interviewed and interrogated in the public arena. The Internet has added to and amplified the discourse. In some cases, friends and families set up websites dedicated to the victim to post messages, appeals, condolences, pictures and videos. In other cases, so-called 'fans' post their own websites though the subject may have been dead for years, as in the case of The Black Dahlia (Elizabeth Short) who was brutally mutilated and murdered in Los Angeles in 1947. These sites often solicit funds and use it to attract the attention of the media to draw and sustain attention to the case. A self-perpetuating cycle is thus set up to feed the vicarious participation of the public.

In many cases, accusations of negligence of the police and lack of protection by the legal system are made by family members. This situation often leads to protective laws being promulgated that are named for the female victim and/or a child, e.g. Amber's Law, Megan's Law, Jessica's Law, Laci and Connor's Law. The last of these laws, officially known as the Unborn Victims of Violence Act of 2004 (Public Law 108-212) is of particular interest and relates to the murder of Laci Peterson who was 8 months pregnant when she disappeared in December 2002. Several months later, her body and that of a newborn male infant were found separately washed up in the San Francisco bay area. Her husband Scott Peterson was found guilty and sentenced to death by lethal injection, but his case is on appeal as of this writing. This law defines the violence against a pregnant woman as two distinct crimes, one against the woman and one against the unborn child. Thus, this law also recognizes the fetus as a distinct person subject to legal protection.

It would seem logical to assume that public and media attention is focused on some of these missing young women, not only because they are young and attractive, but also because there is a prurient interest in their sexual histories. (However, in some cases, such as Laci Peterson, there was no suspicion of sexual assault.) In all these cases, the women were of childbearing age, or potentially childbearing in the future. Laci Peterson's was pregnant, and the subtext in all of these cases may be the subconscious emphasis on female fertility.

It should be borne in mind that immediately proximate to the media frenzy that accompanied the Schiavo case, the cases of Laci Peterson and Natalee Holloway (who disappeared in Aruba in May 2005 after allegedly being picked up by three youths in a bar) were constantly in the news. Prior to these events, there was the still-ongoing media preoccupation with the case of JonBenet Ramsey, a child beauty pageant 'star' found murdered at the age of 6 in 1996, strangled and possibly sexually assaulted. She and other little girls in the US are promoted by their mothers as little princesses at beauty pageants around the country. The grotesque pictures of her with a ligature around her neck are posted on the Internet along with the autopsy report and a television interview on CNN with her parents.

Is this a peculiarly American phenomenon? While the media, in the form of Hollywood films, television, and videos posted on the Internet, have a greater presence in American society, Europe has long seen a preoccupation with the death and sexuality of young white women. There is an extensive literature in folklore and fairy tales extending back to the eighteenth and nineteenth centuries on this topic. Two of the most famous events in European history, much publicized in the media and the subject of several films, both occurred in 1889, and were murder-suicides of young women at the hands of their lovers.

Elvira Madigan, aged 22, eloped with her married lover, a Swedish cavalry officer, who eventually murdered her in Denmark and then killed himself. The other murder was that of the 18-year-old Maria Vetsera at the royal hunting lodge at Mayerling, by the Crown Prince Rudolf, heir to the Habsburg throne, who also shot himself. The public's imagination has been so captivated by the deaths of these two young women for over a hundred years, that a total of 5 films, a few television documentaries and a ballet by Sir Kenneth MacMillan called *Mayerling,* have been produced in the past few decades based on their deaths.

In her excellent book *Lustmord: Sexual Murder in Weimar Germany*, the eminent German scholar at Harvard, Maria Tatar, describes the preoccupation of male lust with female sexuality and murder. She describes an extensive literature from Weimar Germany to the present, with drawings and paintings of that depict the twin themes of sexuality and death in her analysis of cases of sexual murder that aroused wide public interest. Male artists, such as George Grosz openly identified with sexual murderers. He posed as Jack the Ripper in a photograph, creeping up to stab a woman from behind with a knife, the model being his future wife. Tatar suggests the representation of murdered women in visual and literary works functions as a strategy for managing social and sexual anxieties. Tartar also speculates that violence against women can be linked to the trauma of war, to urbanization, and to the politics of cultural production and women's reproductive potential.

Perhaps the most dramatic case of the preoccupation with the idea of the 'White Princess' is the case of Diana, Princess of Wales. The media attention to her death in Paris in 1997 was unprecedented in worldwide coverage and the outpouring of grief, particularly in the United Kingdom. Ten years later, several books, TV specials and commemorations are being held. In June 2007, one TV channel in the UK refused to censor pictures of her taken at the time of her death. The powerful impact that women like Diana have on the public imagination is demonstrated by a study which showed that suicide rates and deliberate self-harm in the UK increased significantly in the three months following her death, particularly in younger females (Hawton et al. 2000). It is likely that the viewing of certain kinds of charged images in repetitive news cycles has negative emotional impacts that are not fully understood.

I believe that in the three cases I have cited above, constant media attention predisposed the public to a situation of *moral panic*. This condition is a mass movement based on an exaggerated and false perception that a certain subculture poses a threat to societal values and interests. In the case of Schiavo, there were opposing forces in the form of right-to-life and the right-to-death movements. There was also the opposition of religious and secular worldviews. Such a moral panic results when the media, causing an increasing spiral of reportage, amplifies a singular event so that the event is transformed into a nationwide concern that goes beyond the event itself. The legal system, the legislature and public activist groups become involved, and new rules and laws are rapidly promulgated. Cohen (2002) has suggested that moral panics (in criminal acts) usually result from what he called a *deviancy amplification spiral*. However, such amplification may also result from legal acts that appear to be morally repugnant, as in the Schiavo case. In the extreme case of Terri Schiavo, the matter went to the Supreme Court of Florida, and then to the Supreme Court of the United States, which refused to hear the case. The US Congress met in late night sessions to debate this one case passionately and it was broadcast live on C-SPAN, a public service cable television channel. The *dénouement* was that President Bush flew from Texas to Washington to sign a special law in the middle of the night, allegedly to protect her right to life. The real intention here was later revealed to be related to the anti-abortion stance of the conservative movement in the US.

In the Cruzan and Schiavo cases, there was a sense of outrage that the medical profession and some family members were callous and disdainful of the right-to-life in coming to the judgment that Nancy Cruzan and Terri Schiavo were not capable of independent existence and therefore needed to have their lives terminated. The right-to-life movement also saw this as an opportunity to conflate arguments about the end-of-life with the beginning of life, to legitimize an anti-abortion stance. In that sense, the Schiavo case gave this movement an opportunity to publicize the value of life at both extremes of life, in order to gain political capital.

The female body in Western culture: woman as a semiotic object

John Locke states in *An Essay Concerning Human Understanding* that there are three divisions to the sciences: (1) *Physica* (2) *Practica* (*praktike*) and (3) *Semeiotike*. We can apply this classification to medical science, as the science and the art of medicine have physical, practical and semiotic aspects. As a physician, Locke understood the interrelationship between these three components. Furthermore, in the *Essay* he also defines the Lockean 'self' as 'the conscious thinking thing' which is self-aware and self-reflective. The key issue here is that the notion of personal identity is rooted in consciousness, and it is the loss of self-awareness with severe brain damage that alters the notion of the self.

In medical practice, patients report '*symptoms*' which are invisible to the observer. During the physical examination, the physician elicits or uncovers '*signs*' that point to a possible diagnosis. In a majority of cases, a preliminary diagnosis of a disease process can often be assessed by evaluating symptoms and signs. Clinical tests often prove the original diagnosis that has already been made and thus, tests are often chiefly of supportive value to validate the diagnosis. Medical technology therefore plays a smaller role in diagnosis than is commonly supposed.

In a comatose patient, however, symptoms are absent, and the only major *sign* available for interpretation – especially by the lay person – is the observation that the person is unconscious and thus, unresponsive. In this situation, a variety of advanced tests are needed to make a diagnosis and track progress of treatment as the patient is unable to give direct feedback. The horror of the situation in an intensive care unit is that the person is connected to snaking pipes, tubes, intravenous lines, tubes, wires attached to sensors, monitors, pumps and computers, and a hissing respirator, all of which seem to spell death. The glass enclosure of the intensive care unit is a simulacrum of a transparent casket. This visual and auditory scenario then becomes the predominant sign on which much interpretation is based.

Caregivers obtain a large amount of observational data (*signs*) and technical data from comatose patients that have to be decoded and interpreted to allow decision-making. The technical data cannot be separated from the fact that the receiver must *decode* the data, i.e. be able to distinguish the data that are *salient* and make meaning out of it. The process of converting signs into meaning (*semiosis*) is different for physicians and the public. Thus, the unconscious state has different connotations for the two groups, so that interpretation is dependent on the observer.

The iconography of the female body is well established in both Western and Eastern cultures. Barthes (1972) connects semiotics and myth, calling them second-order signs, or *significations*. Such *significations* may be seen by laypersons to represent something else, other than what it means to the caregivers. In the case of women, it is likely that there is a connection between the 'sleeping' woman and the many cultural myths that connect death and the seductive image of a recumbent woman. This idea is not new as it extends back to the ancient world. In Greek mythology, sleep, dreams and death are interconnected: Hypnos, the god of Sleep, is the brother of Thanatos, the god of Death, and father of Morpheus, the god of Dreams. Hades, the god of the Dead, abducts the virgin Persephone while she was celebrating her menarche with her mother Demeter and her three sisters. Hades is Demeter's brother, but he abducts Persephone and takes her away to the Underworld. After much negotiation by her mother, Persephone is allowed periodic returns to the living world. On her return to earth, spring blossoms, summer follows and when she disappears into the Underworld, winter sets in.

The Grimms' fairy tales, *Snow White and the Seven Dwarfs* and *The Sleeping Beauty* are stories that deal with fair, beautiful women who die and are revived by the intercession of others (Bettelheim 1976, Tatar 2003). In the case of a temporarily dead Snow White, the dwarfs pull out a poisoned comb to revive her. She then goes into a 'sleeping death' by eating a poisoned apple and is rescued from this state by the intercession of a prince who takes her away in a glass coffin. A jolt of his carriage dislodges the poisoned apple that had killed her and was still lodged in her throat. The Sleeping Beauty's story is more complex. After she falls down dead, she is visited by a Prince who falls in love with her and his kiss revives her. In the Giambattista Basile variant *Sun, Moon and Talia*, Talia is visited by a married King who impregnates her. She gives birth to a son and daughter nine months later and is awakened when one of the infants sucks her finger and removes the piece of flax that caused her death. In all these stories, the woman is only 'temporarily' dead and awaits some magical intercession to revive her. In the modern version of these stories, the recumbent beautiful young white woman lies unconscious, awaiting the kiss of technology to awaken her.

Public policy and the hidden role of women

In this discussion, the three white women I described have unwittingly played a role in shaping public policy. It is difficult to describe the tremendous outpouring of public support played out day after day for months in the press and on television for Terri Schiavo's parents, the Schindlers, who sought to prevent the termination of her life by withdrawing feeding. The estranged husband was vilified and demonized for asking for withdrawal of life support, which he ultimately succeeded in obtaining. There were also battles between and amongst the professions, both legal and medical, and against state and federal legislatures.

Bronfen's critique of woman as a privileged commodity within Western culture, in the Levi-Strauss model, is that there is ambivalence about the act of exchange where a body is transformed into a sign (Bronfen 1993). Women are both valued for their fertility and reproductive capacity and for the survival of the species. But they are also feared and reviled by both men and other women for their sexuality and allegedly predatory and destructive behaviour. In Bronfen's view, the death of a beautiful woman emerges as a requirement for the preservation of existing cultural norms and values and as a focus for debating such cultural norms. It is in this context that we must view the protracted legal battles of the three women discussed in this analysis. The fate of a dying young woman seems to draw on our deepest anxieties and fears about life, sexuality and death. To some extent, the reason why this phenomenon is seen more often in American society than in

European societies may lie in the greater and more pervasive role of the visual media in the US, and in the political machinations that capitalize on societal fears to further political careers and agendas. In the three cases described, in the end, however, it was the medical and legal opinions that prevailed, albeit after protracted social distress over the fates of these young women. And in the process, there was a complex interplay of primitive fears, modern technology, and the iconography of the female body. As Debord has described in *Society of the Spectacle,* there is an 'unconscious history' that builds and modifies the conditions of human existence and survival. In order to understand structuralist categories in the social sciences, these categories express forms as well as conditions of existence that shape the outcome of complex events at the end of life.

Acknowledgements

The author thanks Maria Tatar, Helen Mountfield, Sarah Stillman and Cara Moulton for their discussions, insights and help. I also thank Dr Rob Fisher who allowed the work to be presented in its present form.

References

Barthes, Roland. *Mythologies* (translated by Annette Lavers). Jonathan Cape, London, 1957.
Baudrillard, Jean. *Symbolic Exchange and Death* (translated by I. H. Grant). SAGE Publications, London, 1993.
Baudrillard, Jean. *Simulacra and Simulation* (translated by S. F. Glaser). University of Michigan Press, Ann Arbor, Michigan, 1994.
Bettelheim, Bruno. *The Uses of Enchantment: The Meaning and Importance of Fairy Tales,* Knopf, New York, 1976.
Bronfen, Elizabeth. *Over Her Dead Body: Death, Femininity and the Aesthetic,* Routledge, New York, 1993.
Brooks-Rose, Charlotte. 'Woman as a semiotic object', in *The Female Body in Western Culture,* Susan R. Suleiman, ed. Harvard University Press, Cambridge, Mass, 1985, pp. 305–316.
Cohen, Stanley. *Folk Devils and Moral Panics*, 3rd Edn. Routledge, London, 2002.
Debord, Guy. *Society of the Spectacle* (unknown translator). Black and Red, Detroit, Michigan, 1983.
Derrida, Jacques. *The Gift of Death* (translated by David Wills). University of Chicago Press, Chicago, Illinois, 1995.
Hawton, K., Harriss, L., Simkin, S. et al. 'Effect of death of Diana, Princess of Wales on suicide and deliberate self-harm', *British Journal of Psychiatry*, (2000) 177: 463–466
Locke, John. *An Essay Concerning Human Understanding*. Penguin Books, London, 1997.
Tatar, Maria. *Lustmord: Sexual Murder in Weimar Germany*. Princeton University Press, Princeton, NJ, 1997.
Tatar, Maria. *The Hard Facts of Grimms' Fairy Tales*. Princeton University Press, Princeton, NJ, 2003.

Regis A. DeSilva is Associate Professor of Medicine, Harvard Medical School, Boston, Massachusetts.

5

The Dying Soul: Spiritual Care at the End of Life

Mark Cobb

[...]

Modern medicine developed the power to wrestle with death and attempted to control it with sometimes desperate efforts to maintain somatic life. But at a time when medical advances generated considerable expectations in the ability of doctors to cure and prevent death, people with terminal malignant disease were often denied their diagnosis, afforded poor symptom control and left to die in isolated hospital rooms. Death was a sign of failure in a predominantly curative system; it had become depersonalized, desacralized and a terminal clinical event. It was this type of grim experience, both of the dying and those who witnessed their deaths, that provided a major impetus for the development of the modern hospice movement which has attempted to reaffirm a spiritual aspect of dying and death.

Death is at the margin of life and yet occupies much of its central features. There is an enormous amount of human thought, behaviour, art, religion, finance, science and technology devoted to death: its causes, its purpose, its timing, its place, its consequences and its endless intractable mysteries. Death sets the limit of life, and through this antithesis defines so much of what it means to live, of what it is to be human. Therefore the diagonal of mortal existence, of being and non-being, raises questions about the significance of living and dying and remains *the* permanent existential challenge. Finally, death imposes loss through absence, punctuates familiar continuity with irreversible change, incites severe emotions and presents an unwanted demand to say farewell. In a consequential sense, death happens to the living who have to deal with the dead and who come to interpret it, make meaning out of it, find purpose in it, declare it through ritual and garland it with myth.

Death is fundamental to life, it is a critical determinant of human existence, and it bears a profound significance because it marks the end of what we value as intrinsically precious. This is an important reason why individual human life is understood as sacred because it is irreplaceable, it warrants not just respect and honour, but an absolute sense of sanctity too. This conviction of inviolability is rooted in beliefs about the uniqueness of humankind and in the idea that human life is the result of astonishing natural and human creation and investment. Death matters not just because of the oblivion or salvation it may signal, but also because it is the end of everything we have known and lived. This may explain why most people want their dying and the manner of their death to have some continuity and integrity with their lives (Dworkin 1993). The sacred nature of life finds an unequalled focus in its conclusion, which is why, for many people, dying and death are holy ground because of the intensity they bring to what is precious and meaningful.

[…]

Facing death

A person's comprehension of death and the meaning attributed to death will mediate death's impact. Beliefs and doctrines held about death will also play a part in the way that death is faced and attended to. Personal meanings will influence emotional reactions and shape the way that death is understood.

[…]

To what extent palliative care professionals encounter patients' understanding of death and whether this goes beyond symptoms is uncertain. Few professionals (with the exception of psychological pathology) spend time in their training examining approaches to death and their own feelings and responses. Existential and spiritual issues related to death and dying may rarely surface in time-limited dialogues often aimed at assessments. A patient's attitude to death and that of carers are often presumed in institutional care, which may render the subject unnecessary and avoided. The result may be that such concerns are withheld or learnt to be irrelevant or unacceptable by patients and carers. Facing death takes people to profoundly intimate places which contain fears for most people and may ring alarm bells of vulnerability for professionals. However, being present when patients express their intimate thoughts and feelings provides the opportunity for affirmation and acceptance, challenges the isolation of suffering and creates space for meaning and growth (Barnard 1995). A personal meaning of death is not captured in discrete objective beliefs and values but will include cognitive, somatic, emotional and spiritual aspects. This is not an argument for engineering intimate encounters with patients, but a reminder that, 'Personal meaning is a fundamental dimension of personhood, and there can be no understanding of human illness or suffering without taking it into account' (Cassel 1982: 641).

Death both challenges and reinforces meaning, and people facing death may be challenged to revise the way they understand 'their' world, the way it operates and their place in it. The classic question of 'Why is this happening to me?' may be not only a cry of anguish but an indication that a person's world-view has been contradicted. Beliefs structure a person's world-view and provide familiar and dependable realities upon which life can be ventured. Anticipated and actual loss can threaten the meanings of life and the beliefs by which we interpret it. But beliefs may also enable a person to make sense of loss and find meaning in it. A small study of bereaved people who defined themselves as Christian explicitly related the meaning of their partner's death with their faith and beliefs. It was observed that this provided a predefined understanding of loss, although it did not account for all aspects of it, and there was evidence that discontinuities had prompted some reassessment of what death meant. In addition to feeling supported by their faith, the participants acknowledged uncertainties and doubts but these were understood as being contained within a spiritual framework. It appeared that religious meaning did not lessen feelings of grief and that, for some participants, whilst basic beliefs remained unquestioned, the meaning of death and the purpose of life were uncertain (Golsworthy and Coyle 1999).

The need to make, reform and reassert meaning in the face of death is the human impulse to maintain continuity when life is bereft. Health psychology and oncopsychology have models which encompass meanings and beliefs, few go as far as explicitly incorporating spiritual issues or beliefs. Palliative care is in some state of confusion over this: should it be left to a 'specialist' or is it something that anyone can and should deal with? It is difficult to establish whether or not palliative care services intentionally subordinate spirituality in seeking to help people to face death, but it is equally difficult to understand why something which can have such significant impact upon the way that death is understood is often left to chance.

The rituals of death

Palliative care cannot avoid being involved in rituals: in a general sense, rituals pervade the practice of healthcare professionals, and in an explicit sense they are necessary around the boundaries of life. As anthropology reminds us, no society is devoid of ritual, it is without equivalents and, as a basic social act, is 'requisite to the perpetuation of human social life' (Rappaport 1999: 31).

Rituals allow people to deal with ambiguities of change and give them meaning.

[...]

Rituals of death are ubiquitous, indispensable and possibly one of the most conservative types of ritual. The functional purpose of disposal which they incorporate does not exhaust the use of ritual which interprets death by placing it within a frame of reference. This is frame of beliefs, behaviour, meaning and conventions which allow the bereaved to deal with the calamity of loss in a contained and purposeful way. Rituals enact meaning, express beliefs, evoke emotions, represent ideals; in other words they make the invisible tangible through action and words. Postmortem rituals therefore dramatize and emphasize death, they honour the dead and prepare and commit them to their destiny, they sanction the profoundly intense and ambivalent expressions of grief, and they place the bereaved and the dead within a social and universal context. By enabling and elaborating grief, postmortem rituals express something of the significance of the relationships which have ended and also of the sense of loss which is inherent in the mortal condition, a loss which exists because of the meaning we make of our own life and the lives of others (Marris 1986: ch. 5).

The trivial and inconsequential may be dealt with by routine, convention and repetitive actions, but rituals are used when matters of significance and profound change need to be handled. Therefore, rituals are usually distinguished from other social acts by a number of features, among them: their gravity (solemnity and formality), by the way people are involved in them (participation), by the special places and time at which they occur (context), by their use of an established order (invariance), by the means and content of their communication (formalized utterances and enduring messages), and by their powerful and convincing affect (efficacy) (Rappaport 1999: ch. 3). Rituals accomplish and achieve their purpose not directly through the physical but through the incorporeal by using meaningful words and acts which declare the significance of the ritual and convey deep connotative resonances. Rituals, unlike some other social acts, are not vague, but make explicit and clearly define what is the intention of the performance. Finally, ritual as a social act involves individuals in a collective event, establishing, guarding and bridging the boundaries between the public and private (Rappaport 1999: ch 4).

The way in which the ritual forms are employed in the history of patients and their carers range from the consultation at which the patients and carers receive the terminal diagnosis, the patients' admission for in-patient care, the declaration of death, the last offices, the funeral and memorial service. All of these significant episodes of transition are usually accompanied by the performance of established and formal orders which take place in special settings involving participation which transform that which they are imposed upon. Even if many of the examples offered here fall short of a strict definition of ritual, there are strong resemblances to ritual in that they are acts which articulate, emote, inform and redefine by enacting and communicating meaning. The point here is that palliative care makes use of 'ritual' in order to invest or impose meaning upon that which challenges and dislocates meaning, and in so doing maintains some order in the face of chaos.

At the time of death we find a number of ritual forms converging, not necessarily in any consistent pattern, to facilitate and declare the transition from life to death of the patient, to allow carers and staff to make an acknowledgement of the loss, and to convey at the very least the meaning of life now ended. But rituals of death are increasingly truncated and condensed, a result in part of the professionalization and process of death, which means that they have to carry in concentrated periods that which was once spread out over weeks. The hospice adage of 'live until you die' and the depreciated 'terminal' phase of a life-threatening illness limits the opportunities for the ritual expressions of dying for all concerned. What rituals are allowed and provided, therefore, have to work much harder and cover an area that may have been dealt with in other ways. A contemporary cremation service, in all its brevity, often feels as if it has to pick up from the moment of death, consign the body to its final resting place and take people through mourning towards life adjusted to loss in the space of twenty-five minutes.

[…]

Much of the ritual response to death is a creative declaration that death is more than biological cessation for it has social, symbolic, temporal and spiritual significance. The material facts cannot be excised from more intangible dimensions, and part of ritual's efficacy is its ability to meaningfully represent values, beliefs, states and qualities in ways which substantiate and validate them. The rituals of death do not restrict it to a fatal moment for they also lift it out of its mundane timeframe and can place it in a sacred frame in which all may not be lost:

It is as though human imagination utilizes both the drive for survival and a propensity for hopeful optimism to contradict the visible facts of life. To direct view, death brings people to a decaying end yet, against this cold fact, and in the very face of death, most human societies have asserted that life continues in another world, in a spiritual dimension or amongst the ancestral powers. But not only in an afterlife is death transcended. In this life, too, rites make it possible to lift the individual above the realm of death and decay. The human being may live as one who has died and, through contact with some higher power, now possesses some of that power to ensure that ordinary life is ordinary no longer. The words of the rites are powerful in establishing all these issues. (Davies 1997: 178)

After death

When people face death they face contradictions of finality and continuity, of absence and presence, of decay and redemption, of mortality and immortality. What the nurse pronounces as death may to the carers be a thankful release from 'this life' and to the priest be a passing from this world to the next. The plain facts of death may seem to contravene the facts of experience and the breadth of interpretations evoked by death. In particular, the religious imagination has understood death in most conceivable ways. However, death is not a question to be answered by a single universal response, there is no dichotomy in death, and people can see death both as the consequence of embodiment and the point of its departure to life beyond death, however that is conceived.

Postmortem existence can be understood on many levels but all point to transcending death, whether through personal legacies (objective and subjective), the experiences, feelings or spiritual beliefs of the bereaved and some form of 'survival' beyond the fatal event. A destiny beyond life forms part of the concept of death and may well be a significant factor in people's attitudes and response to death. In essence, a postmortem destiny concerns some future prospect for the dead person which has important consequences most immediately for the dying (in terms of preparation), the dead and those who mourn them, but also for society and the way it deals with death and those who are bereaved. As the present is a point in the human narrative that contains references to the future, any prospects held to follow from death will affect life now and modify its meaning. This has two further interrelated aspects. One concerns the continuity of the person who has died and, in particular, what form of afterlife this will take. The other concerns the 'place' in the universe for those who have died, for, to put it simply, if there is some postmortem survival, it must be 'located' somewhere.

This is not the only possible scenario of what happens after death, although it is a highly prominent one in many cultures. Some people have abolished any future in death and do not believe in any form of life beyond it. Personal immortality is simply an impossibility and there is no place or form of existence beyond the grave, because:

> We are physical beings and we inhabit a physical universe. If we discard the myths of self and soul and spirit, and recognise that all our life and sensation, all our capacity to think and to feel, are inextricably tied up with our bodies – if, in short, we see that we do not have bodies, we are bodies – then we might begin to realise what an extraordinary place we inhabit and what a mystery, in the true sense, life is ... Is not that enough mystery, without your wishing to invent new mysteries of heaven and of hell? (Wilson 1995: 197)

The physicality of the person has long occupied the thoughts of theologians and philosophers, and embodiment has become something of a current preoccupation with sociologists. Death marks the breakdown of the body, and while the body may rest in the grave, it also remains a significant aspect of any postmortem survival, most obvious in the beliefs concerning the resurrection of the body, an idea that can be found in the religions of Judaism, Christianity, Islam and Zoroastrianism. These images of eventual survival beyond death refer substantially to a person's bodily identity, and it is person of gender, appearance, activity and so forth whose presence is evoked in the recollections, memorials and experiences of the bereaved. Bodily identity therefore provides not only continuity but also a reason for a location, something which an abstract and ephemeral spirit may have no need of. More basically than this, as we have been known through our bodies, so it becomes the place of significance and meaning for others, which is one reason why it warrants utmost respect even when it is dead, and why there is usually some form of ritual performed after death even in the absence of religious rites.

Death has for some remained a future fact but without any future scenario and therefore the notion of the afterlife has lost its function. The knowledge of death is accompanied by few, if any, beliefs, but Flowers (1998) suggests that this always leaves an opening for stories and fictions, a space which is, 'even for postmodern minds, still filled with belief, namely the belief that there is no afterlife. This – the story that there is no afterlife – is the one mono-myth left in our culture, when all else is open to revision. This is the bald scenario, a story of nothing' (Flowers 1998: 55). There can be no future in nihilism and no meaning therefore derived from it: death is itself meaningless, it has no consequence, it is empty of implication and representation. Death in this bleak existential version is without a vista and the bereaved are left assuming literally nothing.

It seems reasonable to suggest that this somewhat harsh position is rarely encountered, and that for many people a belief in a form of afterlife is more common. The evidence for this is the persistent use of rituals for the dead that are premised on some form of spiritual belief, or popular expressions of the afterlife in memorials, films and books, and empirical studies. Beliefs in an afterlife are diverse and, as with other beliefs, an individual may hold what appears an incoherent set of notions about the afterlife, acquired unsystematically, and appearing somewhat inconsistent and disorganized. Davies underlines the importance of recognizing this and emphasizes that, 'logical contradiction need not necessarily worry individuals whose varied views are drawn on for different purposes and in different contexts' (Davies 1997: 151). In facing death, a person may for the first time be prompted into formulating their beliefs about death, and have to make choices based upon them: 'Would you like us to call the chaplain to say some prayers before your aunt dies?' 'Do we need to observe any particular requirements in preparing her body?' 'Whom would you like to conduct the funeral service?' These may be questions not only for the deceased but also for the dying who wish to prepare for their death, and may have particularly important consequence for those of certain faiths and traditions. Those who support the dying and bereaved may not have thought through their beliefs either, and a proper reticence that wards against imposing beliefs may frustrate what could be a helpful or necessary exploration of the afterlife.

It is in the religious exploration of death that we discover some of the most significant, enduring and hopeful beliefs concerning what happens after death. As we might expect, what religion implies about 'human nature and its destiny is by no means trivial or ill-considered;

still less is it only a product of abject wishful thinking, or of cynical exploitation of the credulous' (Bowker 1991: 211). [...] Religious exploration also affirms that there is a continuity of a person's identity despite death's disruption. A belief in an indestructible soul, resurrection, rebirth, reincarnation or the attainment of an eternal tranquil state all suggest an ultimate destiny for humanity beyond death (Badham 1995). Differences in these beliefs are not negligible and become evident in the customs and rituals surrounding death, in the concepts used and in the pathways to an ultimate destiny (Bowker 1983: ch. 10). But what can perhaps be made as a more general point is that the religious beliefs about human destiny are remarkably pervasive, durable and adaptable. Reincarnation, for example, is not part of the Christian concept of the afterlife, but Davies has found that 12 per cent of people in Britain claim some belief in the idea of the dead 'coming back as something else' (Davies 1997: 152). Globalization, the lack of a prevailing orthodoxy and the presence of different faith communities have contributed to many people assimilating various postmortem beliefs.

The New Age movement and many of the 'new' religions often have undeveloped although eclectic eschatologies concentrating upon the development and perfection of the true self which is beyond death's destruction. The utopianism of New Age philosophies suggests the transcendence of the ego and attaining a heaven on earth. Death for New Agers is not to be feared but to be mastered, because 'death is a way to life and the subtext is that as god, the individual is responsible for determining the manner and content of both' (Clarke 1995: 136). Death can also be approached from a humanist perspective which does not invoke the sacred or eternal or rely upon metaphysics. The focus of meaning is in the life that has been lived and in the example that can be continued. The ritual form concerns the celebration of the deceased person and is inevitably life-centred. The funeral therefore becomes the concluding chapter of the person's history rather than the rite of transition that the person may have made to another life.

The 'ultimate' destiny of a person with a terminal illness is not something that forms an explicit part of palliative care philosophy. The respect for individual autonomy leaves services open to accommodate almost any personal belief and practice, with in-patient services providing a neutral territory for customs, rituals and views within the limits of tolerance. But the meaning of death to a patient and their carers seems too significant for it to be left unacknowledged and for some unexplored. As with other spiritual aspects this may be another example of professionals maintaining silence because of their own unexplored beliefs and their uncertain comprehension of this dimension. What death means to the professional may be unspoken but it will not be absent in their approach to dealing with death or inoperative from the way they understand the people they care for and witness dying.

[...]

References

Badham, P. (1995) Death and immortality: towards a global synthesis, in D. Cohn-Sherbok and C. Lewis (eds) *Beyond Death*. Basingstoke: Macmillan.
Barnard, D. (1995) The promise of intimacy and the fear of our own undoing, *Journal of Palliative Care*, 11(4): 22–6.

Bowker, J. (1983) *Worlds of Faith*. London: BBC.

Bowker, J. (1991) *The Meanings of Death*. Cambridge: Cambridge University Press.

Cassel, E. J. (1982) The nature of suffering and the goals of medicine, *New England Journal of Medicine*, 306(11): 639–45.

Clarke, P. (1995) Beyond death: the case of new religions, in D. Cohn-Sherbok and C. Lewis (eds) *Beyond Death*. Basingstoke: Macmillan.

Davies, D. J. (1997) *Death Ritual and Belief*. London: Cassell.

Dworkin, R. (1993) *Life's Dominion*. London: HarperCollins.

Flowers, B. S. (1998) Death, the bold scenario, in J. Malpas and R. C. Solomon (eds) *Death and Philosophy*. London: Routledge.

Golsworthy, R. and Coyle, A. (1999) Spiritual beliefs and the search for meaning among older adults following partner loss, *Mortality*, 4(1): 21–40.

Marris, P. (1986) *Loss and Change*. London: Routledge.

Rappaport, R. A. (1999) *Ritual and Religion in the Making of Humanity*. Cambridge: Cambridge University Press.

Wilson, A. N. (1995) Life after death, in D. Cohn-Sherbok and C. Lewis (eds) *Beyond Death*. Basingstoke: Macmillan.

6

Death and Religion

David Webster

Death is one of the fundamental realities of human experience. If we consider religions as phenomena that have, among other things, tried to explain the mysteries we face as humans – it is clear that religions are going to have much to say about death. Much more, indeed, than we can hope to cover here. Nonetheless, what we do offer here is an attempt to understand how some fundamentally important beliefs about death – and what might lie beyond it – influence how religious people might relate to death – most notably when it is imminent in either oneself or someone close to them.

Perhaps the most widespread contribution to our notion of death which is seen as originating in religious traditions is the idea that 'we' might survive death – that some aspect of what we are may not end with the decline and demise of the body (and brain). This notion is one that could lead us into lengthy philosophical speculation as to the nature of what 'we' are – and what there might be in the make-up of a human being that could possibly still exist after death. Some philosophers consider the term 'life after death' to be inherently paradoxical and inconsistent (the very meaning of 'death' being that it is the end of 'life'). Others, most notably perhaps the French philosopher René Descartes (1596–1650), have taken the view that there exists within us something that is able to survive death (referred to as a 'soul' or 'mind'). What this 'something' is remains an area of vociferous debate both within and between religious traditions and in the sometime awkward relationship between faiths and modern science.

What follows is a short survey of the manner in which some key religious traditions have understood the nature of death, and the impact of this on their understanding of what the process of dying involves. It is worth noting that the first three traditions addressed (Judaism, Christianity and Islam) all take what might be best described as a 'linear' attitude to life and death. That is, they tend to believe that we have only one life – with one birth, various incidents in our lives, and then a single death – leading to our permanent post-death fate. Religions such as Buddhism and Hinduism, having a belief in some notion of karma and rebirth, see this life as one of many: we have lived many times before and will come to be born and die many more times yet. This approach to life and death is often described as 'cyclical'. The more 'linear' of these traditions are often those that see human life as in the gift of God (perhaps because of its unique and singular occurrence) and are most likely to be uncomfortable with euthanasia.

It is also worth quickly addressing a common misconception related to the relation between religion and death. In an age where faith is often, and not without cause, subject to a critical interrogation, some take the view that death is somehow easier for people with a religious belief. We may have heard the phrase: 'I wish I was able to believe that …'. This view is drawn from the notion that the belief in some kind of survival removes the fear and anxiety from death – and hence lessens its 'sting'. This is an error. Not only does the unknown of death make religious people as frightened and anxious as anyone else – their faith may even bring greater fears: such as that of judgement for their misdeeds. Indeed, the approach of death can itself trigger in some a crisis of faith itself – as old certainties fade and the end nears. Whatever other impacts religious belief has on death and the way we approach it, it does not make it easy.

Judaism

Jewish beliefs date back around three and a half millennia – and yet what is notable with relation to its post-death beliefs is the apparent reluctance of Jewish traditions to enumerate these beliefs in detail. Traditional Jewish belief sees some existence continuing after death: death is not the end. While there are some conclusions we can draw about Jewish views of life after death, the Torah itself says relatively little. However, as the traditions developed two important ideas emerged.

First, there is the idea of the eventual resurrection of the dead during a messianic end-time. This intra-historical time is sometimes referred to as *Olam Ha-Ba* (in Hebrew) – but this term is sometimes used in another sense, which brings me to the second idea: that of *Olam Ha-Ba* as the 'world to come' in the sense of the afterlife. This afterlife may include aspects of reward and punishment related to our life here, but is not clearly divided into those who are 'saved' and those who are 'damned' as you find in some Christian and Islamic traditions.

Although all Jews are considered morally accountable to God, the reason most often cited as to why Jewish thought has not dwelt in detail on the nature of the afterlife is two-fold. First, for the rabbinic Judaism of late antiquity and the medieval period, it was considered unnecessary to speculate about matters inaccessible to human knowledge and reason. Second, post-Enlightenment Judaism's primary focus is on life in the here and now: it is a life-affirming tradition. This focus on the vitality and value of human life leads traditional Judaism to, mostly, oppose euthanasia and assisted suicide – although it may permit the withdrawal of treatment. While there is a set of specific post-death rituals that demonstrate absolute respect for the dignity of the corpse, these might be seen as being as much for the benefit of the bereaved as for the deceased. What is noteworthy is the mandatory use of burial as opposed to cremation for the most Orthodox traditions, namely those affirming the bodily resurrection of the righteous, whose bodies must therefore be buried whole. This sense of the preservation of the integrity of the body may lead some Jews to be uncomfortable with the notion of an autopsy – although if it benefits the lives of others this may prove of overriding importance.

In Judaism, the idea that our story, the narrative of ourselves, does not end at death, can be seen as a source of reassurance, and a reason not to fear death.

Christianity

Christianity has, perhaps almost as much as any other religion, speculated on the nature of death and where it may lead us. We could argue that this stems from the Christian claim that Christ 'conquered death' with his crucifixion and subsequent resurrection. With a much described (although often without theological or biblical basis) view of heaven and hell, with a final day of judgement, Christianity demonstrates that death is an arena for a moral reckoning. After death we shall be called to account – and so the time approaching death can be one of anxiety regarding past misdeeds. Of course, alongside this is the Christian tradition of divine forgiveness – which states that all have failed to attain the moral standards required – and that salvation is therefore only available through the forgiveness offered by the death and resurrection of Jesus Christ. For some traditions this forgiveness is obtained through private prayer between the believer and God – while some, such as Roman Catholicism, have more formalised aspects to this process – notably including the notion of 'last rites'.

While for many Christians the post-death world is clearly divided into heaven and hell, there are also those who look to a final resurrection of the body during the end-times, as also found in Judaism. For most Christians, though, the primary notion of death relates to the death of the body and the survival of the soul. The Christian understanding of the nature of the soul has varied over time – although most contemporary popular understandings are heavily influenced by the 'dualism' of René Descartes. His view of the non-physical part of us – which survives death – was that it had no 'extension' into the physical and was indestructible: unlike the body which, although has a worldly presence, is temporary and mortal.

The notion of the soul can be troubling – as it raises many philosophical questions. Among these are issues as to whether we retain our memories, whether our souls are re-embodied or exist separately, and whether heaven are places where time passes (or even exists) and the manner and extent of our conscious awareness in such a state. In the face of such complexity – and partnered with an absolute lack of guidance as to the answers to these questions – Christianity (in line with many of the other traditions mentioned here) has often presented a post-death world rather analogous to this one: with people, places, bodies and life not dissimilar to our pre-death existence. It is important to understand that most traditions, Christian and other, that offer such a view, predominantly do so as a metaphor, or symbol, which stands in for our lack of knowledge. Many would stress that life beyond the grave will be so different to this life as to be inconceivable to us in our present: leaving us to live not with knowledge, but with faith and, perhaps most importantly of all, hope.

Islam

Islam clearly places itself in the tradition of religions which we might refer to as Abrahamic, indeed seeing itself as the correction and completion of the religious journeys undertaken by Judaism and Christianity. It should not surprise us then to see something not wholly dissimilar to Judeo-Christian traditions in the Islamic view of what happens after death. Two key areas can seen as pertinent here. First there is the notion that reward and punishment will be administered – which ties in with the central Islamic tenet of the justness of God: Allah would therefore not leave sins unpunished and virtue unrewarded. Second, there is a notion of heaven and hell (it has become popular to refer to the Islamic view of heaven as 'paradise' in some Western contexts). Throughout the Quran, there are numerous depictions of heaven and hell – although many Muslims would understand these as allegorical in character: no one can be sure what it will truly be like after death (although Surah 55 of the Quran talks of 'two gardens' – often taken to mean a lower and higher form of heaven). We also find notions of a day of judgement in the end-times, and as we might expect in a 'linear' tradition, some sense of an end to all things.

With regard to death itself, certain key points are of note. The Quran has much to say on death, and talks of it being like sleeping – and that at the moment of death each of us knows our fate as to whether we are bound for heaven or hell. In a sense that has great significance: the good Muslim, the righteous believer, does not die – but continues in heaven. However, death is indeed to be feared by the wicked, and while the unbelievers may not fear death they truly ought to.

In preparing for death, Muslims remember that in a sense all life is preparation for what lies beyond. One of the most important aspects of this preparation is the remembrance of God – to have Allah in one's thoughts. For example, for very ill patients having someone read the Quran to them can be a great source of comfort when approaching the end of life. Islam has a clear preference for burial as opposed to cremation – which it usually forbids.

Hinduism

'Hinduism' is a relatively modern term (19th century in its wider application) for an ancient set of traditions. There is often lively debate as to whether Hinduism constitutes an individual religion, or is better understood as an umbrella term for a broad set of religious traditions. While this debate is not one to explore here, it is worth being aware of the vast diversity one is likely to encounter with relation to Hinduism. Not only are there differing sects and traditions, but practices vary hugely by region of origin (in the Indian subcontinent) and by social class (or caste – *jati* or *varna*). Hinduism also represents probably the oldest of the faiths which believes in some form of rebirth, reincarnation or at least cyclical approach to human life and death.

Despite this diversity, some common threads can be seen as tying together Hindu beliefs – and their attitudes towards the process of death and its approach. A word regarding the nature of the divine in Hinduism will be useful before moving on to more practical matters. While Hindus may well appear to worship many gods (and may wish to have statues, pictures, incense and other religious equipment to hand – especially during longer stays in health facilities – to enable *puja* – acts of worship) the most common understanding is that Hindus believe in one God who has many forms or expressions.

As previously indicated, Hindus believe in the idea of rebirth – and that our future lives are determined by our karma. While the Sanskrit word 'karma' literally means 'action' it usually represents the consequences of action – and the approach of death is a time to reflect on one's past – and the impact it may come to have on our futures. It is worth noting that Hindu beliefs in rebirth (or 'reincarnation' as it is sometimes referred to) sit alongside the idea of heavens and hells. This indicates that rebirth may be somewhere other than in this realm. The approach of death will turn a Hindu's thought to the future, and a number of factors become important (in addition to karma) in determining the future journey of the inner-self (the Atman – the true self which is indestructible and eternal). The state of mind of a person at death is seen as of deep significance. The preference is a for a calm, reflective, contemplative even, state of mind at the moment of death, and preceding it. Some traditions believe that the detailed contents of the mind at death have a much more deterministic impact – but overall the priority is to have time to make sure any tradition-specific rituals or practices are carried out, that family is allowed access, and that people have a sense that they have completed their duties (a very important notion in Hindu thought).

Since earliest times, Hindus have cremated their dead (preferably on the banks of a sacred river such as the Ganges). There is a complex set of mythic imagery representing the aspects of the person returning into the wider cosmos, while the inner-self (the Atman) continues onwards its journey into the next life.

Buddhism

Buddhist thought shares the notion of karma with Hinduism, and also features the idea of rebirth. Due to not believing in the Atman or inner-self, some Buddhists avoid the term 'reincarnation'. What is perhaps important to understand, though, is the manner in which reflection on the transience of life and imminence of death runs through Buddhist thought. Many Buddhists have written critically of the Western attitude to death – and point to Buddhist traditions as a more 'healthy' alternative.

Of central importance to most of the diverse traditions within Buddhism is the notion of impermanence: that all that exists is finite, temporary and in a state of constant flux or change. Many traditions include meditations on the transitory, ever-changing and fragile nature of human (and indeed, animal) existence within their practices. Given that meditation plays such a central role in most Buddhist traditions, it is not surprising that the practice is of importance in our final days. Many specific meditation practices exist which pertain to the person who is dying, in pain or very ill. However, meditation requires a quiet and calm place to be successful. What is worth noting is that, contrary to some Western stereotypes, meditation is a vigorous and draining form of mental exertion – and many seriously ill people will struggle with marshalling the necessary resources. What is of serious concern to patients (and their families) is that a person should die in as calm a state of mind as possible. While some traditions of Buddhist thought may wish for the recitation of prayers or sutras at the close of a person's life, the maintenance of calm, dignity – and even serenity – is vital, and seen as a key factor in ensuring a peaceful transition to the next life.

Within Buddhist cultures, cremation is common (in some places it is believed that burning the body allows for the passage onwards to the next life). Many Buddhist traditions stress that the funeral should not be a time of sadness, but of reflection. The Buddha, in the earliest account of his own death, admonished monks present for 'wailing and moaning' – and told them to cease.

Conclusion

Many other traditions exist in the UK, such as Sikhism, Jainism, Rastafarianism, new forms of paganism and countless sectarian offshoots of the major religious traditions previously discussed. While it is not feasible to enumerate the death-related beliefs and practices of them all, some general concerns are worth keeping in mind. Given the wide variation even within a single religious tradition, when dealing with the imminent death of a person the best practice would be to ask. In doing so, individuals will be given permission to discuss this often difficult topic, and may feel able express their preferences. Secondly, it is worth noting the great significance virtually all religions attribute to the manner of dying – and the subsequent impact on this. Alongside many rituals of remembrance that pertain to bereaved people, maintaining a quality of life that permits a person time for reflection and consideration of their life is to be seen as a gift of profound import to the dying person.

Religion does not see death as the end – but rather as a transition – albeit one often associated with loss, sadness and difficulty. The person approaching death is in a liminal state: they stand at the threshold of the unknown. While we all have to cross that threshold alone, people of faith often stand at it with hope. Even where hope falters, many feel they still are able to face death with a grace born from doing that most vital of things – having lived well.

7

Mortality: World Variations in Death and Dying

Cathy E. Lloyd

Across the world there are wide variations in the experience of death and dying. Death occurs at different times and places according to many factors including age, gender, ethnicity, wealth and environment. Demographers and epidemiologists, who study, among other things, the prevalence and causes of diseases and death, have helped those concerned with who dies to better understand the association between social and environmental factors and death. In this reading these relationships will be considered through comparison both within and between countries, for example, between developed and developing parts of the world. Globally, causes of death have changed over time as has the age at which death occurs, however many developing countries have high mortality rates and their citizens continue to die at a much younger age than those living in more developed countries. International data show how those living in poorer countries have a lower life expectancy than those living in wealthier regions of the world. Comparing mortality rates between countries can be problematic however, and a brief critique of the way in which mortality statistics are collected and how they can be interpreted will also be offered.

Measuring mortality

Epidemiologists and demographers are both involved with counting the population according to particular social characteristics such as age, gender, ethnicity and social class, and this includes reporting morbidity and mortality data (Sidell and Lloyd, 2007). Epidemiologists use this data to show how the causes of death have changed over time and make comparisons of death rates between different groups of people or populations, examining potential reasons for any differences. In order to do this, mortality rates are calculated on the basis of an analysis of completed death certificates. In the UK registration of deaths has been compulsory since 1836, and include the name, age and sex of the deceased as well as (since 1874) cause of death. The latter has provided important epidemiological information for decades, but its usefulness depends on the use of standardised methods of reporting when death certificates are completed (Sidell and Lloyd, 2007). There are variations in both accuracy and the completeness of records within and between different countries, as will be discussed below. It is the 'underlying' cause of death, as reported by the attending doctor on the death certificate, that is used by the Office of National Statistics in the UK to generate rates of death and causes of death. It is possible, if the same recording and calculation procedures have been followed for all those populations involved, to make comparisons between different sections of the population at area, regional, national and international levels. Mortality rates can be compared between men and women, rich and poor, or between different ethnic groups. Indeed, mortality rates are deemed to be so important as to be a vital indicator of the health status of a population.

Variations in mortality in the UK

In the UK, variations in death rates can be examined because the procedure for recording deaths is standardised across the four nations. Although death certification is not without its limitations, it is possible to demonstrate differences in mortality according to a number of factors, including age, gender, ethnicity and area of residence. For example, in 2006, Glickman and colleagues compared overall infant mortality rates for the four nations of the UK, and demonstrated variations between the nations, with Wales having the lowest rate compared to England, Scotland and Ireland (see Figure 7.1).

Infant mortality rates are used as an indicator of overall health because this rate correlates well with young adult mortality, and is sensitive to socio-economic and environmental changes as well as improvements in health care (Sidell and Lloyd, 2007). Factors associated with infant mortality have been examined in the past and have shown that low socio-economic status is a strong contender for explaining variations in rates. For example, in a study in London, UK (Bowles, Walters and Jacobson, 2007), among the most important factors associated with infant deaths were mothers living in the most deprived parts of the capital, babies born to particular minority ethnic parents, and infants born to parents working in manual occupations. Although this research only reported findings from London, the authors of the report argue that these trends are similar to the picture for the whole of the UK. They go on to state that:

> In the longer term, collective effort needs to be focussed on tackling the wider causes of infant mortality such as reducing child poverty, reducing the gap in educational attainment and improving employment opportunities. These measures, combined with well-targeted approaches via Sure Start and Children's Centres, will also impact positively on wider infant and child health. (Bowles, Walters and Jacobson 2007: 6)

In the Glickman report (Glickman et al., 2006), differences in overall mortality rates between the four nations of the UK were highlighted, with England having the lowest mortality rate and Scotland the highest. People living in Scotland were more likely to die from heart disease and lung cancers, whereas deaths from breast cancer were highest in Northern Ireland. Scotland also had a greater proportion of heavy smokers compared to England and Wales (no data were available for Northern Ireland). Alcohol-related and drug-poisoning deaths were also highest in Scotland compared to the other countries of the UK. This report does not discuss the reasons why there might be variations in mortality rates or in causes of death across different nations of the UK. However an earlier study

**United Kingdom
Rates**

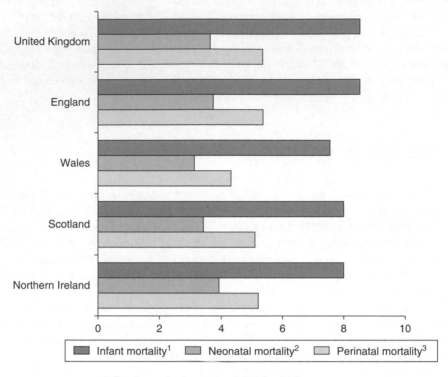

1 Deaths under 1 year per 1,000 live births.
2 Deaths under 4 weeks per 1,000 live births.
3 Stillbirths and deaths under 1 week per 1,000 live and stillbirths.

Figure 7.1   Infant neonatal and perinatal mortality rates, 2003
(Glickman et al., 2006: 33)

focusing specifically on differences in mortality from coronary heart disease (CHD) in Scotland, showed that the risk of dying from a heart attack was two and a half times greater in those living in more deprived areas compared to the less deprived parts of Scotland, particularly for those under the age of 65 (McLaren and Bain, 1998). Although deprivation was not a significant predictor of mortality from heart attacks in those over the age of 65, older individuals from more deprived areas were less likely to undergo coronary bypass operations than those from the wealthier parts of Scotland. Earlier death from CHD was associated with deprivation as was a higher prevalence of smoking. The authors of this report highlighted concerns over access to treatment for heart disease and this research showed a clear association between the absence of wealth, or living in a deprived neighbourhood, and an increased risk of mortality from CHD. They state that:

Reduction of socioeconomic inequalities in mortality from coronary heart disease is likely to be mainly achieved by appropriate and effective primary and secondary preventive measures matching need wherever people live. (McLaren and Bain, 1998: online)

This report highlights the complex associations between different indices of deprivation and mortality. The concept of deprivation should not only be thought of as a marker of personal level of wealth, but also the type of environment in which we live, whether we smoke, the level of access to health services and so on. As such, the mechanisms via which deprivation (however it is measured) might influence mortality are often difficult to untangle (and outside the scope of this reading). However, the relationship between poverty (in its broader sense) and mortality has been debated for decades (Wilkinson, 1986; 1997). Differences between as well as within countries around the world have illustrated how deprivation or lack of wealth has a strong influence on life expectancy and mortality.

International variations

The relationship between what Wilkinson (1997) calls 'relative poverty' and mortality that has been observed within countries can also be found when comparing different parts of the world. For example, the UK Health Statistics report (Glickman et al., 2006) compared the mortality rates within the four nations of the UK with other countries within the European Union (EU). The report states that infant mortality in the EU as a whole has declined overall – from 8.5 per 1,000 live births in 1992 to 4.6 per 1,000 live births in 2003. In spite of this overall decline, some countries still have high rates of infant mortality, for example, Latvia had the highest rate in 2003 of 9.4 per 1,000 live births, followed by Slovakia, Hungary and Poland (Glickman et al., 2006). In the UK, Wales was the only country with an infant mortality rate lower than the overall rate for the EU.

The World Health Organization (WHO) describes mortality statistics as 'the most basic health outcome' (WHO, 2007: online). The WHO collects data from nearly 200 countries across the world, and is thus a key source of mortality data. The International Statistical Classification of Diseases, version 10 (ICD-10) provides the basis for mortality statistics as it provides a unique code number for each cause of death. In this way data both within and between countries can be standardised and compared. WHO mortality data enables the comparison of mortality rates between these countries and can illuminate the influence of socio-economic status on rates of death as well as inequities in health status in general. Mortality rates, as reported by the WHO *World Health Statistics* report (WHO, 2007) include the probability of dying under the age of five, compared in terms of place of residence, income level and educational level of the mother. Not all countries report comprehensive and accurate mortality rates, however these data are a powerful reminder of the association between mortality and socio-economic status.

In 2000, The Millennium Declaration was adopted by the United Nations, promising to 'uphold the principles of human dignity, equality and equity at the global level' (UN, 2000). The UN Millennium Development Goals (MDGs) were developed from the Millennium Declaration and this included two targets for reducing mortality: Goal 4 aims to reduce by two-thirds the mortality rate among children under five, and Goal 5 aims to reduce by three-quarters the maternal mortality ratio (UNDP, 2006: online).

The under-five's mortality rate has been described by the WHO as 'a leading indicator of the level of child health and overall development in countries' (WHO, 2007: online). Two other MDGs also identify mortality rate reductions as a key indicator of health

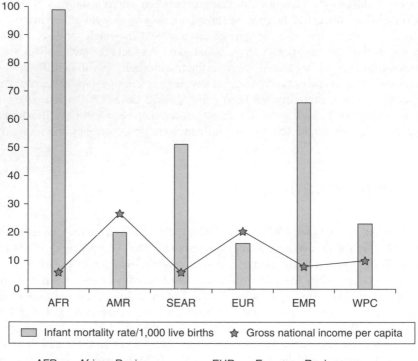

AFR : African Region   EUR : European Region
AMR : Region of the Americas EMR : Eastern Mediterranean Region
SEAR: South East Asia Region   WPC : Western Pacific Region

Figure 7.2   Variations in infant mortality compared with variations in socio-economic status – indicated by gross national income per capita

outcome. The above targets for reducing child and maternal mortality have strengthened the impetus for the collection of robust data on mortality, not least because developing countries depend on funding that is based on these targets.

The WHO *World Health Statistics* report on mortality in 2007 showed wide variations in infant mortality not just in Europe but across the world. WHO statistics on the economic status of these countries (as indicated by gross national income per capita) demonstrate similarities between the experiences of countries according to both mortality and to deprivation, some of which are illustrated in Figure 7.2. As the figure suggests, those regions of the world where infant mortality is high are more likely to be those regions where there is lower gross national income per capita. It is important to remember, however, that these data mask the within- and between-country variations in relation to mortality and deprivation.

Causes of death have changed over time and this is illustrated through the comparison of death rates in developing and developed countries as societies change and become more affluent. It also gives further support to the evidence of a relationship between death and socio-economic circumstances. The concept of 'health transition' has become widely used to encompass the changes in the patterns of health, disease and death that occur within a society as it becomes richer. For example, as a country becomes more affluent 'diseases of poverty' become less prevalent and 'diseases of affluence', such as coronary heart disease and cancer, become more common. This in turn leads to changes in the most common causes of death. For example, in the developed world, where people are more likely to live longer, the most common causes of death are heart disease and cancer, whereas in the developing world people are more likely to die from malnutrition or communicable diseases, such as chest infections and diarrhoea. The concept of health transition is not a simple one however, and it has been argued that many developing countries face a double burden – of both non-communicable and communicable diseases (Kapoor and Anand, 2002). Kapoor and Anand use the example of Brazil, a country undergoing rapid transition, to demonstrate this double burden. They report high rates of obesity (a disease of affluence) as well as marked thinness or underweight cases – examples of over-nutrition and under-nutrition, coexisting in the low income population of Brazil, which pose unique challenges to public health interventions to reduce mortality rates (Komaromy, 2006).

Interpreting mortality statistics

The use and interpretation of mortality statistics is not without difficulties as there are variations between countries in terms of the degree of surveillance undertaken, that is the completeness of death registration data. This often makes comparisons between as well as within different sections of a population problematic. Accurate data is particularly difficult to collect in parts of the developing world such as sub-Saharan Africa and South East Asia, as medical personnel are often not present to record cause of death (Adjuik et al., 2006). Furthermore, data from low-income countries is often based on historical trends or household surveys rather than the use of internationally agreed methods for monitoring trends (Child Mortality Coordination Group, 2006). In 2005 a report indicated that little or no data was available on mortality for 66 per cent of the world's population and only two countries of sub-Saharan Africa (the region with the highest mortality rates) were able to provide data on causes of death for at least half of their deaths (Mathers et al., 2002). Particular underlying causes of death may also be problematic or may be under-reported, for example, deaths due to suicide or HIV/AIDS which may be stigmatised in particular societies.

In recent years the use of 'verbal autopsy', where information is gleaned from the relatives of the deceased person in order to reconstruct the events that preceded death so as to identify a probable cause of death, has been promoted (Fauveau, 2006). Although there remain problems in terms of accuracy, particularly in terms of reporting the underlying cause in diseases such as HIV/AIDS or malnutrition, verbal autopsy has become recognised as a viable option to death certification where there are no medical personnel involved. Indeed, the WHO has now recommended a standardised method for using verbal autopsy in infant and child deaths (Fauveau, 2006). In spite of the continuing uncertainty with regard to the validity of verbal autopsy, in recent years there has been an increase in its use, with a greater range of contexts in which it is used. As Fauveau (2006) notes, this technique is now used:

> to determine priority diseases and identify areas of programmatic attention, to approach cause-specific mortality rates, to compare different age groups or different regions of a country, different countries of the two sexes, to assess the effect of

public health programmes focusing on specific diseases, or to conduct rapid assessments in emergency situations (such as cholera outbreaks, earthquakes and displaced populations). (Fauveau, 2006: 247)

In 2007, the Health Metrics Network, under the auspices of the WHO, launched a new drive to encourage civil registration of births and deaths. At the time of writing, only 31 of the 193 WHO member states reported reliable cause-of-death statistics (WHO, 2007).

Conclusions

Mortality statistics can provide a useful and informative way of identifying differences in causes of death and explanations for who dies. Data on death rates remain a powerful indicator of the overall health status of a population and it is clear that there is a strong association between social deprivation and death. However, the limitations of such information must be taken into account. In order to monitor progress towards the UN's Millennium Development Goals, which include targets to reduce infant and maternal mortality, standardised accurate data collection must take place. The WHO predicts that while infant and maternal death rates will continue to decline, deaths caused by cancer, heart disease, stroke and HIV/AIDS will increase (WHO, 2007). These changes in causes of death reflect both the increasing ageing population as well as the changes within societies as they develop and become more affluent.

References

Adjuik, M., Smith, T., Clark, S., Todd, J., Garrib, A., Kinfu, Y., Kahn, K., Mola, M., Ashraf, A., Masanja, H., Adazu, U., Sacarlal, J., Alam, N., Marra, A., Gbangou, A., Mwageni, E. and Binka, F. (2006) 'Cause-specific mortality rates in sub-Saharan Africa and Bangladesh', *Bulletin of the World Health Organization,* 84 (3): 181–8.
Bowles, C., Walters, R. and Jacobson, B. (2007) *Born Equal? Inequalities in Infant Mortality in London. A Technical Report.* London: London Health Observatory.
Child Mortality Coordination Group (2006) 'Tracking progress towards the Millenium Development Goals: reaching consensus on child mortality levels and trends', *Bulletin of the World Health Organization,* 84 (3): 225–32.
Fauveau, V. (2006) 'Assessing probable causes of death without death registration or certificates: a new science?', *Bulletin of the World Health Organization,* 84 (3): 246–7.
Glickman, M., Corbing, T., Tortoriello, M. and Devis, T. (2006) *United Kingdom Health Statistics.* London: Office of National Statistics.
Kapoor, S.K. and Anand, K. (2002) 'Nutritional transition: a public health challenge in developing countries', *Journal of Epidemiology and Community Health,* 56: 804–5.
Komaromy, C. (2006) *Working for Health: Health on Wider Agendas.* Milton Keynes: Open University Press.
Mathers, C.D., Stein, C., Ma Fat D., Rao, C., Inoue, M., Tomijima, N., Bernard, C., Lopez, A.D. and Murray, C.J. (2002) *Global Burden of Disease 2000: Version 2 Methods and Results.* Geneva. World Health Organization.

McLaren, G.L. and Bain, M.R.S (1998) *Deprivation and Health in Scotland: Insights from NHS Data*. Edinburgh: ISD Scotland Publications. Available online at: www.show.scot.nhs.uk/publications/isd/deprivation_and_health (last accessed 23 November 2007).

Sidell, M. and Lloyd, C. (2007) 'Studying the population's health', in S. Earle, C.E. Lloyd, M. Sidell and S. Spurr (eds), *Theory and Research in Promoting Public Health*. London: Sage/The Open University. pp. 231–72.

United Nations (UN) (2000) *United Nations Millennium Declaration*. Available online at: http:/www.un.org/millennium/declaration/ares552e.htm (last accessed 23 November 2007).

United Nations Development Programme (UNDP) (2006) *Millennium Development Goals*. Available online at: www.undp.org/mdg/goallist.shtml (last accessed 23 November 2007).

World Health Organization (WHO) (online) www.who.int/whosis/mort/en/ (last accessed 1 June 2008).

World Health Organization (WHO) (2007) *World Health Statistics 2007*. Geneva: WHO. Available online at: www.who.int/whosis/whostat 2007. pdf (last accessed 1 June 2008).

Wilkinson, R.G. (1986) 'Socio-economic differences in mortality: interpreting the data on their size and trends', in R.G. Wilkinson, (ed.), *Class and Health: Research and Longitudinal Data*. London: Tavistock. pp.1–20.

Wilkinson, R.G. (1997) 'Socioeconomic determinants of health. Health inequalities: relative or absolute material standards?', British Medical Journal, (7080): 591–5.

Part II
Caring at the End of Life
Introduction

Sarah Earle

This part of the reader focuses on caring at the end of life, exploring the role of individuals, organisations and health systems in ensuring appropriate and timely care.

In the final reading in Part I, Cathy E. Lloyd explored the wide variations in the experience of death and dying, concluding that there remains a strong association between social deprivation and death. The first two readings in this part of the book explore end-of-life care within this wider context. In Reading 8 Allan Kellehear argues that while contemporary technological innovations enable the delay and timing of death, poverty and ageing are the two global exceptions which serve to deny such privileges to the majority of people who live on the margins of society (see also Reading 33). Exploring what he defines as 'shameful deaths', Kellehear argues that changing the circumstances of dying people relies not only on institutional change but on the role of a wide range of individuals, organisations and governments.

Reading 9 continues with this theme. In this reading, Peter A. Singer and Kerry W. Bowman argue that, although it has not traditionally been viewed as such, quality end-of-life care is a global public health issue. The reading begins by outlining the underlying premise of this position before exploring how and why quality end-of-life care is a global health systems problem. The authors highlight the lack of knowledge related to end-of-life care in a global context suggesting that quality end-of-life care is a health systems problem in so far as it is a problem of health information. The final section in this reading outlines the importance of cultural sensitivity, acknowledging the importance of religion and other belief systems in improving end-of-life care (see also Reading 6).

Central to the provision of end-of-life care is the way that the 'end of life' comes to be defined. In the next reading, Carol Komaromy explores the definition of dying by drawing on an ethnographic study of death and dying in care homes for older people (see also Reading 8). Komaromy highlights the importance of making temporal predictions of death but notes that the period of dying is often determined by a range of seemingly arbitrary markers. The privileged status of dying, Komaromy argues, enables care staff to prepare for a death – particularly important in homes where resourcing is scarce – but also ensures that residents can benefit from routine care reserved only for those near death.

In Reading 11, Mercedes Bern-Klug, Charles Gessert and Sarah Forbes explore end-of-life care in relation to social work practice. They argue that dying is more than a medical event and is one which can have devastating effects – both financial and emotional – on all concerned. As such, Bern-Klug, Gessert and Forbes suggest that social workers should work with people who are dying as counsellors, advocates and 'context interpreters'. They also highlight the important role of social workers in working with the families of those who are dying as well as with other colleagues who are caring for people at the end of life.

Reading 12 also focuses on the importance of emotions at the end of life (see also Reading 30). In a sociological analysis of reproductive loss, Sarah Earle, Carol Komaromy, Pam Foley and Cathy E. Lloyd focus on the care provided by midwives when a baby dies. In this reading the authors argue that the expression of emotions is socially and institutionally determined. This means that emotions are regulated and that feelings are managed according to what is seen to be a 'normal response' to death. As noted by the authors of the previous reading, caring at the end of life is emotionally demanding. However, Earle, Komaromy, Foley and Lloyd conclude by arguing that when midwives (and other care workers) are themselves supported, they are often better placed to provide appropriate and timely care for others.

While Readings 11 and 12 have focused on the role of professional carers, Reading 13 turns its attention to the needs of informal carers. In this reading Richard Harding and Irene J. Higginson report the findings of a systematic review of interventions designed to support informal carers. Focusing specifically on informal care-giving in cancer and palliative care, they argue that while informal carers are known to have significant psychological needs there are, in fact, very few targeted interventions and many of these have not been effectively evaluated. The reading outlines a range of interventions including: home nursing care, respite services, social networks and activity enhancement, problem-solving education, and group work.

Reading 14 also discusses the role of evaluation in end-of-life care, and in this final reading Jacqueline H. Watts focuses on the role of the creative arts. Watts explores the creative arts as a medium for communication and expression, as well as its role in motivation. The role of the creative arts as a tool for managing emotions is also critically explored. However, the author argues that while the potential benefit of such practice is widely acknowledged, its evidence base is lacking. Watts concludes by arguing that although artistic practice is positively encouraged in many end-of-life settings, attention must be paid to issues of power, evaluation and resource distribution.

8

A Social History of Dying

Allan Kellehear

[…]

Late and early dying, from AIDS or frail ageing, can take many years, sometimes over a decade. Like state detainees everywhere, this is further complicated by the fact that the people inside these experiences are not always clear about their destination, or if they are, even when it might be reached.

Certainly in the anthropological literature this is a rare example of 'liminal' status indeed. 'Bare life' now signifies a new and proliferating social category of dying and living. It points to the shameful death: a dying characterised by an inability to successfully time death in clinical and biographical terms and to make that timing 'good' through redemptive social practices such as organ donation, economic continuity or political inclusion.

The power of timing

Nowotny (1994: 152) observes that 'knowing the right moment is useful; determining it confers power and promises control'. This comment is fundamental to the contemporary challenge of timing death. With major improvements in public health and medical technology there is a widespread desire and optimism that the timing of death can be controlled. Life support technology is merely one example of how death can be delayed almost indefinitely. Public health screening, with all its emphasis on prevention, is also, at least in part, a storyline about the potential to delay death. But at the time of our greatest optimism about our abilities to time death two global exceptions stare down that optimism – ageing and poverty.

Our public health successes in the prosperous parts of the globe have created life span overruns, with more and more people paradoxically outliving their bodies or minds. And in the streets and alleyways of those prosperous countries and in the towns and villages of poor nations everywhere the conditions of rural and urban squalor conspire to smash the hopes and health of millions. These populations have little or no access to life-saving technologies or liberal ideas about tolerance towards the contagious.

The desire to at least time death, the realisation of which promises practical benefits at the deathbed, or power and control over one's family and community relations during the life course, is cancelled in the shame, stigma and loneliness of death in institutionalised old age and in poverty-related contagion. Both in the uncertainty of the terminal phase of dying, and in the social redundancy inherent in a spoiled identity unable to redeem itself through other rites of community contribution, the challenge of timing asks the seemingly impossible.

Furthermore, both the interpersonal and broader institutional changes that might alter these circumstances in favour of these dying people are mostly dependent on other people – not these at the centre of shameful dying. It is other people who will hold the key to reversing or rehabilitating shameful deaths: the carers in nursing homes, transnational pharmaceutical industries, wealthy countries and their governments, international and national health policy-makers concerned with international aid but also the social alternatives to institutionalising the elderly.

After some two million years of human death and dying history we find ourselves at the beginning again, but with some reverse characteristics. The dying in the Cosmopolitan Age find themselves dependent on the community of others to assist them, not in some challenging otherworld journey but in an uncomfortable or distressing this-world journey. Inheritance is once again to come from survivors rather than the dying as it once did.

But it is not weapons, charms or food that the dying require now. It is rather the technical and social challenge of recognising dying itself among those for whom the task of detecting dying can be difficult and ambiguous. The 'weapons' and 'food' we must offer up to the dying now are the less tangible but no less real products of social support, tolerance and courage to sit with the contagious or the unrecognising dying. This is the inheritance we would seem to owe the dying, yet in these matters of obligation it is no longer easy to gain consensus, even less cooperation.

For in the Cosmopolitan Age, unlike the Stone Age, men and women do not make decisions from small wandering groups but in international consortiums of nation-states and global financial and trade organisations. Even within a single country, decisions about aged care policy are taken in the broader context of rival political parties, rival social and medical priorities, competing vested interests and the bureaucratisation and dilution participatory democratic institutions. The desire for managed dying in properous countries commonly eclipses concern for hidden forms of dying that are stigmatised, and therefore of marginal social interest and worth, as well as those at the international margins.

And as each year passes, the prevalence of shameful deaths in aged care facilities and poor countries rises. The challenge of their timing fuels a growing interest and recruitment into anti-heroic forms of dissent and resistance. The desire to take control of the timing of death grows stronger in this context as the fear of losing that control grows globally. There is more interest in suicide, assisted or otherwise; greater resentment towards those with control and power – both interpersonal and institutional, both domestic and international. These forms of dissent create further divisions within moral and social debates everywhere about quality of life, the meaning of life, and control and social inclusion at the end of life.

In the otherworld journey death was a form of dying. In the Cosmopolitan Age dying has become a form of social death, a living without supports and a dying frequently unrecognised. The growing global desire to avoid this kind of dying continues to fuel the obsession with timing. And there seems no end in sight for these forms of dying and these timing strategies to avoid them.

Personal control and impersonal death

There are strategies to avoid shame and to recapture control. There are ways to undermine the prospect of a shameful death. Some of these strategies are socially respectable, others less so. But all these strategies, whatever their moral features, should be understood in terms of time. According to Shneidman (1973: 82–90) a dying person who wishes to commit suicide is someone who wishes to choose the time and place and simply refuses to wait for 'nature' to take its course. He or she might also be a 'death ignorer', someone who believes that death will only end his or her physical but not mental and spiritual existence.

The dying person who wishes to die might also be someone who hastens their own death through risk-taking or failure to safeguard themselves. Shneidman has also suggested that many people who wish to die may give little psychological and perhaps physiological resistance to death, making them more vulnerable to infection and other disease. These attitudes and actions may all constitute a certain control over the timing of one's death under shameful and stigmatising social conditions (DeSpelder & Strickland 2005: 422–8).

Another strategy to control the timing of death is the rising interest in 'advanced directives'. Advanced directives, also known as 'living wills', are written directives left by people who are well and psychologically competent to indicate their desires in case of a catastrophic medical event that does not allow normal communication to occur. Accidents or medical emergencies, such as massive stroke, may leave a person gravely and irreversibly ill and uncommunicative. Under conditions of this kind some people will leave a set of 'directives' that advise medical staff and family that they do not want cardiac resuscitation, mechanical respiration, artificial feeding or hydration, or antibiotics. Only pain relief, even pain relief that might kill them, is requested (DeSpelder & Strickland 2005: 245–52).

In a terminal phase of dying, some patients may also request a do-not-resuscitate (DNR) order. This is an advice to emergency services personnel that if the dying person is found to be dead at home, or even in hospital, they are not to be resuscitated. The dying patient wishes the fatal disease and dying to take their natural course.

Advanced directives, DNR orders and some suicides can be seen as examples of the rise in interest and anxiety over timing death in modern industrial contexts. All these strategies are designed to undermine or to outright avoid a shameful situation of 'living death' – a set of circumstances where a dying person is repeatedly brought back from death, is kept in a biological space between living and dying, or where failed medical interventions leave the ageing or dying person vulnerable to an indefinite period of nursing home or life support care.

In poor countries of the world, the strategies to avoid shameful forms of death create, not careful contingency plans for the future, but rather contingency plans for the present. Rifkin (1987: 166–7) reviews some of the literature on time-usage by the poor. He demonstrates that people in poverty have a present-directed time approach to life because their futures are often uncertain. This is a rational response to the time-cultures of poverty due to the precariousness of their health and illness experiences, the vagaries of their labour market experiences, a lack of economic resources to invest, and their lower thresholds towards economic, social and political adversity.

Wood (2003: 455) argues that poor people are dominated by a 'dysfunctional time preference' behaviour where people pursue short-term goals of security and forgo or have little
interest and confidence in long-term prospects. Often the reason for this lack of confidence
is found in the simple fact that long-term plans have seldom worked for them. Why plan
for a farming future when two tribes have been warring over your lands for the last two
decades? Why plan for retirement when you are HIV-positive and have no antiviral drugs
to help you plan even for a single decade of your remaining life?

In sub-Sahara Africa, a large region of assorted so-called nation-states, vast areas are
ruled by 'warlords' – a network of quasi-military chiefs who control militias and food lines
and dispense rough justice in crude life-and-death terms (Wood 2003: 467). Under these
conditions, the state does not guarantee protection or any safety net in health or welfare.
There is no future except cooperating with such local networks of militia, so land, family
and loyalty are paid in return for meagre food and protection.

Part of the offering from these modern forms of 'client' relations includes 'opportunities' for cheap labour but also military service. These short-term risk management strategies offer livelihoods that work. For an alternative sociology of dying they also offer other
forms of death that are possibly more 'honourable' and timely. Death in war, against an
'outside' rather than 'inside' evil, may he preferable to a slow, stigmatising dying. These
death also have the advantage of offering a social future morally more competitive than a
biological one controlled by a shameful virus. Choosing a political and economic lifestyle,
in the context of poverty and the prospect of AIDS dying, is also choosing a time strategy
that might avoid both, and remove the prospect of shame into the bargain.

The future of dying: a time for change

Within the modern experience of the well-managed life, people who live with life-
threatening illnesses are able to 'buy time' from an array of medical, surgical and pharmacological interventions. For children, young adults, and other people in mid-life these
interventions are among the many blessings and wonders of living in a technically complex and wealthy society. But without money political influence or well-functioning memory there is no power to 'buy' time. Shameful deaths of the present Cosmopolitan Age do
not represent a failure of technological achievement but rather – and there is no delicate
way to express this – a moral and social failure to provide satisfactory models of social
care for dying people at the economic margins of our world.

Our domestic priorities continue to target the laboratory pursuit of new cures without an
equally serious eye on the end-of-life consequences of these successful medical cam-
paigns. Our international priorities continue to target poverty and health without an equally
serious recognition of the inevitable end-of-life experiences of people who are dying now
and will continue to die in the future *without community supports*.

There remains a longstanding failure to recognise that greater health and welfare bring
us greater life-expectancy and therefore greater end-of-life care challenges that are not
adequately addressed in any wealthy country by current social policies and practices. The
nursing home is a location greatly feared by people in the wealthy countries that paradoxically love to build them. There is little effort in designing, experimenting or even

debating the alternatives. While this period of policy paralysis exists, more populations move towards these institutional destinations with their communities neither socially, financially nor politically prepared for any other options.

The tiresome Cosmopolitan tendency to focus on health, along with wealth, youth and beauty, continues to threaten the social reciprocity at the core of the dying experience. Although such social values sometimes disguise a deeper fear of decay and difference, the tendency we are witnessing is to concentrate most of our community, policy and media attention on well-managed dying as part of the well-managed life. We of the wealthy countries have a public reputation to keep and a cultural morale to maintain in this regard.

This results in an over-attention and romantic obsession with heroic storylines of people dying of cancer, receiving palliative and hospice care, of fighting for the right to die 'with dignity and choice'. These images and storylines obscure the less glamorous but more numerous marginal experiences of dying among the elderly and the poor of the world. Furthermore, such images and storylines distract people from placing the problems of long-term care on equal footing with their obsessions with short-terms cures.

Care of the dying, as we have witnessed throughout human history, is a complex challenge, never more so than today. There is no magic bullet; there will be no quick fix here. People yearn for their dying as otherworld journey, or as good death, or as a well-managed dying. They hope to die with the support of their communities, anticipating and preparing for death, dying in basic comfort afforded them by their healers – and at the right time. At all levels in today's societies these different desires, values and ideals of dying undergo great challenge.

Grave doubts now confront the idea of the otherworld journey. In other quarters of the world, new ideas and experiences near death provide serious questions and revisions about the otherworld. Preparing for death has become uncertain; often it is simply detached now from the prospect of death itself since no one is absolutely sure when death might come.

Managing dying is becoming increasingly easier for the wealthy few who can afford the best medical and palliative care and, anyway, many people die suddenly of circulatory disease or accident and avoid a period of social and psychological dying. In other parts of the health system, death is being tamed so strongly by health services that it is now indistinguishable from emergency, acute and community care of the sick. The idea of dying would almost slip away from modern view save for one major development – the rather public mistimed and embarrassing dyings of the Cosmopolitan Age that do not respond to high-tech interventions and routine hospital care.

The presence of AIDS among us reminds most of us that the engine room for these problems lies among our international economic and foreign policies more than simply a failure of laboratory science. The presence of dementia among us reminds us that successful public health and medical programs have a disturbing nemesis that we must face as an equally urgent but domestic social challenge. What both of these demographic trends in mortality and social experiences of dying ironically tell us is that dying is not, and never was, solely a medical challenge.

The human problem of dying has always been a set of social and moral choices about care, and about how those choices are negotiated between dying persons and their community – whatever form that community has taken in the past. In this precise way, the study of dying is like gazing into a reflecting pool. The waters there reflect back to us the kinds of people we have become. More than ever before then, it is timely to ask the question: what kinds of people *have* we become?

References

DeSpelder, L.A. & A. Strickland (2005) *The Last Dance: Encountering death and dying*. McGraw-Hill, New York.

Nowotny, H. (1994) *Time: The modern and postmodern challenge*. Polity Press, Cambridge.

Rifkin, J. (1987) *Time Wars: The primary conflict in human history*. Henry Holt & Co., New York.

Shneidman, E.S. (1973) *Deaths of Man*. Quadrangle Books, New York.

Wood, G. (2003) Staying secure, staying poor: The Faustian bargain. *World Development* 31(3): 455–71.

9

Quality End-of-Life Care:
A Global Perspective

Peter A. Singer and Kerry W. Bowman

[…]

Why is quality end-of-life care a global public health problem?

[…] There are 56 million deaths per year in the world, 85% of which are in developing countries. One can assume that each also affects five other people in terms of informal care-giving and grieving relatives and friends – a very modest estimate, particularly in the developing world. The total number of people therefore affected each year in the world by end-of-life care is about 300 million people, about 5% of the world's population [1]. This makes quality end-of-life care a global public health problem on the grounds of numbers of people involved.

To put this problem in perspective, there are 36 million people living with HIV, 8 million people become sick with TB annually, resulting in 2 million deaths [2] and 300–500 million cases of malaria result in 1.5–2.7 million deaths [3]. Admittedly, we do not conceptualize quality end-of-life care as a public health problem in the same way we conceptualize HIV, malaria and TB as public health problems. But this difference may have more to do with the social constmction of these problems rather than any intrinsic difference between quality end-of-life care and these other problems. Like HIV, malaria, and TB, quality end-of-life care threatens the health and well being of a large population of people. The fact that we do not traditionally view end-of-life care as a public health problem is perhaps more a symptom of Western death-denying culture than any intrinsic difference between quality end-of-life care and these other global public health problems.

In addition to the sheer numbers, quality end-of-life care is a global public health problem because of the nature of the interventions that could be used to improve the problem. Improving end-of-life care will require improvements in health systems as discussed

---

Excerpts from 'Quality end-of-life care: A global perspective' by Peter A. Singer and Kerry W. Bowman, *BMC Palliative Care*, 1(4): 3–10.

below. However, other needed interventions are more in the realm of public health, such as large-scale educational programs for public health workers and for the public, population-based strategies to destigmatize death and mainstream it into health systems, and changes in social policies in relation to, for example, orphan care.

[...]

Why is quality end-of-life care a global health system problem?

End-of-life care is a health systems problem in the sense that – at least in some countries – the majority of deaths occur in hospital [4]. It is a health system problem because [...] much research in palliative care has involved the organization and delivery of palliative care services [5]. It is a health systems problem because quality improvement techniques, such as repaid cycle change, have been applied in an effort to improve the quality of end-of-life care. Finally, it is a health systems problem because of the need to introduce quality end-of-life care into the education and accountability of health system managers and health care professionals.

However, there is a more fundamental sense in which quality end-of-life care is a health systems problem. [...] Improving quality end-of-life care is a problem of health information. Information about quality is recognized as a central health system concern, as exemplified by the report card movement. We have never seen information on quality end-of-life care on quality report cards. Why? Just as clinicians once put dying patients in the room at the end of the hall and never made rounds on them, health policy makers have kept the issue of quality end-of-life care outside the mainstream of their concerns. For example, despite data on mortality, and on other measures of quality of care, there is no information on quality indicators for end-of-life care in the statistical appendices of WHO's World Health Reports. There were also no measures related to quality end-of-life care among the health system performance measures in the 2000 World Health Report.

The lack of knowledge related to the end-of-life experience represents a health information deficit. It is remarkable that such a significant element of health care delivery is so poorly understood. Health systems may not want to be known as good places to die, since this may counteract the cure-oriented message underlying much of acute care. Yet the conditions of the dying are often unacceptable, and more and more people are calling for change.

[...]

The cultural context of quality end-of-life care

Because culture significantly influences how we see the world, any effort to understand or improve quality end-of-life care in the world must be sensitive to cultural considerations. Cultures are much deeper than their traditions, extending to fundamental differences in modes of reasoning grounded in the way the world is perceived. Furthermore, it is known that attitudes toward end-of-life care is relative to particular cultures, societies, and times [6]. Often, when people planning or providing health care and recipients of health care come from different cultural backgrounds, they interact under the influence of unspoken assumptions that are so different that they prevent effective communication and initiatives may break down all together [7–9]. Simply applying Western perspectives on end-of-life care to developing nations is unrealistic, and apt to fail.

Although Western culture is diverse, evolving and increasingly views health and illness in a broader context, Western medicine remains largely based on scientific, rational and objective principles. Ultimately this is as much a cultural construction as any non-Western philosophic or health-related belief system. Disease is perceived as being largely under the control of science [10]. Because of the institutionalization of death, many people may expect medical solutions at the end-of-life. Death is often perceived as a failure of medical care. Demand for aggressive treatment at the end-of-life can become extreme and unrealistic. Research in North America shows that 18 percent of lifetime costs for medical care are apt to be incurred in the last year of life [11].

[…]

Some of the early hospices were founded by people with Christian beliefs, or in religious institutions. Therefore, some aspects of the palliative care/hospice care movement are rooted in Christian heritage and have philosophic underpinnings that may be foreign to many people in the developing world who see the world from a different philosophic or religious perspective. The direct application of traditional hospice/palliative care programs to the developing world may therefore be problematic.

An important cultural distinction in Western medicine is that it is assumed that the person experiencing the illness is the best person to make health-care decisions. However, many non-Western cultures perceive the family or community as vital in receiving and disclosing information necessary to decision making and to the organization of patient care. Furthermore significant differences exist in gender roles. Particularly in the developing world, caregiving has been and continues to be overwhelmingly the responsibility of women [12]. Although men may also be caregivers, these roles are not culturally perceived as significant aspects of their lives. Unfortunately, because much discussion and policy formation have been from male perspectives the individual and social significance of female procreative and caregiving roles has often been ignored. These differences require respect, understanding and careful cross-cultural consideration.

Many people in developing countries hold profoundly different views of the nature, cause and meaning of health, illness, death and dying than those in the developed world. The concept of explanatory models of illness reflect the cultural understanding of what illness is, how it occurs, why it exists and what measures can be taken to prevent or control it [13]. In Western medicine, the primary explanatory model of illness focuses on abnormalities in the structure and function of body organs and systems. Most non-Western cultures tend to perceive illness in a much broader and far less tangible manner – for example, some Africans may perceive health and disease as separate entities, influenced by external forces such as witchcraft, revenge or other social causes [14]. These belief systems are often referred to as traditional belief systems. Western culture however is ubiquitous, the vast majority of explanatory models of illness are now intricately blended between Western and traditional perspectives.

For many people in developing countries stronger religious and cultural observances and community support may ameliorate much of the need or expectation for 'specialized' approaches to end-of-life care. In many societies in the developing world many people are barely exposed to other views – traditional beliefs of death being the will of God or a natural consequence of the cycle of life may be profoundly comforting and nurture a fatalistic acceptance and stoicism toward death. Introducing death as a 'specialized' service – by viewing suffering as a treatable, medical phenomenon – raises a profound ethical questions as to whether in the developing world would it be at odds with existing cultural and religious perspectives on suffering, death and their meaning [15].

The health care infrastructure of some developing countries may be minimal, and focused on disease prevention. Discussions of death, in this context, may be shunned as they are a reminder of the gross inadequacies of the health care system. As with Western nations effective pain control is problematic, although the roots of the problem are different. In developing nations pain control is impeded by a lack of opioids and a fear of Western style drug problems, which may greatly limit the use of analgesics.

These cultural considerations lead to the conclusion that any effort to improve quality of end-of-life care in developing countries must be carefully tailored, and include people from developing countries, who will be sensitive to the cultural context. Bringing end-of-life care into the main stream may fit well with the worldview of many developing cultures, as life and death are more often viewed as integrated [16].

Capacity for end-of-life care in developing countries

[...]

Health care initiatives in the developing world must deal with inadequate infrastructures, poor administrative systems, the extreme poverty of many patients, restricted opioid prescribing and minimal educational opportunities for health care staff [17]. Clearly, these are not the conditions for building specialized programs. Aggressive high-tech approaches at the end-of-life are not feasible. A further impediment to improving end-of-life care in the developing world is that a majority of health care spending, both public and private, goes to curative efforts – hospitals in urban areas often account for more then 80% of total health care costs. Although changing quickly, the majority of the population in the developing world continues to live in rural areas [18].

'Grass roots' palliative care initiatives in developing nations such as Zimbabwe and South Africa [19] are funded at a very low level and are often left to deal with assisting social needs which arise out of the effects of extreme poverty exacerbated by illness. Yet these are early encouraging results from *The Foundation for Hospices in Sub-Saharan Africa* which has the mandate of helping the existing hospices sustain and expand their programs. Additionally, the program teaches basics of HIV/AIDS care and prevention. Family members are instructed in care-giving techniques, and are also given an essential orientation of how HIV/AIDS is and is not transmitted [20]. [...]

The urban elite of many developing nations are often the only recipients of Western style palliative care. This group and the rural masses live in different worlds. In India, and other developing nations, palliative care for cancer patients exists often for the privileged and reaches only a minority of cancer patients [21]. Again, small local initiatives in the area of pain control have shown encouraging results [22].

Views of illness and help-seeking behaviour in the developing world are in rapid transition. A study done in Northeast Thailand on the experience of villagers dying at home revealed that biomedical theories of disease coexisted or have been supplanted by traditional beliefs about illness [23]. When patients involved with the minimal health care system are diagnosed with terminal disease they are quickly sent home to die. Family and community provided ample psychosocial care – fortunately the developing world often has three generation families which are able and willing to care for the dying (although this may no longer be the case in countries that have been devastated by AIDS). Community and traditional healers, however, are on their own to consult and provide diagnosis, treatment and palliative care.

An excellent example of how the end-of-life can be improved without high-tech solutions is the WHO Cancer program [24]. This initiative works with local governments to establish national cancer control programs (NCCP) to address the cancer problem at the country level in accordance with the epidemiological, social and economic situations. This comprehensive approach assesses the cancer burden and defines priority objectives within the areas of prevention, treatment and palliation. With careful planning the establishment of NCCP offers the most rational means to achieve cancer control, even where resources are severely limited.

[...]

Death in the developing world is most often seen as an integral part of life. Consequently, the Western 'specialization' of death may already be a contributing factor to why traditional Western approaches to end-of-life care have had so little effect in the developing world. Integrating local, culturally based perspectives of health, illness and dying in combination with building national consensus to changes in policies, and procedures, are apt to have a greater effect on improving end-of-life care in the developing world than implementing contemporary Western medical advances.

[...]

References

1   World Health Organization: 'World Health Report annex table', 2000, 164–167 [http://www.who.int/whr/2000/en/statistics.htm]
2   World Health Organization: *Fact Sheet #104* [http://www.who.int/inf-fs/en/fact_104.html]April 2000
3   World Health Organization: *World Health Statistics. Geneva* 1998
4   Heyland DK, Lavery JV, Tranmer JE, Shortt SED, Taylor S: 'Dying in Canada: is it an institutionalized, technologically supported experience?' *Journal of Palliative Care* 2000, 16: S10–16

5   Higginson IJ: 'Evidence based palliative care: there is some evidence and there needs to be more'. *BMJ* 1999, 319: 462–463

6   Bowman KW: 'Culture, ethics and the biodiversity crisis of Central Africa', *Advances in Applied Biodiversity* 2001, 2: 167–174

7   Kleinman AM: *Patients and healers in the context of culture.* Berkeley: University of California Press; 1980

8   Hahn RA, Kleinman AM: 'Biomedical practice and anthropological theory: frameworks and direction', *Annual Review of Anthropology* 1983, 12: 305–333

9   Harwood A: *Ethnicity and medical care.* Cambridge: Harvard University Press; 1981

10   Bowman KW, Hui C: 'Bioethics for clinicians: 20. Chinese bioethics', *Canadian Medical Association Journal* 2000, 163: 1481–1485

11   Fuchs VR: 'Though much is taken; reflections on ageing, health and medical care', *Milbank Memorial Fund Quarterly: Health and Society* 1984, 62: 143–166

12   King-Patricia A: 'Helping women helping children: drug policy and future generations', *Milbank-Quarterly* 1991, 69(4): 595–621

13   Kleinman AM: *Patients and healers in the context of culture.* Berkeley: University of California Press; 1981

14   Chipfakacha V. 'The role of culture in primary health', *South African Medical Journal* 1994, 84(12): 860–862

15   Seale C: 'Changing patterns of death and dying', *Social Science and Medicine* 2000, 51: 917–930

16   Olweney CLM: 'Quality of life in developing countries', *Journal of Palliative Care* 1992, 8: 25–30

17   Haber D: 'New themes in palliative care: book review', *Social Science and Medicine* 1993, 48: 1301–1303

18   World Health Organization: 'Cities and the Population Issue', *44th World Health Assembly, Technical discussion 7, background document* Geneva 1991

19   Hockley J: "The evolution of the hospice approach," *New themes in palliative care. Buckingham: Open University Press*; 1997, 84–100

20   Chermack JA: 'Assisting hospices in Sub-Saharan Africa', *Lost Acts Electronic Newsletter,* January 2001

21   Seale C: 'Changing patterns of death and dying', *Social Science and Medicine* 2000, 51: 917–930

22   Guha R: 'Living with cancer', *The Hindu* 19 August 18, 2000

23   Bennett E, Salazar F, Williams A, Himmavnh V, Charerntanyarak L: 'Dying at home: the experience of four villages in northeast Thailand', *Annual Conference of Australasia Society of HIV Medicine* 123: November 3–6, 1994

24   World Health Organization: '*World Health Report annex table 3*', 2000, 164–167 [http://www.who.int/whr/2000/en/statistics.htm]

10

The State of Dying

Carol Komaromy

Dr. Riley[1] told me that Elsie was in what he considered to be 'a state of dying'. He added that she had surprised everyone by pulling through on Thursday night, but 'she won't recover. She may last a few more weeks, but she's terminally ill. She's had a CVA[2] and this is the cause of her sudden deterioration last week'. (Komaromy, 2005: 151)

This reading is based on the findings of an ethnographic study into the management of death and dying in care homes for older people. The quote above sets the scene for the discussion that follows on how 'dying' was diagnosed. The data were drawn from participant observations over a 12-month period and interviews with care staff, general practitioners, care home residents and relatives of deceased residents in eight care homes in England.

Glaser and Strauss (1976) highlight the importance of being able to make temporal predictions of death for those people who work in the area of death and dying. They claim that this is explained by the need to reduce the uncertainty associated with death. Certainly my findings showed that such 'temporal predictions of dying trajectories' enabled care home staff to prepare for death and, this preparation included the expressed aim of affording the benefit of terminal care to residents. Senior home staff members with experience of death and dying were more likely than less experienced colleagues to be able to assess whether or not a resident was 'dying' and, if so, how imminent the death might be. However, while staff often speculated about the significance of particular signs of dying, this dying status had to be confirmed, or conferred onto specific residents by a doctor, most often the resident's GP. I would argue that by formalising the period of dying, doctors acted as imprimaturs. They also decided whether or not to launch a rescue for those residents whose lives were considered to be worthy or capable of being 'saved'. As a last resort, general practitioners might also decide to transfer residents when it was agreed that it was beyond the home's capacity to care for them in this terminal phase. However, in my study, despite the fact that it was usually the resident's general practitioner who made any formal diagnosis of dying, the senior staff members were the people who orchestrated the management of death and dying. In practice, this meant setting up a routine of terminal care, usually through a care plan. The privileged status of dying afforded a routine of care that was distinct from other forms of care. This involved residents being nursed in the private space of their own bedroom and no longer sharing the communal spaces of the home.

The rhetoric of a 'good' death, expressed so often at interviews, was not always the reality. My observations revealed that the main focus of end-of-life care was on the physical needs of residents. In particular, keeping residents clean and free from pressure sores was the main aspect of this care. For example, the matron of Regis House set up a care plan for Alice (one of the residents whose dying and death I observed), that included the need to avoid pressure sores by changing Alice's position every two hours and also offer her liquids. I observed that the staff visited at least every hour, and when the aforementioned two-hourly care was due, care staff spent longer with Alice (but not ever more than ten minutes) performing the tasks of physical caregiving. Therefore, while staff expressed the aim of avoiding a 'lonely' death by sitting with dying residents, this seemed to be compromised by staff shortages and different priorities. If relatives were not available to keep a bedside vigil, then I noted from observations that care staff would look in on a dying resident at regular intervals.

In what follows, I explore in more depth how the status of dying was awarded to residents. Throughout, I argue that the way in which the category of dying was constructed served to produce a good death as it was interpreted within institutional life.

Awarding a status of dying

The combination of changes in policy that result in later admission to care homes, and the shift away from the dangers of institutional care (Booth, 1985), have resulted in the need to 'keep residents going' in care homes. Therefore, despite their frailty and chronic illnesses this has resulted in a blurred boundary between living and dying, and, within this, I argue that the dying phase is narrowly defined as days or weeks. I argue further that a narrow dying trajectory minimised the risk of identifying dying too early and inappropriately.

While the transition into the category of dying allowed for material privileges associated with terminal care to be awarded to residents such as being kept in bed and receiving bodily care and pain-relieving drugs (often tokenistic) my data showed that, as with 'living', the 'dying' period also fulfilled symbolic functions. For example, fieldwork observations revealed the extent to which the boundaries between life and death were maintained and the strategies that staff deployed in order to do so. The literature on boundaries and rituals is useful to this type of exploration and van Gennep (1960) identified crucial stages of life as rites of passage, including birth, puberty, marriage and death. He argued further that, through ageing and illness, individuals withdraw from active life and social contact. The arguments by Douglas (1984) also help to explain the symbolic significance of boundaries and thus the need to categorise and keep distinct and separate living and dying residents. Douglas argues that by maintaining boundaries that carry high levels of significance such as that between life and death, the rituals and actions that maintain a distinct boundary can, as in this case, serve to avoid contamination of life by death. It seemed to me that in care homes rites and customs served important psychological, sociological and symbolic functions that contributed to the need to separate living and dying residents.

However, while the short duration of the period of dying, allowed for a more sustained intense period of terminal care, my data showed the arbitrary nature of these categories. In a spiral of gradual but uneven decline, which is the case for many older and frail residents, the boundary between living and dying was not easily demarcated and, therefore, predictions were difficult to make. Furthermore, I argue that making an overt and explicit separation between living and dying residents was problematic in settings where death was viewed as the 'natural' and timely outcome of a long life (Komaromy and Hockey, 2001).

In the following section, I consider how the dying trajectory for older people in care homes was narrowly defined, and illustrate the qualities of dying and the way certain features served as signs of the beginning of the dying trajectory. While there was some variation between homes, they all shared the practice of changed routines for a resident once the status of dying was afforded.

The separation of living and dying residents

When residents were considered to be dying, I was keen to explore any existence of the practice of moving them into a separate part of the home, which had been the case in Hockey's study (1990). However, in one interview with Meg Johnson, the head of Poplar Court, she told me that the practice of moving sick residents into bedrooms on the same corridor, so that care staff could more easily observe and attend to their needs, had ceased. She went on to explain how she had discovered that the surviving residents referred to this corridor as 'death row'. In none of the homes in my fieldwork did I observe the transfer or separation of dying residents into special spaces set aside for their care. However, it was clear from talking to care staff that, when a resident who was thought to be dying shared a room, the non-dying resident might be moved out of that bedroom, either at the terminal phase of dying or at the moment of death. Furthermore, several members of staff suggested that having a 'sick bay' would be one way of overcoming the problems of having to care' for dying residents in the home.

While my data suggest that the practice of separating living and dying residents by moving such categorised residents into dying spaces had largely ended, living and dying residents continued to be kept spatially apart. For example, I noted that dying residents no longer shared the public spaces of the home and instead were kept in the more private space of their bedrooms. Separating residents categorised as dying from those who were considered to be living was the first significant change in the routines and practices of care homes that marked the beginning of the dying process. For example, I would argue that the absence of the qualities of living, and the exclusion from the community of living residents that followed and sometimes extended into a sustained lack of presence in public spaces of homes, could be interpreted by other residents and visitors to the home as a sign of dying. In other words, this transition from the status of living to that of dying was marked by absence rather than being able to observe the physical signs of dying.

During my fieldwork, I heard staff and residents refer to vacant chairs as belonging to a particular resident. In this way, the surviving home residents were marking the space of an absent resident and participating in the activities associated with the production of dying. I argue that the absence of dying residents from public spaces not only separated 'dying' from 'living' residents, but also signalled to those residents who were 'living' what was taking place. Since making predictions about death and dying was in the interests of everyone in care homes, I argue that the interpretation was something that was co-produced by staff and residents. A resident's absence from the public spaces of the home was something that living residents remarked upon. For example, Lucy, a resident in Autumn Lodge, told me about the first time that she noticed something was wrong with another resident, called Mary, with whom she was friends:

> She didn't come down to breakfast which was not like her, you know? Then she didn't make it for her lunch and I thought to myself, like, oh erm, there's something wrong here. I asked Jane [the care assistant] and she said, 'She's not so good today Lucy.' I knew it were *more* than that, though!

(Komaromy, 2005)

This brief extract from Lucy suggested to me that Mary's absence from her usual space in the home, in this case, the dining table, was something that Lucy interpreted as being significant and more than 'not so good' as the care assistant explained to her.

It might seem to be self-evident that part of the task for care staff was in distinguishing between living and dying, and the outcome would be the development qualities that could be attributed to each living and dying category. However, while there is a clear distinction to be made between those residents who were able to get up and dress themselves, and those whom the staff had to help, this degree of ability did not in itself define one of the qualities of living. The reality was that for a resident who usually got up out of bed and who could no longer do so, this change could be interpreted as a sign of dying, as the following quote by Lin, the head of Peacehaven Home, illustrates. I asked Lin how she knew that a particular resident – Florence – was dying:

> Possibly about a month before she actually died, she just lay in bed really; she didn't want to do anything. It was just a case of wanting to keep her fluid intake up. We just didn't want to get her into hospital because we didn't feel she would benefit from that. We did speak to the niece and say that she was deteriorating; do you want us to get her into hospital? And she said, 'No. She's been here so long.' Obviously we called the doctor in.

(Komaromy, 2005)

The head of home indicated that because Florence 'just lay in bed' she was dying. This was significant as it marked a change for someone who had been a relatively active participant in living activities. Also in that account, the head of home used the word 'obviously' as if sending for the doctor was an uncontested part of confirming the process of dying, even though, from what she had told me, she did not think that the hospital could do anything for Florence. I would argue that, for Florence, the medical diagnosis served to confirm the staff's own prediction of the beginning of the dying phase.

Medical diagnosis as a marker of dying

By contrast, Danny, a comparatively young male resident aged 67 years at Regis House, had been considered to be dying over a period of months. Eight months after Danny died,

I visited Danny's wife, Lauren, at her own home and talked to her there about his death. There were several events during his illness trajectory that made Lauren think that Danny was dying. The following example from Lauren describes the first of a series of markers which she interpreted as significant:

> And I thought then, I don't know he's going, you know, and that he was going down. And I thought, 'Oh golly, you do look frail' – you know, because he was a strong person. But I thought then that he wasn't getting much better, you know? But he seemed to go down from then.

> (Komaromy, 2005)

Lauren described how Danny had changed his routine from sitting in the residents' lounge to going to bed to lie down in the afternoon, marking a change in his routine behaviour. She followed this account with a description of the moment at which she knew that Danny was definitely going to die and used pneumonia as a metaphor for death. Lauren's retrospective account of Danny's death in the nursing home also shows how the signs that marked dying were not universal since the staff and Lauren placed different interpretations on their significance as features of dying:

> Well, I didn't think he was getting any better because they said he had a chest infection. But when I looked at him, I thought it was pneumonia and I thought, 'Oh golly, I bet he's' – you know – this is the end – or the beginning of the end. Because, you know, people that are ill, or been ill for a long time, they don't always die of the – of what they're ill with. They die of pneumonia, don't they? … And I sort of guessed that he hadn't long to live, you know. But they made him very comfortable. In the last period, they came up every half hour. And they were feeding him liquid drinks.

> (Komaromy, 2005)

This account from Lauren conflicted with those accounts from the home staff who considered that Danny might live. For example, home staff told me that they did not think that Danny was dying because, as the youngest resident in the home, he was *too* young. Chronological age, as timeliness, was an essential feature of a 'natural' death at the end of a long life. Lauren's translation of the term 'chest infection' into 'pneumonia' and, for her, its associations with death, suggested to me that there were different signs being read from similar information. I would emphasise the difference in opinion between the staff and the wife of a resident about what counted as a sign of the beginning of the dying period, and the power which conferring a medical diagnosis had on confirming bad news as Lauren anticipated.

For many residents, it was difficult to discover clear bodily signs that they were dying, since theirs was a path of general deterioration. I argued earlier that the deaths that occurred in homes often followed a slow deterioration and, as such, residents were not subjected to the diagnostic medical tests that a younger person might receive. The pronouncement of a doctor, even in the absence of any medical evidence was a common marker of the beginning of a period of dying. In this way, for Lauren, it seemed that she was part of the negotiation of dying, in that the interaction between the information which she received, combined with her own interpretation of what she looked for, persuaded her that her husband was dying. This suggests that on one level, information, although carrying a high level of significance, was still subject to interpretation. On another level, the medical information, in the form of the doctor's announcement, seemed to carry a lot of weight and made Lauren use the information to confirm her fears.

The following example is taken from an interview with the head of Church House. She described a medical diagnosis that she interpreted as a marker of dying:

> She had a stroke, CVA and – a very large one – and unfortunately she lingered for about a month. Full nursing care, similar to Ted.

(Komaromy, 2005)

There are several interesting points about this brief extract. First, while it is the case that many people make a recovery from a stroke, for this resident the stroke, which was called 'a very large one', served to indicate that a catastrophic event had occurred. The head of the home's assertion was underpinned by an assumption that after a 'large' stroke, which qualified as an acute episode and, as such, a clear marker of dying, there would be a rapid decline into death. Second, the use of the word 'unfortunately' suggests regret that this resident's period of dying was protracted. The regret could also refer to the amount of care that this resident required, 'full nursing care', which would have been difficult to sustain in such a small home. Furthermore, because this death followed Ted's death, another resident who also needed a lot of nursing care, there would have been no respite for the staff. Deaths in care homes were not necessarily spaced over a period of time and even in small homes, with a comparatively low death rate, two deaths close together could make considerable resource demands. The need to be able to marshal scarce resources, and the timing of deaths so that they did not consume all of the resource, further explains the staff's reasons for their preoccupation with the prediction of dying and their desire to avoid defining dying 'too early' and thus have a more extensive period of giving terminal care.

Conclusion

The examples of markers of dying discussed above which included being absent from the public spaces of the home, having a care plan, becoming immobile and having a medical diagnosis confirmed, have provided brief illustrations of how the period of 'dying' was negotiated. The markers also include not eating and other withdrawals from activities associated with living, which were likewise negotiated and not intrinsic signs. In my data, I noted how in the retrospective accounts from staff and other residents, those residents who had been able to move around and who were no longer capable of independent movement were marked as having suffered a severe and possibly irreversible change. I argue that this change from an established way of behaving served as a marker of dying. Furthermore, the way in which dying was produced could be seen as a circular process whereby certain qualities of dying were attributed to individual residents and their condition was then interpreted on this basis. The boundary between life and death which is maintained through such practices requires care home staff to make complex and seemingly arbitrary judgements. The price for getting this wrong is high. Predicting dying sets in motion activities that are difficult and embarrassing to reverse.

Notes

1   The names of care home staff, residents and care homes have been changed to pseudonyms to protect their identity.
2   CVA – Cerebro-vascular accident refers to either a clot in the brain which deprives a large area of brain tissue of oxygen and causes this to die, or a bleed which can have the same effect. Both types of CVA are more commonly called a stroke and result in a one-sided paralysis and depending on the site of the cerebral event, a loss of speech.

References

Booth, T. (1985) *Home Truths: Old People's Homes and the Outcomes of Care*. Aldershot, Hants: Gower Publishing Company.

Douglas, M. (1984) *Purity and Danger: An Analysis of Concepts of Pollution and Taboo*. London: Routledge and Kegan Paul.

Glaser, B.G. and Strauss A.L. (1976) 'Initial definitions of the dying trajectory', in E.S. Schneiden (ed.), *Death Current Perspectives*. California: Mayfield, Palo Alto.

Hockey, J. (1990) Experiences of Death: *An Anthropological Account*. Edinburgh: Edinburgh University Press.

Komaromy, C. (2005) *The Production of Death and Dying in Care Homes for Older People: An Ethonographic Account*. Unpublished PhD thesis. Milton Keynes: The Open University.

Komaromy, C. and Hockey, J. (2001) 'Naturalising death among older adults in residential care', in J. Hockey, J. Katz and N. Small (eds), *Grief, Mourning and Death Ritual*. Buckingham: Open University. pp 73–81.

van Gennep, A. (1960) *The Rites of Passage*. London: Routledge and Kegan Paul.

11

The End of Life and Implications for Social Work Practice

Mercedes Bern-Klug, Charles Gessert and Sarah Forbes

During the 20th century the experience of dying changed dramatically. At the beginning of the 1900s, dying and death were integral parts of the life experience of most people at any age. Many deaths occurred at home following a short course of illness largely unaffected by the limited medical care available. At the beginning of the 21st century, in many cases, the process of dying has become invisible. Today, most deaths occur in old age. Social workers have a key role as 'context interpreters' in helping people at the end of life and their families understand the natural course of the illness, the process of dying, and the advantages and drawbacks of medical interventions. An expanded role for social workers in helping people comprehend the medical and social contexts within which they face end-of-life decisions is discussed.

As a nation we can take great pride in the dramatic improvements in mortality trends achieved during the course of the 20th century. Premature death – death before old age – has been reduced greatly. Indeed, for the majority of people born in the 20th century, death has been postponed. Over the past 100 years we have traded in an early death following an acute illness for a death decades later associated with chronic illness. However, we also have traded in a dying process that was straightforward and recognizable for a dying process that is often unrecognized, invisible, and confounding. All too often contemporary dying is accompanied by limited patient and family understanding of the medical care being provided, poor communication between the patient (or his or her proxy) and the medical team, and unrelieved physical pain and psychospiritual suffering. Most contemporary deaths do not occur at home, but rather in an institution. Many have devastating effects on the family, both emotionally and financially.

[...]

Excerpts from 'The need to revise assumptions about the end of life: implications for social work practice' by Mercedes Bern-Klug, Charles Gessert and Sarah Forbes, *Health and Social Work*, 26(1): 38–47, including Table 3, Copyright © 2001, National Association of Social Workers, Inc., Health & Social Work. Reprinted with permission

Table 11.1 Selected clinical social work roles in end-of-life practice

Role	Major Tasks
Counselor	Works with individuals who are dying and their loved ones on issues related to values clarification, emotional assessment, crisis intervention, goal setting, decision making, dealing with transition and loss, active pursuit of interpersonal growth, and the pursuit of peace of mind.
Context interpreter	Works with other health professionals to ensure that the medical prognosis is understood (by the client, family, and team) within the client's social context. Facilitates consensus building among all parties vis-a-vis goals toward a meaningful end-of-life experience. Assists with advance care planning.
Advocate	Helps clients gain access to medical care in the location of their preference. Advocates for aggressive pain relief. Advocates for financial relief. Helps with negotiations with authority figures. Helps clients gain access to mental health services and care for spiritual concerns.
Team member	Coaches clients and loved ones to identify and communicate physical pain, symptoms, and suffering. Assists clients in achieving a good dying process. Helps fellow team members with their emotional concerns related to providing end-of-life care.

Implications for social work

Social workers in hospital, hospice, home health, nursing home, and assisted-living settings can assist families in visualizing the dying and death of a loved one in the broadest and most meaningful terms (Table 11.1). Skills in values clarification, emotional assessment, crisis intervention, goal setting, decision making, active listening, bereavement counseling, advocacy, and interpersonal communication can be helpful in working with client and families. The process should include a discussion of what constitutes peace of mind for the person who is dying and for the family.

It is difficult to develop peace of mind when perspective is lacking. Social workers can strive to be 'context interpreters' by providing individuals and families with the information they need to understand the natural course of the illness, the likely dying trajectory, and the medical decisions that they are likely to face. Social workers can help people understand what is known and indeed what is knowable about these factors. Social workers with basic medical background can help families put the factual information into context and deal with the emotions provoked by the information or the lack thereof. Most people who are dying—or at increased risk of dying—benefit from a 'big picture' of the end-of-life journey they are making, including discussions about the possible paths to dying and death. The fact that dying may proceed invisibly (that is, without being acknowledged) should be introduced and explored. Families should be encouraged to recognize that with some illnesses there may not be a period when they will be told, or it will otherwise be obvious, that their loved one is 'dying.'

Without a well-developed understanding of the context, families may approach the end of a loved one's life with an unrealistic sense of control over, and responsibility for, the death. With all the progress made in postponing death during the 20th century, the face that we have not abolished death is sometimes overlooked in the heat of a medical crisis.

Death happens. If families develop a realistic understanding of the possible ways in which dying may occur, they improve their chances of making decisions that are consistent with the kind of end-of-life experience they prefer. Social workers can help families understand that when death is approaching it may be desirable for the patient and the family to consider how and where they would prefer to have the death take place. They should be made aware that in some cases the 'natural' path to death (that is, with aggressive medical care voluntarily withheld) may be the most peaceful and painless. For example, even the treatment of reversible conditions such as pneumonia in patients with advanced dementia should be weighed in light of the values and end-of-life goals of the patient and family.

Social workers have plenty of opportunities to use their advocacy skills when working with clients who are at the end of life. Social workers can help clients anticipate that may have to deal with powerful authority figures who 'weigh in' on what should or should not be done medically (personal communication, Michael J. Klug, director, Heartland Medicare Help Program, January 26, 2000). These interactions can be highly guilt provoking and emotionally explosive. Authority figures may be found among well-intentioned family members, physicians, and other health professionals; members of the clergy; friends; and even people unknown to the family. Social workers should assure clients that there are different ways of thinking about the appropriateness of interventions such as feeding tubes, respirators, CPR, and antibiotics (Dunn, 1994) and that it is appropriate and healthy to examine each medical intervention in light of their own values and goals. Families may benefit from validation and support in pursuing the type of dying experience preferred.

Social workers can help other members of the health team understand the dying individual's hopes, desires, and fears. They also can use interpersonal skills to help fellow staff members deal with their own feelings related to end-of-life experiences.

Social workers should develop skills in assessing physical pain. Workers need to be able to help individuals and families articulate the intensity, duration, and quality (for example, aching, sharp, numbing, or cramping) of pain and to request help from physicians. Social workers can help counsel people on common misconceptions about pain (such as the likelihood of addiction at the end of life), the right to pain relief, and locating help to pay for pain medications (Glajchen, Blum, & Calder, 1995; Miller, Hedlund, & Murphy, 1998). Workers and families also need to be vigilant about seeking relief for treatable symptoms such as nausea, shortness of breath, dizziness, and intense itchiness. Health professionals and families should recognize that some patients will opt for more medical treatment at the end of life, even at the risk of physical discomfort (Finucane, 1999; Lynn et al., 1997). This in no way diminishes the importance of pursuing good pain control.

Social workers have an important role in the recognition and relief of suffering that is caused by factors other than physical pain. Helping clients recognize the source of their suffering and decide what to do in response to suffering can fall within the domain of social work. Social workers can help facilitate the process of finding meaning in the end-of-life experience.

Osman and Perlin (1994) discussed the role of the social workers in relation to advance directives. This role can be expanded to work with fellow team members to encourage families to participate in an advance care planning process (Gessert, Bern-Klug, & Forbes, 2001). Such planning need not be limited to medical decisions. Workers can help families anticipate the need for social support, community resources, and financial help. There is also a role for social workers in assisting families with learning about funeral and burial options (Bern-Klug, Ekerdt, & Nakashima, 1999).

Even when clients state that they want to begin preparing for the end of life, it is not always easy to know where to start. Social workers can encourage families to use tools that have been developed to facilitate family discussions, such as the five messages of relationship completion for families to share and individualize (Byock, 1997) and 'caring conversations' (Midwest Bioethics Center, 1999).

Workers also should realize that despite the potential for a 'good death,' including inter-personal growth and meaning making at the end of life, some people and families will not have a positive experience. Wasow (1984) cautioned that in some cases expectations for a good dying experience are unrealistic and can provoke a new set of anxieties for the person who is dying and the survivors.

Despite the postponement of death for the majority of people in the United States, some people will face the end of life before they reach old age. These people have special needs. Social work skills are called on to assist individuals and families of people who experience dying and death 'off-time,' including individuals dying from AIDS, parents of babies dying a neonatal death, and survivors of accidental and suicidal deaths. Some of these 'premature' deaths also are associated with 'disenfranchised grief'—grief not validated by the community (Doka, 1989).

Miller, Hedlund, & Murphy (1998) reminded us that the sense of helplessness that can occur at the end of life can be compounded for people who are socially vulnerable as a result of poverty, bias, oppression, or prejudice. Social workers should strive to identify and then work to change the factors in the social environment that contribute to these burdens at the end of life.

Conclusion

During the 20th century important gains were made in the eradication of the causes of early death. We now have medical interventions that can reshape the dying experience, even in old age. Death has become 'forbidden' in Western societies (Ariès, 1974). To a large degree, dying has become invisible. It has become difficult to recognize who is dying – or who could be dying. This can make it much harder for families to honor the wishes of those who are near the end of life and to achieve peace of mind. As a society we are struggling with a new type of dying experience. Social work has an important role to play in the efforts to match services provided at the end of life with the new realities of dying.

References

Ariès, P. (1974). *Western attitudes toward death: From the middle ages to the present.* Baltimore: Johns Hopkins Press.

Bern-Klug, M., Ekerdt, D., and Nakashima, M., (1999). Helping families understand final arrangement options and costs. *In B. DeVries (ed.), End of life issues: Interdisciplinary and multidimensional perspectives* (pp. 245–262). New York: Springer.

Byock, I. (1997). *Dying well: Peace and possibilities at the end of life*. New York: Riverhead Books.

Doka, K. (ed.). (1989). *Disenfranchised grief: Recognizing hidden sorrow*. Lexington, MA: Lexington Books.

Dunn, H. (1994). *Hard choices for loving people: CPR, artificial feeding, comfort measures only and the elderly patient*. Herndon, VA: A&A.

Finucane, T. (1999). How gravely ill becomes dying: A key to end-of-life care. *JAMA, 282*, 1670–1672.

Gessert, C., Bern-Klug, M., & Forbes, S. (2001) Planning end-of-life care for patients with dementia: Roles of families and health professionals. *Omega: Journal of Death & Dying 42*(4): 273–291.

Glajchen, M., Blum, D., & Calder, K. (1995). Cancer pain management and the role of social work: Barriers and interventions. *Health & Social Work, 20*, 200–206.

Lynn, J., Teno, J.M., Phillips, R.S., Wu, A.W., Desbiens, N., Harrold, J., Claessens, M.T., Wenger, N., Kreling, B., and Connors, A.F. (1997). Perceptions of family members of the dying experience of older and seriously ill patients. *Annals of Internal Medicine, 126*, 97–105.

Midwest Bioethics Center. (1999). *Caring conversations: Making your wishes known for end-of-life care* (Online). Available: www.midbio.org.

Miller, P.J., Hedlund, S.C., and Murphy, K.A. (1998). Social work assessment at end of life: Practice guidelines for suicide and the terminally ill. *Social Work in Health Care, 26*(4), 23–36.

Osman, H., Perlin, T. (1994). Patient self-determination and the artificial prolongation of life. *Health & Social Work, 19*, 245–252.

Wasow, M. (1984). Get out of my potato patch: A biased view of death and dying. *Health & Social Work, 9,* 261–267.

12

Understanding Reproductive Loss: The Moment of Death

Sarah Earle, Carol Komaromy, Pam Foley and Cathy E. Lloyd

At a time of stillbirth and neonatal death, the role of the midwife is central to the way that women and families experience that loss. Providing care and support is part of what midwives do – and yet, at a time when the outcome is death instead of life, this requires an additional set of skills to those that are taught to midwives. While it is the case that training in these skills is a crucial aspect of helping midwives to develop the high level of competence that is needed at this time, anecdotal evidence suggests that training and development in this area is often limited and uneven (Ball et al 2002).

Taking a sociological approach to understanding the experience of professionals at the time of stillbirth and neonatal death, we consider the nature of emotional support and how this is framed by social expectations. Furthermore, while individual behaviour is often explained by psychologists and located within that discipline, a sociological approach offers a challenge to assumptions about the intrinsic nature of emotions that tend to dominate 'normal responses' to death. The sociological theories used here are those from the discipline of 'symbolic interactionism' – an area of sociology that considers the relationship between the individual and society.

Read what Claire says about her emotions (Vignette 1) and consider the extent to which you agree with her.

Claire's story of becoming a midwife highlights the key issues in this article that are focused on the emotional demands of managing feelings in midwifery, and also the way that these demands set up expectations in midwives of how they ought to feel. While you might have been surprised by the expectation that the experience would be mainly positive, it is probably fair to recognise that expectations rarely match reality. Perhaps the expression of boredom is the one that is most likely to elicit feelings of discomfort or shame in midwives.

The management of emotions is only one aspect of the debate. It is also the case that not only is the display of emotions regulated by institutional and social expectations, but they also change over time.

Originally published in *The Practising Midwife*, 8(10).

Sociological theories of emotion

There is a large body of literature on the sociology of emotions, especially within health and social care. The seminal work, which focused on the airline industry, was that of Hochschild (1983), who argued that people employed to work in commercial companies need to do more than the tasks that are required of them; they also need to regulate their emotions according to the expectations of that organisation. She argued that this is what was being sold as much as the service that airline staff delivered to passengers.

These ideas have been applied to nursing more than to other professional groups mainly because the work is considered to be both emotionally demanding and also one that requires a professional demeanour – see Mitchell and Smith (2003) on learning disability nursing, Smith and Gray (2000) on nursing and McQueen (2004) on negative emotions. It is interesting to note the extent to which this demeanour has changed over time, but the argument here is that, regardless of what is expected of the role in terms of the professional demands, nurses (and many other professional groups) need to develop and present a professional demeanour that involves the management of their own feelings.

If it is the case that emotional rules are developed by institutional norms, then offering support to women and families during labour and childbirth in a way that recognises the authenticity of feelings is particularly challenging. Sociological theory and research can help by challenging the assumptions on which these expectations about the management of feelings are based, and also by highlighting the dangers inherent in any generalisations – see Hunter (2001) for a discussion of the theories of emotional labour.

Vignette 1   Becoming a midwife: Claire's story

I did my training when my children had flown the nest. By that time, I had been a nurse for many years and I had a degree. I thought that being a midwife would be the most rewarding work that anyone could do. I was attracted to the fact that midwives were practitioners in their own right, and that midwifery was concerned with supporting women during 'normal' life events. I told friends that I had had enough of sickness, and wanted to work with healthy people.

I was not prepared for the downside of the job. I frequently felt bored, sometimes happy, occasionally terrified and at other times completely powerless. I was worried that I did not feel the excitement that I had expected to feel at every birth. Yet, I was also aware that I had to control these emotions and be professional. For example, I had to act as if I was delighted with every birth; behave as if instrumental deliveries were not horrific events; that I was pleased to be with someone who had an epidural for eight hours with very little happening and not bored. I needed to be able to convey the right emotions for each situation, and this was more challenging than I had anticipated.

Earlier than this, Goffman (1959), the person associated most with the discipline of symbolic interactionism, argued that the impression people make is shaped by the expectation that others have of them in a particular role. This 'creation of the desired impression', as he called it, means that individuals manipulate their efforts in order to achieve certain ends and try to live up to the standard by which they think they will be judged. In institutions, he argued, the regulations, structures and roles clearly define the performance that is expected by 'inmates' and members of staff. An important aspect of the performance in terms of emotional demeanour would also reinforce established professional identities and behaviours.

Applying this to settings that deal with stillbirth and neonatal death, midwives and bereaved family members have to negotiate how they select certain feelings for display and how these fit in with what they understand to be the institutional expectations and norms. It is not just the task of professionals who are trying to help bereaved parents to cope with their emotions and in doing so manage their own emotions appropriately – although there are reasons why having to do this so often and consistently might be particularly challenging – but families also are required to behave in particular ways.

Death and dying, even for the seasoned professional, is still a social process and, as such, is guided by expectations of appropriate conduct (Glaser and Strauss 1965). Goffman might argue that the professional scripts adhered to by midwives are successful because of their clear obligation to perform well in their professional role.

Changes in the responses to stillbirth and neonatal death

In hospital, the primary obligation to save lives sometimes fails and presents serious challenges to those whose job it is to cope with this failure. In a comparative study of the responses to stillbirth between the 1970s and 1990s in Belgium, the social anthropologist Bleyen (2006) highlights the way that stillborn babies, acting as reminders of the fragility of the boundary between life and death, historically were hidden from the parents and how midwives followed unwritten rules about not showing their own emotions and not talking about the death.

A professional performance of death at a distance, he argued, in some ways reduced the baby to an object. The contrast between this and more recent practice of what he calls 'intimate' death. Where close family members are expected to see and hold their babies after death, is striking. In this way, Bleyen argues, the different ways of making sense of death change over time.

In sociological terms, it is society, through its hospitals as social institutions, that shapes the needs of people at times of loss; furthermore, the expectation is that these needs will be the same for everyone. Even when professionals embrace the need for individual diversity, the expectation of what people ought to do and say in order to grieve in a healthy way is the standard by which judgements are made.

This is not to deny that this change from concealing babies was brought about in part by the expression of the needs of bereaved families since, as Bleyen highlights, not allowing mothers to see their babies left many women feeling emotionally damaged. Rather, it is to suggest that a 'one-size-fits-all' approach to any type of loss presents even more challenges to those professionals with support roles such as midwives.

Usha's story (Vignette 2) is based on practice, and highlights some of the challenges to midwives when women do not want to see their stillborn babies. What do you think the midwife is feeling about responding to Usha and her husband's needs?

Maria appears to be left feeling quite helpless in this situation and does not know what to do to help Usha and her husband. It seems that she is left hoping that Usha will change her mind and do 'what is best' and even what has become 'normal'. The scenario highlights the way that changing norms shape the expectations of behaviour on the part of the bereaved parents and how these expectations can become embedded in professional practice.

Vignette 2   Stillbirth: Usha's story

Usha was born in India, and moved to a town in the Midlands in England after her marriage. She was learning to speak English, and found this quite challenging. Her husband was fluent, however, and acted as her interpreter.

After being married for a short time, Usha became pregnant. All was going very well until she was 32 weeks pregnant and noticed one day that there was a reduction in her baby's movements. She got her husband to ring her midwife who arranged for Usha to go to the local hospital for fetal monitoring.

Usha's husband took her there immediately, and after the monitoring and a fetal scan they were told that the baby had died. Despite the suggestion that they should go home and try to come to terms with the loss, Usha wanted to be delivered straight away. Following a scan later that evening to confirm the lack of fetal heart beat, her labour was induced.

Maria was their named midwife, and she found it particularly difficult not to be able to communicate directly with Usha. She was also worried that Usha did not want to have an epidural and was going to experience a painful labour and tried to persuade her to reconsider, to no avail.

The following morning, when the baby was delivered, Maria washed her and wrapped her in a blanket and handed her to Usha, who immediately turned away. Usha's husband told Maria that he did not want to see the baby.

Maria talked to her colleagues after the delivery, and they reassured her that she should give Usha more time to recover from the trauma – both of the bed news and the labour – and then she might "come round", and want to see her baby. Maria found this advice helpful.

It could be argued that, in this situation, it is the expectation of how Usha and her husband ought to respond that has reduced the resources that Maria seems to have available to her. In other words, with a fixed model of how to help parents best respond to death, there does not seem to be room for Maria to use her own judgement. Maria's moral demeanour might be more geared to trying to persuade Usha to do what is best for her and her emotional and mental health.

The case study also highlights the difficulty that midwives and other professional groups face in increasing awareness of the need for different responses to death that might arise out of cultural and individual diversity. The danger is in making assumptions about particular groups in society rather than recognising that, within a culturally framed response, individuals might have different needs that sometimes over-shadow the traditional response associated with a belief system. Usha's midwife might have been more effective if she had been able to find out from Usha and her partner about their wishes, recognising that each might have had different needs which might have been in conflict. Negotiating how to respond in a culturally sensitive way requires good communication skills much more than an awareness of the traditions and belief systems of particular groups in society. The latter has been called a fact-file approach because it loses sight of individual diversity.

Vignette 3   Neonatal death: Margaret's story

...There is this picture of me with this dead baby in my arms looking at Laura [her daughter] and we just look like this little happy family group, and when the midwife showed it to me I said to her quite firmly, "Put that away, just put that away, don't show it to her!". It was just so awful, I found it so shocking to see this, and I was sort of looking at Laura and we just, really... there we are with a new baby – you know? – and the experience wasn't – it certainly wasn't unpleasant or frightening – but it wasn't real somehow.

But there was this immense sense of just awfulness as well – and sadness – so there wasn't any joy in this little thing, but it was quite comforting at the same time. It was a strange mixture of feelings, of not really engaging with the idea of a dead baby but somehow being comforted by him.

In the scenario provided by Margaret's story (Vignette 3), the opportunity to hold the baby provides great comfort, but there are different challenges to being able to respond appropriately. The scenario highlights how the power of protocols and training can both enable and limit the options that are available to midwives

Elliot was born at full term following a normal labour. He died suddenly and unexpect-edly a few hours after birth, and Margaret (his grandmother) describes her feelings and how she needed to protect her daughter from what she perceived as an unhelpful response to coping with this loss. The scenario highlights a more subtle reaction to deriving com-fort from holding and handling the baby after death.

In the interview, part of which is highlighted, Margaret described the details of the death and how her daughter had been encouraged to hold Elliot and the comfort that she had derived from feeling his 'life-like' body. Then how, after a while, a midwife came into the room and took several photos.

In this scenario, being professional involved the midwife in managing the birth and death as a significant event. Taking a photograph is one way of being able to provide evidence of the existence of a baby who had died unexpectedly shortly after his birth. Also, this mid-wife would have had to control her own emotions so that she gave the appropriate response.

What is interesting in this example is that while this management might be skillfully pulled off by the midwife in what Goffman (1959) would describe as performance man-agement, Elliot's mother and grandmother did not know how they ought to respond. The interview extract highlights the ambiguity that Margaret felt, and how she did not think that the photograph that is normally associated with and becomes the record of a happy event should be shown to her daughter. Indeed, she stopped the midwife from doing so.

The guidance given to midwives – the professional group that mostly has to manage this schism between life and death – includes preparation for coping with the silence that accompanies such events. However, it would seem that, even though midwives can talk about death with the family following the death of a baby, there remains no script for death when there was only one for life.

Sociological theories can help to explain the management of emotions. These explanations help professionals to examine their own practice in ways that challenge the assumptions that underpin the routines and protocols that have been set up to prescribe appropriate responses. Theories of emotional labour and performance management suggest that whatever is deemed to be the right professional demeanour requires midwives to be able to manage their own feelings. Furthermore, training in supporting bereaved parents would need to take into account how helpful these strategies really are to everyone in this situation of emotional distress.

Reponses to death at the time of birth are not universally appropriate and helpful. A more authentic level of engagement on the part of professionals might require them to be able to engage at a level that allows for a more nuanced and diverse range of experiences to be shown and expressed, and which is less about what ought to be helpful and more about accommodating any emotional expression of the reality of the experience.

The challenge for midwives is in creating a space that has room for them to be able to hear the feelings of bereaved mothers, fathers and families and to respond to those needs according to what they are. This suggests that the culture of care needs to shift to one that also provides space outside of this support for the feelings of midwives to be expressed and shared – and is valued as part of continuing development and support for each other.

By being supported and having their own emotions acknowledged, midwives are better placed to improve practice. Many midwives in practice will have found informal systems of support and will be attempting to do this already. Like the uneven delivery of skills training in supporting people at a time of loss, 'being with woman' – the essence of midwifery care – might require a challenge to the care of midwives and women and families in an institutionalised system. As Lock (2000: 235) states, 'Whatever form death takes, it conjures up that margin between culture where mortality must be confronted.

References

Ball L, Curtis P and Kirkham M (2002). 'Why do midwives leave?' http://www.rcm.org.uk
Bleyen J (2006). *Hiding Babies: Birth Professionals Making Sense of Death and Grief, University of Leuven, Belgium.*
Glaser and Strauss (1965). *A Time For Dying,* Chicago: Aldine.
Goffman E (1990[1959]). *The Presentation of Self in Everyday Life,* Harmondsworth: Penguin.
Hochschild A R (1983). *The Managed Heart: the Commercialisation of Human Feeling.* Berkeley, CA: California University Press.
Hunter B (2001). 'Emotion work in midwifery: a review of current knowledge'. *Journal of Advanced Nursing,* 34(4): 436–444.

Lock M (2000). 'Death in technological time: locating the end of meaningful life'. *Medical Anthropological Quarterly*, 10(4): 575–600.

Mitchell D and Smith P (2003). 'Learning from the past: emotional labour and learning disability nursing'. *Journal of Learning Disabilities*, 7(2): 109–17.

McQueen A (2004). 'Emotional intelligence in nursing work'. *Journal of Advanced Nursing*, 47(1): 101–8.

Smith P and Gray D (2000). 'The emotional labour of nursing: how student and qualified nurses learn to care', South Bank University London, cited in Mann S (2005): 'A health-care model of emotional labour'. *Journal of Health Organisation and Management*, 19(4/5): 304–317.

Resources

Antenatal Results and Choices, http://www.arc-uk.org/

Centre for Death and Society, University of Bath, http://www.bath.ac.uk/cdas/index.html

Kohner N (1995). *Guidelines for Professionals: Pregnancy Loss and the Death of a Baby*, Sands.

Kohner N (2000). 'Pregnancy loss and the death of a baby: parents'choices', in D Dickenson, M Johnson and J S Katz (eds), *Death, Dying and Bereavement*, 2nd edition, London: Sage/ Buckingham: Open University.

Miscarriage Association, http://www.miscarriageassociation.org.uk/

Moulder C (2001). *Miscarriage: Women's Experiences and Needs*, 2nd edition, Routledge.

SANDS, http://www.uk.sands.org/

13

What is the Best Way to Help Caregivers in Cancer and Palliative Care?

Richard Harding and Irene J. Higginson

Introduction

Current provision for informal carers (i.e., those unpaid carers providing one or a combination of physical, practical and emotional care and support) has been described as crisis intervention, in that services ignore successes and reward failure.[1] Those carers who appear to be coping in their role and do not request services are assumed to have no unmet needs, and it is only in the crisis situations of imminent or apparent breakdown of informal care that services respond. The carer can be seen as holding a unique position of both providing and needing support, and it has been suggested that it is sometimes unclear who is 'the patient'.[2] Towards the end of life needs are high. During the last two weeks of life, both patients and carers identify the anxiety effect on the nearest carer as one of their biggest problems, and the needs of the family may exceed those of the patient.[3, 4]

Although the systematic psychosocial assessment of carers has been proposed, and comprehensive assessment schedules developed,[5] it is not yet clear how to meet assessed need. The service conceptualization of the carer as coworker rather than client is problematic and leaves unmet support needs.[6] Support models need to carefully consider how they provide services for carers, as it may not be appropriate to simply incorporate carers into existing home care nursing support.[7] A broad range of needs must be met; therefore, a single approach will not be adequate.[8] Intervention studies are needed to provide evidence for the most useful supportive services.[9] The literature has begun to identify which carers are likely to experience negative outcomes (particularly younger carers, women and those caring for patients at diagnosis and end stages). Beyond the identification of specific needs, we are as yet unsure as to the format and content of acceptable and effective interventions.

'What is the best way to help caregivers in cancer and palliative care?' by Richard Harding and Irene J. Higginson, *Palliative Medicine*, 17, excerpts from pp. 63–74. Reprinted by kind permission of the publisher and authors.

Outcomes that may be affected by interventions

The range of carer's needs is vast, incorporating domestic help, informal support, fatigue, financial difficulties, anxiety, isolation and information.[10] Studies generally conclude the priorities are information and psychological support.[8, 11] Provision of supportive interventions to carers may also improve outcomes for patients, particularly in terms of the quality and duration of home care.[12] Optimum home care for patients depends in a large measure on adequate care for the carers to sustain them in their role.[13] [...]

Methods

Search strategy

Database searches were undertaken in August 2001, and these were supplemented with hand searches of journals (including journal alerting services for cancer and palliative care journals and hand searches of tables of contents of same journals, and reviews of reference lists of all identified papers). The databases searched were Medline (1966–2001), Cancerlit (1975–2001), PsycInfo (1967–2001) and Cinahl (1982–2001). Keywords used for the searches were carer(s) caregiver(s), palliative and cancer. Papers that reported interventions for adults actively providing informal care (including family members) for non-institutionalized cancer and palliative care patients were included. Descriptions of interventions as well as evaluations were included in the review. Data were extracted regarding the target population of the intervention (i.e., carers, patients or both), patient population (cancer or palliative care), service description, evaluation design and study findings.

Analysis

Study details were entered into common tables where the interventions, methods, limitations and findings were contrasted and compared to determine common results and differences for common interventions. Because of heterogeneity in outcomes and study design it was not possible to combine studies further in a meta-analysis. The evidence (where provided) was graded according to the rigour of the study design and analysis. [...]

Results

A considerable body of knowledge was identified with respect to need, but little on interventions and their evaluation. This review identified 22 papers related to interventions in cancer and palliative care which included/targeted carers. Of these, nine were services specifically for carers, and six had been evaluated. Of the evaluation, two had used a randomized control trial (RCT; grades IB), three employed a single group methodology (two prospective grades IIIC and one retrospective IIIC) and one was evaluated using facilitator feedback.

[...]

Home care

Home care services generally include carer support in their aims. Carers report high satisfaction with such services,[14, 15] and describe them as useful.[16] However, the high levels of psychological morbidity and unmet need reported in samples of carers of patients using home nursing care services in both cancer[8] and palliative care[6] demonstrate that such generic supportive nursing care does not meet all of carers' needs.

Carers of those using hospice care ($n = 83$) reported a greater reduction in anxiety and higher satisfaction compared with conventional care ($n = 69$) in an RCT.[17] However, the data does not distinguish between those using inpatient and home hospice care. An RCT of a hospital at home service for the terminally ill, concentrating on the last two weeks of life, importantly found low uptake of the intervention due to the carer feeling unable to cope. No significant difference was reported between intervention ($n = 152$) and standard care ($n = 33$) by carers on perceived support, suggesting that further specific interventions are needed for carers. However, carers in the intervention arm did report having a better perception of the patient care provided.[15]

A formative qualitative evaluation of a community palliative care service (incorporating home care, day care and respite, evaluated as a single service) found carers valued specific elements of the service, particularly that the service offered a single point of contact, that it felt like a 'home from home', that it helped them overcome reluctance to access services and that familiarity was achieved between patients, carers and staff.[18] A prospective single group evaluation of a home hospice service (service not described, $n = 118$) found that from entering the service to four weeks, carers' quality of life scores remained stable.[16] This stability is attributed to home care provision.

Respite care provision

The importance of respite services lies in providing time away from the caring role.[2] Respite can take many forms, and may prove unacceptable to those carers unwilling to leave the patient. Great ambivalence has been identified among this caring population, and respite care may not be accessible to those who wish to remain in the home.[43]

A 'sitting service' designed to provide practical and emotional help to both cancer patients (624 referrals in one year) and families was evaluated using retrospective postal questionnaires.[19] Respite for carers was the most common reason for referral (42 per cent). Eighty-six per cent of respondents felt able to go out and leave the sitter with the patient, and 70 per cent found the service to be 'very important' to them. Descriptive data from carers emphasized the importance of talking and having someone to listen. However, high costs and lack of funding options for mixed health and social care interventions made the service unfeasible. Elsewhere, the costs of such sitting service were reduced through the use of volunteer sitters.[20] However, issues of boundary maintenance, high stress and early burnout among sitters were experienced. This volunteer sitting service was evaluated using a single group retrospective questionnaire study ($n = 190$). It found over 90 per cent satisfaction among carers, though 33 per cent felt the service had been offered too late.

Massage has been provided as a form of respite, aiming to enhance physical caring abilities and sleep, and reduce physical and emotional stress.[21] The single group prospective evaluation ($n = 13$) reported improvements in single items of emotional stress, physical stress, physical pain and sleep difficulty.

Social networks and activities

An 'activation programme' for relatives of cancer patients aimed to promote increased active caring on behalf of carers, with the aim of also increasing social activity patterns.[22] The evaluation comprised a controlled trial with an age and sex matched comparison group from a control ward. Data were collected monthly and one and two months into bereavement ($n = 50$ for invention and $n = 45$ for control at baseline, $n = 22$ and $n = 19$, respectively, two months post-death). The activity group reported a significantly higher proportion of activities involving friends during treatment, and data from the last interview preceding death found the activity group were significantly more involved in their own activities. However, the patients in the study were using both inpatient and home care services, and the data does not distinguish between places of care.

The Well Spouse Foundation promotes the wellbeing of carers of the chronically ill through peer rather than professional support.[23] This national network provides telephone, letter and group support, providing information and practical sharing of ideas. The advantage of this organization is that the 'round robin' letters ensure that those who are unable to attend services are still able to access support. [...]

One-to-one interventions

One-to-one interventions, where feasible, are proposed as a means to provide support, education and build problem solving/coping skills. However, these interventions are time consuming and costly, and such psychological- and/or individual-based services may prove to be unacceptable to many carers.

An RCT of six one-hour sessions focusing on carers' problem solving skills ($n = 40$) versus standard management ($n = 38$) among cancer carers found that the intervention appeared effective only for a distressed subsample of the cancer carers in the study. This burdened subsample was better at dealing with pressing problems following intervention ($n = 11$) compared with controls ($n = 18$). This may be explained by the fact that the caregiving activities of the sample were low, and that carers of patients with high Eastern Co-operative Oncology Group (patient physical performance) scores or recent diagnoses were excluded from the study.[24]

A family cancer pain education programme consisting three one-hour sessions on the management of cancer-related pain was delivered in the home to patients and carers ($n = 50$).[7] Data were collected (by the same nurse who had delivered the intervention) at baseline and one week following the intervention's completion. Significant improvements were found on all scores (knowledge/attitudes to pain, pain management and carer burden).

An RCT of psychotherapy for the spouses of newly diagnosed lung cancer patients evaluated the service aim of assisting the carer in fulfilling their support function, i.e., to maintain patient social support, promote patient autonomy, advocate for patients in the medical system, encourage patient communication and facilitate mutual expression of feelings.[25] It is noteworthy that only the latter two aims can be seen as providing direct benefits to the carer. Twenty-three per cent of the eligible population refused to participate, and 35 per cent were deemed ineligible.

Ongoing weekly support counselling was provided for the 27 carers in the intervention arm, and 21 were allocated to the control. The outcome analysis was of those interviewed at the third point of data collection (six months after diagnosis): 10 carers in group 1 and 13 in group 2. No significant difference was found on the outcomes of emotional, social or physical function.

Group work

Group work interventions in cancer and palliative care are widely suggested as an appropriate format to deliver the necessary support and information to carers, and have been used successfully in this way for cancer patients.[26]

Although carers groups may not be appropriate for all carers (particularly those psychologically vulnerable carers who may have their needs best met elsewhere[27]), it is postulated that the benefits of information requesting and giving, sharing practical and coping skills, and social comparison processes[28] may be great. The sharing of experiences underpins most group work interventions, with other carers being seen as the most natural form of support.[29] Carers groups appear to favour a format of mixed content, combining information on care and group discussion, with an emphasis on promoting self-help.[30] However, research into the effectiveness of these interventions is needed, particularly the format and optimum length of interventions.[12]

An RCT of a six-week stress and activity management group of patients and carers ($n = 26$) versus standard management ($n = 25$) found that spouses who had attended the intervention had significantly higher knowledge scores, achieved activity goals, coped better with medical situations and were more satisfied with the care provided. However, psychosocial adjustment did not alter between the two groups.[31]

A descriptive evaluation of eight weekly combined patients ($n = 73$) and carers ($n = 54$) group session in cancer care found that the provision of information and education promoted understanding and facilitated coping, and that familiarity with the facts and feelings involved reinforced confidence.[32] Although anxiety was not reduced it was better recognized, therefore making it easier to deal with.

A retrospective single group questionnaire evaluation of a monthly group (one hour plus socializing) designed for both cancer patients and families found that opinions were divided on whether bereaved carers should be allowed to return to the group after a patient's death. The evaluative questionnaire explored negative feelings experienced after having attended the intervention. Twenty-six per cent reported feeling more anxious, worried and 29 per cent sadder. This is an interesting aspect of the study although it lacks comparison group data. Uptake of the group was low at 18 per cent, and one of the reasons cited for not attending was a fear of finding the experience of listening to others too depressing.[33]

An observational study evaluating the impact on quality of life in cancer patients and their families compared a control ($n = 12$), six group sessions plus individual/family counseling

($n = 12$), or ongoing support group having previously attended the group ($n = 8$).[34] No significant differences were found in quality of life or coping strategies. However, scores of patients and carers were combined, and comparative baseline or post-intervention scores between these groups were not presented, and the number of participating carers is not identified.

The development of a multidisciplinary group model has been described, aiming to alleviate the carer stress that stems from lack of knowledge in implementing necessary caring skills.[35] Three two-hour multidisciplinary sessions are proposed, though no evaluation is presented. A similar description of the development of a group intervention for family cancer carers describes the content focus as being on communication, symptom management and community resources.[36] The intervention combined lectures, group discussions, case studies and written materials over a period of six hours of education and interaction, with allowance for regional variation to meet local need. The group was evaluated using a single group prospective design with measures taken at baseline and 6–8 weeks after the intervention. However, neither the outcomes measured nor the data are reported, although attendees are reported as being less overwhelmed and more able to cope. Further descriptive evaluation data reported recruitment difficulties. The major issues preventing attendance by potential attendees were being in employment and having family obligations, having concerns about leaving the patient alone and the carers' own physical restrictions.[37]

An ongoing group for spouses of patients with brain tumours, aiming to enhance physical and emotional capabilities and provide education, met for 90 minutes per week for two years, with an average of 10 spouses attending. Evaluation was undertaken using only data from facilitator feedback, stating that the group provided social support and transition between phases of caring.[38]

The feasibility of an education and support group for patients with gynaecological cancer and their family carers was explored in terms of content and projected uptake.[39] Those with formal education were most interested in attending, and topics prioritized were cancer and its treatment, living with cancer, treatment side effects, pain and psychological reactions.

Ongoing family group therapy has been described, although not evaluated.[40] The group (for both patients and carers) aimed to enhance communication, deal with the intrapsychic conflicts of serious illness and enhance communication with physicians. The group ran for two hours per week, was not closed (therefore membership varies each week) and families of the recently deceased were permitted to attend.

A retreat/workshop approach has been taken in an attempt to meet the needs of all generations of cancer family members.[41] The weekend retreat consists of parallel sessions (separating adults, teenagers and children) using a multidisciplinary approach to education, relaxation and family/communication, with additional social activities.

[…]

Implications for research and practice

Currently there is a small body of evidence on the effectiveness of interventions for carers in palliative and cancer care. There are a handful of unevaluated descriptions of interventions, which are valuable in terms of providing information about the design and format of interventions. However, evaluations (especially rigorous ones) are rare, with only two (quasi-) experimental evaluations identified in the present review.

The provision of supportive interventions may be detrimental to carers,[42] and this proposition has as yet not been refuted due to the lack of evaluation data in services for carers. Supportive interventions need to consider acceptability in the early design stages.[43] Despite carers' recognition of unmet need, they report self-reliance and independence as important values,[44] and the barriers to accepting or making extensive use of services need to be more fully understood.

No single service model will be acceptable to the population of carers, or meet all needs for individual carers. A range of models have been identified in the present review, although only nine papers referred to interventions designed specifically for carers. The evidence for home care highlights the satisfaction with patient care on behalf of carers. However, the evidence of unmet need among carers using home palliative care services highlights the limited scope of this type of intervention. The expansion of such services to include multiprofessional support for families and carers independently of patient care would offer opportunities to meet unmet carer need.

Respite services aim to provide carers with the time away from caring and rest needed, although the literature has rarely answered questions of acceptability among a population noted for its ambivalence toward leaving the patient.[46]

The challenge of supportive provision may be greater in rural areas, and therefore it is important that carers and families are informed of informal peer support (such as the US model of postal networks).[23] Existing social networks should be maximized, and the present evidence from controlled trials is positive for such interventions in both individual and group formats. The evidence for one-to-one therapeutic interventions for carers is currently unclear. From the two published trials, only one found benefits for the intervention group and this was for a significantly depressed subsample. Although larger trials and evaluations of different styles of interventions may find benefits, at present there is no evidence for the general provision of this high cost intervention.

The only controlled trial of group intervention invited patients to attend the intervention with their carers. However, the outcome data from carers in attendance showed benefits gained in information and social activities. The development and provision of group work entails many variables regarding aims, format and content, and is largely chosen as a vehicle for the provision of information and support. However, group work interventions usually have fairly low uptake and tend to be acceptable to carers with particular demographic profiles. It would be worth running outcome evaluations of groups specifically for carers, as the current evidence suggest benefits in several domains, including support, coping and information giving.

Each of the models of provision described offered formats to meet the needs of carers, and there is as yet little proof that they have met their aims. Practitioners planning to develop interventions for carers must 1) ensure that their service is theory based, 2) focus specifically on the needs of carers (i.e., not a generic care service), 3) address issues of access and acceptability in the initial stages, 4) have clear and modest aims (which should not necessarily be multidimensional) and 5) ensure that these aims are evaluated using rigorous evaluation methods (using repeated measures from base-line and employ comparison groups).

Conclusion

The growing bodies of evidence of carers' needs in cancer and palliative care consistently call for the development and evaluation of targeted interventions. The evidence for unmet need is clear. Ethically, the time is overdue to apply this data and to build on what has been begun in the development of accessible and acceptable interventions. Carers interventions should aim to be feasible (grounded in the theory and evidence of interventions), acceptable (in a format seen as useful and appropriate by carers), accessible (carers must be able to access services should they wish to do so) and effective (shown to improve intended outcomes for carers using rigorous evaluation methods). But feasible and robust evaluation methods are needed. The unanswered questions that must be addressed are 1) which interventions (or combination of interventions) best meet carer needs, 2) what outcomes might we hope to improve and 3) what is the effectiveness of such services?

Notes

1   Clark D. Evaluating the needs of informal carers. *Prog Palliat Care* 1993; 1: 3–5.
2   Northouse LL, Peters-Golden H. Cancer and the family: strategies to assist spouses. *Semin Oncol Nurs* 1993; 9: 74–82.
3   Wingate AL, Lackey NR. A description of the needs of noninstitutionalized cancer patients and their primary care givers. *Cancer Nurs* 1989; 12: 216–25.
4   Higginson IJ, Wade A, McCarthy M. Palliative care: views of patients and their families *BMJ* 1990; 301: 277–81
5   Powazki RD, Walsh D. Acute care palliative medicine: psychosocial assessment of patients and primary care-givers. *Palliat Med* 2001; 13: 367–74.
6   Payne S, Smith P, Dean S. Identifying the concerns of informal carers in palliative care. *Palliat Med* 1999; 13: 37–44.
7   Ferrell BR, Grant M, Chan J, Ahn C, Ferell BA. The impact of cancer pain education on family caregivers of elderly patients. *Oncol Nurs Forum* 1995, 22: 1211–18.
8   Hilleman JW, Lackey NR. Self identified needs of patients with cancer at home and their home caregivers: a descriptive study. *Oncol Nurs Forum* 1990; 17: 907–13.
9   Rabins PV, Fitting MD, Eastham J, Fetting J. The emotional impact of caring for the chronically ill. *Psychosomatics* 1990; 31: 331–36.
10 Neale B, Informal palliative care: a review of research on needs, standards and service evaluation. Occasional Paper No. 3. Trent Palliative Care Centre, 1991.
11 Hileman JW, Lackey NR, Hassanein RS. Identifying the needs of home caregivers of patients with cancer. *Oncol Nurs Forum* 1992; 19: 771–77.
12 Holicky R. Caring for the earegivers: the hidden victims of illness and disability. *Rehabil Nurs* 1996; 21: 247–52.
13 Cull AM. Studying stress in care givers: art or science? *Br J Cancer* 1991; 64: 981–84.
14 Fakhoury WKH, McCarthy M, Addington-Hall J. Carers' health status: is it associated with their evaluation of the quality of palliative care? *Scand J Soc Med* 1997; 25: 296–301.
15 Grande GE, Todd CJ, Barclay SIG, Farquhar MC. A randomized controlled trial of a hospital at home sevice for the terminally ill. *Palliat Med* 2000; 14: 375–85.

16   McMillan SC. Quality of life of primary care givers of hospice patients with cancer. *Cancer Practice* 1996; 4: 191–98.

17   Kane RL, Klein SJ, Bernstein L, Rothenberg R, Wales J. Hospice role in alleviating the emotional stress of terminal patients and their families. *Med Care* 1985; 23: 189–97.

18   Ingleton C. The views of patients and carers on one palliative care service. *Int Palliat Nurs* 1999; 5: 187–95.

19   Clark D, Ferguson C, Nelson C. Macmillan carers schemes in England: results of a multicentre evaluation. *Palliat Med* 2000; 14: 129–39.

20   Johnson IS, Cockburn M, Pegler J. The Marie Curie/St Luke's relative support schema: a home care service for relatives of the terminally ill. *J Adv Nurs* 1988; 13: 565–70.

21   MacDonald G. Massage as a respite intervention for primary caregivers. *Am J Hospice Palliat* Care 1998; 14: 43–47.

22   Haggmark C, Theorell T, Ek B. Coping and social activity patterns among relatives of cancer patients. *Soc Sci Med* 1987; 25: 1021–25.

23   Randall T. Spouses of the chronically ill help each other cope [news] *JAMA* 1993; 269: 2486–86.

24   Toseland RW, Blanchard CG, MCallion P. A problem solving intervention for caregivers of cancer patients. *Soc Sci Med* 1995; 40: 517–28.

25   Golberg RJ, Wool MS. Psychotherapy for the spouses of lung cancer patients: assessment of an intervention. *Psychother Psychosom* 1985; 43: 141–50.

26   Cella DF, Sarafian B, Snider PA, Yellen SB, Winicour P. Evaluation of a community-based cancer support group *Psychooncology* 1993; 2: 123–32.

27   Ell K, Nishitimo R, Mantell J, Hamovitch M. Longitudinal analysis of psychological adaption among family members of patients with cancer. *J Psychosom Res* 1988; 32: 429–38.

28   Molleman E, Pruyn J, van Knippcnberg A. Social comparison processes among cancer patients. *Br J Soc psychol* 1986; 18: 135–13.

29   Slaby AE. Cancer's impact on caregivers. *Adv Psychosom Med* 1988; 25: 1–53.

30   Hunt RW, Bond MJ, Pater G. Psychological responses to cancer: a case for cancer support groups *Commun Health Stud* 1990; 14: 35–38

31   Heinrich RL, Coscarelli Schag C. Stress and activity management: group treatment for cancer patients and spouses *J. Consult Clin Psychol* 1985; 53: 439–46.

32   Grahn G, Danielson M. Coping with the cancer experience. 2. Evaluating an education and support programme for cancer patients and their significant others. *Eur J Cancer Care* 1996; 5: 182–87.

33   Plant H, Richardson J, Stubbs L, Lynch D, Ellwood J, Slevin M. Evaluation of a support group for cancer patients and their families and friends. *Br J Hosp Med* 1987; 317–22.

34   Reele BL. Effect of counseling on quality of life for individuals with cancer and their families. *Cancer Nurs* 1994; 17: 101–12.

35   Cawley MM, Keendey Gerdts E. Establishing a cancer caregivers program. *Cancer Nurs* 1988; 11: 267–73.

36   Robinson KD, Angeletti KA, Barg FK, Pasacreta JV, McCorkle R, Yasko JM. The development of a family caregiver cancer education program *J Cancer Educ* 1998; 13: 116–21.

37   Barg FK, Pasacreta JV, Nuamah IF, Robinson KD, Angeletti KA, Yasko JM, McCorkle R. A description of a psychoeducational intervention for family caregivers of cancer patients. *J Fam Nurs* 1998; 4: 394–413.

38   Horowiz S, Passik SD, Malkin M. 'In sickness and in health': a group intervention for spouses caring for patients with brain tumors. *J Psychosoc Oncol* 1996; 14: 43–56.

39   Carlsson ME, Strang PM. Educational group support for patients with gynaecological cancer and their families. *Support Care Cancer* 1996; 4: 102–109.

40   Wellisch DK, Mosher MB, Van Scoy C. Management of family emotion stress: family group therapy in a private oncology practice. *Int J Group Psychother* 1978; 28: 225–31.

41   Johnson JL, Norby PA. We can weekend: a program for cancer families. *Cancer Nurs* 1981; 4: 23–28.

42   Siegel K. Psychosocial oncology research. Special Issue: research issues in health care social work. *Soc Work Health Care* 1990; 15: 21–43.

43   Harding R, Higginson IJ. Working with ambivalence: informal caregivers of patients at the end of life. *Support Cancer Care* 2001; 9: 642–45.

44   Grande GE, Todd CJ, Barclay SIG. Support needs in the last year of life: patient and carer dilemmas. *Palliat Med* 1997; 11: 202–208.

14

Illness and the Creative Arts: A Critical Exploration

Jacqueline H. Watts

For most people their sense of who they are assumes a healthy fit body with which they pursue their daily lives. However, when illness occurs (particularly serious or life-threatening illness) the way that people see themselves and envisage their future can be radically altered. Bury (1982) describes the identity change brought about by illness as a 'biographical disruption' which impacts on a physical, psychological and emotional level. In contemporary society, disease and sickness are increasingly positioned as issues of personal responsibility with lifestyle choice (for example, diet, exercise and safe sexual behaviour) central to constructions of well-being. People who are sick and unable to work have a responsibility to 'get better' and, therefore, occupy a different status from economically productive citizens. The development of sophisticated medical interventions and effective drug therapies, as part of a general improvement in prosperity in the West, has led to good health being regarded as a social right (Turner, 2004) and illness and disability as stigma (Goffman, 1964). The polarisation of life and death as success and failure within curative medicine is simplistic and, increasingly, concerns about harsh invasive treatments and related loss of independence and marginal quality of life, have entered discourses of health care.

This reading discusses the role of the creative arts in end-of-life care and begins by considering art as a medium for communication and self-expression. This is developed in the context of the use of the creative arts within palliative care, focusing particularly on the issues of motivation and changes in the meaning of time for those nearing the end of life. The discipline of art therapy, as a tool for managing emotions, is the subject of the next section, raising questions about its utilitarian value in light of its increasing use with people who are chronically or terminally ill. The chapter concludes with a discussion of the ethics of formal institutionalised artistic practice with those who are terminally ill calling attention to issues of evaluation and resource distribution within a regulated and cash-starved health care system, such as exists in the UK.

Art as communication and expression

The demonstration of art as a particular form of communication and self-expression is central to what has come to be known as 'hospital art'. In 1973 Peter Senior established a multidisciplinary arts team to work in hospitals and health centres in the Manchester area, signalling the start of Hospital Arts Manchester that has since developed into the internationally recognised Arts for Health (Senior, 1998). Many hospitals now display the work made by clients alongside that of local artists and schools. The aim of 'brightening up' potentially frightening and dull surroundings is one underpinning value of this practice and benefits clients, staff and visitors. Recognition of the worth of aesthetic improvement to public health care spaces such as walk-in clinics, GP surgeries and hospitals has underpinned the establishment of Fosterart for Health that acts as a sponsored art-lending facility for the NHS. Similar recognition of the need for more congenial environments for health workers and clients has led hospices to mount art displays. Indeed, within the hospice movement, arts and craft activities are offered to clients as an important and essential component of care (Kennett, 2001: 67) and it is to the issue of the role of the creative arts in the lives of people who are chronically and terminally ill that the discussion now turns.

Creative arts and the management of temporality

Artists working within a range of health care settings have sometimes been reluctant to engage in audit and evaluation of their work. Many health care institutions have been equally reluctant to undertake initiatives to explore the efficacy of the creative arts, leaving us with a barren 'evidence landscape' in this area. Yet, the power of the creative arts used with people in times of trauma and distress is documented elsewhere (Bolton, 2008), and discussion of the connection between artistic genius and severe mental illness, for example, continues to feature in the popular press (Linklater, 2007). Because creativity is subjective and difficult to measure, its formal place within the bureaucratic systems that underpin health care provision in the UK continues to be contested and its contribution to the lives of people who are chronically or terminally ill remains a topic of sceptical debate. The hospice movement, however, takes a proactive institutional position on the potential positive contribution that a range of creative activities can make to client well-being. The movement particularly promotes the use of music and art as a celebration of life and, in many hospices these are incorporated as an integral part of a holistic care programme. Bertman (1991) claims a particular role for the arts within palliative care arguing that they increase understanding of psychosocial and existential issues related to death and dying, and help to create alliances between the medical community and social sciences and the arts.

Hospices use the creative arts in a variety of ways to give clients 'space' to concentrate on an activity that is unrelated to the 'work' of being terminally ill. Also, the opportunity to create something to leave behind can be significant. One feature of terminal illness is the re-framing of temporality, where life (perhaps formerly organised around family and work) becomes governed by the practicalities of hospital visits and treatment and medication regimes (Armstrong-Coster, 2004). With the profound 'biographical disruption' (Bury, 1982) for those with a life-limiting condition, temporality acquires a more strongly present-bound orientation with constructions of the future a fragile and uncertain prospect (Lawton, 2000). Thus, bodily deterioration experienced as lower energy levels and reduced physical strength can act as a potent 'temporal filter' with the temporal perceptions of the dying gradually moving out of synchrony with those of family and friends (Lawton, 2000). Against this background, being motivated to do even the simplest of things can be greatly diminished, with disappointment at one's disobedient body a powerful emotion. Illness and dying can be isolating, especially for older people (Armstrong-Coster, 2004), so participation in shared creative activity can foster what May (1975) refers to as the courage to make 'doing' possible. Where this takes place as an organised communal activity within hospice day care, an 'alternative reality' (Lawton, 2000: 61; 67) is constructed that coheres with the 'alternative potential' within individuals.

Acknowledging and exploring alternative potential emerges as an underpinning focus of much of the discussion in the literature of the use of creative artistic activity with those who have a limited survival time. This is the central theme of recently reported findings of small-scale Swedish research that investigated the meanings that people with advanced cancer ascribe to engaging in creative activity in palliative occupational therapy (La Cour et al., 2007). Benefits of engagement were seen in terms of better coping with declining physical abilities, specifically using their hands and bodies in craft sessions that, for some, afforded an opportunity to 'present a gift to oneself' (Osamu, 2005: 2727). The therapeutic value of arts and crafts in maintaining enriching aspects of life for participants in this study was seen as a counter to the often negative focus in palliative phases of cancer. However, the extent to which this 'alternative reality' is an artificial substitute reality but one preferable to the vacuum of 'waiting for death', remains unclear from research in this area.

When faced with a terminal illness, people may surrender their jobs and lose their sense of purpose and it is the creation of a new sense of purpose that lies at the heart of Rosetta Life, a charity which places artists in residence in hospices around the UK. This artist-led organisation enables those with life-threatening illness and their families to express and channel their experiences through the arts. In 2004, a week-long festival of music, poetry, film, dance and fine art took place in London to celebrate the creativity of hospice users from across the UK. The work of the project continues and advances in technology mean that people who are terminally ill can find creative solace on the Internet and, following the trend of increasing online expressionism, Rosetta Life now runs a series of Web events to engage client with client and client with doctor (Jarrett, 2007).

The literature also reveals that artistic practice can be a source of support for those caring for dying people as well as a tool for enhancing health care practice. For example, Robinson (2004) argues that sharing the writing of poetry with terminally ill clients can help enable expression of individuals' deepest unspoken concerns, those of both the client and the carer. Coulehan and Clary (2005) take a similar view arguing that reading and writing poetry enables clinicians to develop a compassionate presence and empathic connection within the clinical encounter. This, they argue, is a far cry from the rational world of hard data, diagnostic testing and pharmacological developments that frames so much of the work of the modern medic.

Art therapy and the management of emotions

Art therapy is a form of psychotherapy that uses art for therapeutic purposes. Art therapists work with both individuals and groups in a range of institutional and community settings that include child and family centres, schools, prisons, hospitals and hospices. Using visual and tactile materials, art therapists work with clients to enable them to create an outlet for complex emotions that cannot always be voiced (Sibbett, 2005: 65). There are aspects of the human experience for which spoken language is insufficient in capturing the rawness of fear and suffering (May, 2002) and some proponents of art therapy argue that this form of creativity can provide a metaphorical arena within which these emotions can be faced and managed through multisensory re-portraying of the self.

The expression by clients of deeply felt anguish and pain may also be distressing for health care workers. Mason et al. (2008) argue that arts in palliative care can help staff deal with difficult and sensitive care situations, helping to maintain a culture of 'institutional niceness' and an atmosphere of calm and peace which has come to be seen as the 'hallmark' of hospice care and the 'good death' (Sandman, 2005). In some settings, a client's strong emotional behaviour in the form of tears, anger and physical agitation can be distressing for other clients too. Some art therapists argue that the medium of creative artistry can enable the non-verbal expression of rage and anger that has positive benefits and cathartic effects, with the potential for growth and insight on a personal level.

Art therapists work with a variety of media to support clients adapting to the changed circumstances of their lives. Unlike the creative arts undertaken in hospice day care discussed above, art therapy is not simply a diversionary recreational activity (Waller and Sibbett, 2005), although both sets of art practitioners claim the healing power of all the arts. The art therapist enters a therapeutic relationship with the client as part of a holistic and social model of health, working with the client towards insight and integration of her/his fears into a manageable and meaningful reality. Arguably, this model of therapeutic practice is predicated on the concept of healing; what heals is the relationship between the client and the therapist in which the client is wholly valued and accepted and their unique experience fully attended (Mason et al., 2008: 64). Bolton (2008: 15) describes this as 'healing art' that offers reflective processes upon memories, hopes and anxieties in a creative self-revelatory but non-directive way.

The effectiveness of art and similar therapy, such as music for example, is part of the wider debate about the evaluation of the range of artistic practice within health care, with some practitioners addressing the question of why art therapists choose to work in a health context characterised by the extremes of illness. Duesbury (2005), for example, discusses his reactions to his work in a palliative setting noting both the rewards and frustrations of the role. He highlights the privilege of entering the emotional space of clients at such a significant life stage. The expressed juxtaposition of pain and pleasure, as part of this process, suggests a form of emotional colonisation on the part of the therapist who, because of a position of therapeutic privilege, can exercise high levels of control over vulnerable people. Codes of professional and ethical practice within art therapy, however, draw attention to the importance of power relationships and to the need for art therapists to have the support of regular clinical supervision as part of continuing professional development (see www.baat.org). The emphasis given within formal training programmes to the importance of the relationship between the therapist and the client, that is itself central to the project of creating an image or artefact, contributes to a highly collaborative process. The making of art uses symbols and metaphor that are subject to interpretation and therapists enable clients to understand what they have created in her/his own terms (Mason et al., 2008: 65). The responsibility of working through the inner terrain of individuals, that is often a painful process, requires ongoing scrutiny of practitioner values and the professional regulatory body acknowledges this.

Evaluating the role of creative arts

The role of the creative arts as a support to people who are chronically or terminally ill is subject to a range of disciplines, applications and settings and some of these have been discussed above. However, central to all these practices is the issue of cost and effectiveness – irrespective of the particular art form. This is a difficult area, not least because the approach of profuse and intense 'niceness' within wider cancer culture, and hospice culture in particular, conveys an impression of the uncontested value of creative art (Myers, 2001). However, the question remains: 'How do we know?' Where is the empirical evidence for the effectiveness of this work and what counts as 'effective' in the newly arrived evidence-based world of health care? These questions now frame the closing discussion that considers how the cost of artistic provision within health care services can be evaluated and justified.

The application of the creative arts within palliative day care forms part of a model of psychosocial care informed by Maslow's (1968) hierarchy of needs and Roger's (1951) person-centred approach. As discussed above, artistic practice in this context has undergone very little evaluation, though Sheldon (1997) summarises an evaluation of projects by Hospice Arts, which highlights the need for clients to be involved at the start in helping shape activities. Hearn (2001) offers further insight from a small-scale evaluation of arts and craft activity that is integral to palliative day care at St Christopher's Hospice in London. This evaluation revealed that the benefits to clients of creating pottery, painting, textiles, digital art, stories and poetry were enjoyment, enthusiasm, pride, surprise, achievement, sense of purpose and incentive to work towards a goal. A phenomenological approach was used to underpin this evaluation and Hearn (2001) postulates that the essential phenomenon observed was hope. But what does 'hope' mean for those facing their death? This phenomenon may have multiple properties but Twycross (2003) argues that all hope needs an object involving realistic goal-setting that contributes to quality of life – a contested concept that is best defined as subjective well-being (Cohen, 2003). For those near death, hope of recovery is replaced by alternative hopes that still hold a sense of direction for the life that remains, though Twycross (2003) argues that hope in these circumstances becomes focused on being rather than achieving and on relationships with others.

This leads to ask how is it possible to place a rationally costed economic value on the phenomenon of hope, particularly in light of Mason et al.'s contention that 'every person's approach to their death is unique' (2008: 63). Enabling those with advanced disease to transcend the circumstances of their illness and find new ways of maintaining quality of life and enhancing well-being, which may include participation in a range of artistic creativity that provides short-term goals and an opportunity to express without words what has been achieved and lost, does not readily lend itself to economic scrutiny. The benefits are experienced at an individual level and, as such, cannot be easily measured as part of a business model of health care delivery, with its primary focus on the allocation of scarce resources for the collective good. With the growing rationalisation of services in all areas of health care, this type of provision may increasingly be seen as a valuable, but unjustifiable, luxury.

References

Armstrong-Coster, A. (2004) *Living and Dying with Cancer*. Cambridge: Cambridge University Press.

Bertman, S. (1991) *Facing Death: Images, Insights and Interventions*. Washington, DC: Taylor and Francis.

Bolton, G. (2008) 'Introduction: dying, bereavement and the healing arts', in G. Bolton (ed.), *Dying, Bereavement and the Healing Arts*, London: Jessica Kingsley.

Bury, M. (1982) 'Chronic illness as biographical disruption', *Sociology of Health and Illness,* 4 (2): 167–82.

Cohen, S.R. (2003) 'Assessing quality of life in palliative care', in R.K. Portenoy and E. Bruera (eds), *Issues in Palliative Care Research*. Oxford: Oxford University Press.

Coulehan, J. and Clary, P. (2005) 'Healing the healer: poetry in palliative care', *Journal of Palliative Medicine,* 8 (2): 382–9.

Duesbury, T. (2005) 'Art therapy in the hospice: rewards and frustrations', in D. Waller and C. Sibbett (eds), *Art Therapy and Cancer Care*. Maidenhead: Open University Press.

Goffman, E. (1964) *Stigma: Notes on the Management of Spoiled Identity*. Englewood Cliffs, NJ: Prentice Hall.

Hearn, J. (2001) 'Audit in palliative day care: what, why, when, how, where and who', in J. Hearn and K. Myers (eds), *Palliative Day Care in Practice*. Oxford: Oxford University Press.

Jarrett, L. (2007) 'Voicing change: online not in line', in L. Jarrett (ed.), *Creative Engagement in Palliative Care*. Oxford: Radcliffe Publishing.

Kennett, C. (2001) 'Psychosocial day care', in J. Hearn and K. Myers (eds), *Palliative Day Care in Practice*. Oxford: Oxford University Press.

La Cour, K., Josephsson, S., Tishelman, C. and Nygard, L. (2007) 'Experiences of engagement in creative activity at a palliative care facility', *Palliative & Supportive Care,* 5: 241–50.

Lawton, J. (2000) *The Dying Process*. London: Routledge.

Linklater, A. (2007) 'You don't have to be mad', *Guardian Weekend,* 7 July 2007.

Maslow, A. (1968) *Towards a Psychology of Being*. Second edition. Toronto: Van Nostrand.

Mason, C., Davis, C., Langley, G., Lee, B. and Verduci, C. (2008) 'Healing arts in palliative care', in G. Bolton (ed.), *Dying, Bereavement and the Healing Arts*. London: Jessica Kingsley.

May, M. (2002) 'It's the way my spirit speaks', in B. Rumbold (ed.), *Spirituality and Palliative Care*. Melbourne: Oxford University Press.

May, R. (1975) *The Courage to Create*. New York: W.W. Norton and Company.

Myers, K. (2001) 'Future perspectives for day care', in J. Hearn and K. Myers (eds), *Palliative Day Care in Practice*. Oxford: Oxford University Press.

Osamu, T. (2005) 'Arts therapy in palliative care', *Clinic All-round,* 54 (10): 2727–8.

Robinson, A. (2004) 'A personal exploration of the power of poetry in palliative care, loss and bereavement', *International Journal of Palliative Nursing,* 10 (1): 32–9.

Rogers, C.R. (1951) *Client-centred Therapy*. Boston: Houghton Mifflin Co.

Sandman, L. (2005) *A Good Death: On the Value of Death and Dying*. Maidenhead: Open University Press.

Senior, P. (1998) *Arts for Health Information Pack*. Manchester: Manchester Metropolitan University.

Sheldon, F. (1997) *Psychosocial Palliative Care*. Cheltenham: Stanley Thornes.

Sibbett, C. (2005) 'Liminal embodiment: embodied and sensory experience in cancer care and art therapy', in D. Waller and C. Sibbett (eds), *Art Therapy and Cancer Care*. Maidenhead: Open University Press.

Turner, B. (2004) *The New Medical Sociology: Social Forms of Health and Illness.* New York: W.W. Norton and Company.

Twycross, R. (2003) *Introducing Palliative Care.* Fourth edition. Abingdon: Radcliffe Medical Press.

Waller, D. and Sibbett, C. (2005) 'Introduction', in D. Waller and C. Sibbett (eds), *Art Therapy and Cancer Care.* Maidenhead: Open University Press.

www.baat.org The British Association of Art Therapists website.

Part III
Moral and Ethical Dilemmas in Practice

Introduction

Mary Twomey

The range of ethical dilemmas and problems that arise in palliative care is enormous. As medical technologies advance, new dilemmas emerge and as palliative care becomes more widely available, more health care professionals will grapple with decisions about what is right and wrong in end-of-life care. Ethical practice is something that concerns everyone. It isn't unusual, for example, to hear someone express the opinion that certain procedures or certain actions aren't ethical, and this is often uncomfortable. Ethical theory on the other hand can be difficult and obscure and sometimes seems to have little to do with the practical realities faced by those who are dying and those who are caring for them. The contributions to this part of the reader explore some of those realities and ask questions about how decision making in these areas should be approached.

This part begins with Reading 15 by Eve Garrard, entitled 'What is ethics?'. Here Garrard explores the way in which moral theory can help to decide what actions are the most justifiable in difficult situations. Just as there will be disagreements in practice so, too, there will be disagreements about which moral theory provides the right guide, but Garrard shows that there is value in considering different theoretical approaches as each will provide useful insights that might otherwise be overlooked. Having considered the two theories that have carried much weight in traditional moral theory, consequentialism and deontology, Garrard focuses her discussion on the approach developed by W.D. Ross which has gained wide recognition in medical and health care ethics through the work of the ethicists Beauchamp and Childress.

Some of the most difficult ethical dilemmas which are encountered in caring for people who are dying arise when dying people themselves are not able to participate in decisions about their treatment and care. In Reading 16, Anne-Marie Slowther discusses the complex question of how much weight should be given to the views and concerns of family members in such circumstances. There are both legal and moral issues to consider in resolving possible conflicts between respecting someone's autonomy, seeking to do what they might wish for themselves, and acting in their best interests. Conflicts between principles need not imply conflict between professional carers and families, however, and as Slowther suggests, ethical perspectives which emphasise relationships and negotiation have much to contribute here.

The conflict between respecting someone's autonomy and acting in a person's best interest is brought sharply into focus in Reading 17 through Vince and Petros' case study of an adolescent boy facing imminent death following the planned withdrawal of his life support. The question of whether or not the boy should be woken in order to be informed of his situation and to consent to the withdrawal of treatment highlights the very real and distressing dilemmas faced by those involved in caring for dying children and young people. As this case shows, the very nature of these dilemmas means that there is no single 'right' answer, and that a paternalistic approach, while much criticised by those who feel that respect for autonomy should be paramount, might in some circumstances be appropriate.

In Reading 18, Jane Seymour introduces a sociological perspective to decision making in intensive care units and suggests that decisions about the withdrawal of treatment are part of a social process which is partly shaped by hospital organisation. By requiring immediate decisions about short-term problems, Seymour suggests, the distress and confusion of those accompanying the dying person are increased. By focusing on a series of 'potentially soluble puzzles', she claims, the contextual details of someone's dying can be lost. When thinking about ethical considerations such as best interests, or the social practices surrounding someone's death, however, context is clearly of great importance. Continuing the focus on intensive care, Allan Kellehear, looks at brain death in Reading 19, arguing that the emphasis on technical rather than social understandings of death is a problematic feature of current criteria for determining when death occurs. By ignoring the understandings from the social sciences about social perceptions of death, argues Kellehear, it is likely that there will continue to be resistance to clinical definitions of brain death, and misunderstandings about the reactions of both staff and families to 'death' will persist.

As Kellehear points out, while social scientists have been excluded from debates about brain death, philosophers have engaged in these and similar debates. One such debate is about the validity or otherwise of the doctrine of double effect, which is explored by Stephen Wilkinson in Reading 20. Wilkinson focuses on the role of intention in situations where achieving a desired outcome, such as relief of pain, also has an unlooked-for outcome, such as the hastening of death. This discussion of intention leads into controversial discussions about issues such as euthanasia, areas where philosophers and clinicians disagree among and between their respective disciplines. Such disagreement is not restricted to debates about euthanasia, of course, but extends to the range of ethical debates not only in the field of palliative care but also in the wider field of moral philosophy. As Garrard suggests in the opening reading, moral theory can assist in thinking about which actions are justifiable but difficult decisions, and therefore disagreements, will remain.

15
What is Ethics?

Eve Garrard

Ethics is the study of morality, and morality is a central part of all of our lives[1]. We're constantly thinking and making judgements about what we ought to do and what we ought not to do, and also about what others ought to do or not do. Should I go for the interesting and demanding new job which would be a really good career move, or should I stick with the more boring work so that I can spend more time with the children? Should I cover up for my colleague's petty theft from the cashbox, because she really loves the patients and is always very good with them? Should we tell the grieving parents that their loved daughter died in pain and fear as they were rushing to the hospital to be with her, or should we protect them from that terrible truth? Even when we don't think of ourselves as morally high-minded people we usually turn out to have quite strong views about the rightness or wrongness of at least some of the things that human beings do. Think of the great debates about abortion, or euthanasia, or racial discrimination, or war – these are topics which many people feel very strongly about. All these concerns are moral ones: morality is about good and bad, right and wrong. And it's a central part of being human – those (very few) people who have absolutely *no* sense of right or wrong are very unusual indeed, and very difficult for others to deal with.

One of the most notable features of morality is that people often disagree about it. In fact there's also a great deal of agreement about morality – people and cultures can disagree, for example, about whether killing is ever morally permissible, but everyone thinks that it's impermissible to kill just anyone you want to. But there's no doubt that moral matters are ones where people's views often differ very markedly indeed. What are we to think about these strong disagreements, and how should we try to handle them? Some people think that we can deal with them by appealing to our conscience to tell us what's the right thing to do. But unfortunately different people's consciences may tell them different things – the problem of moral disagreement arises again about consciences. Some people think that we should appeal to moral authorities to help resolve our disagreements about moral matters. But who are we to count as a moral authority? People who disagree about major moral issues are quite likely to disagree about who to count as morally authoritative. For example, people with religious commitments who feel strongly about the issue of abortion may regard their religious leaders as moral authorities on this matter, as on others; but those who lack religious beliefs are unlikely to accept the appeal to religious leaders as in any way authoritative.

A third possible response to the fact of moral disagreement is to come to the conclusion that in morality there's no truth of the matter, apart from people's opinions. This view about morality is known as relativism, and relativists think that a moral view is right for the person (or in some versions, the society) who believes it, but not necessarily right for others. So we can all have different moral views without any of us being really wrong. One person may think she should give much of her money to charity, and in that case, it's right for her to do so. But another person may think he has a duty to use his money to provide for his nearest and dearest, in which case, according to relativism, that's the behaviour that's morally right for him. In the societal version of relativism, one society may think women should stay at home and confine themselves to the domestic sphere, in which case it's morally right for people in that society to restrict women's occupational choices. But in a different culture, one which regards women as equal in every way to men, then it's right for women to compete on equal terms with men in the job market. The practices of each society are right for that society, according to relativism – there's no objective moral truth of the matter to which every society should conform.

In some ways, relativism seems to be an attractive solution to the problem of moral disagreement, since it sounds as if it will encourage tolerance. If what you believe to be morally right is indeed right for you, and if what I believe to be morally right is right for me, then there seems to be no reason for either of us to object on moral grounds to what the other one does. Each of us seems, on a relativist understanding of morality, to be just as morally justified as the other, and so there's no reason for either of us to be intolerant. But in fact, this view of morality has some very unattractive implications. If moral views are right just so long as you believe them to be right, then it looks as if we never have any good reason for criticising other people's beliefs. But this means that we'd have no way of criticising people, or societies, who think that it's right to harm children, or to discriminate against women or members of ethnic minorities, or to enslave the weak for the benefit of the strong. And if we have no reason to criticise them, then we'd also have no reason to try to improve them in any way – indeed the very idea of moral improvement wouldn't make much sense, since people's moral ideas are right for those who believe them. But that means that the victims of those societies would be left unsupported and unaided, and morality itself could have no objection to this. Many people find this implication of relativism about morality a deeply unappealing one.[2]

Another way of thinking about moral disagreement is to regard it as resulting from the fact that moral problems are *hard*. We are complicated creatures leading complicated lives, so it shouldn't surprise us that questions about how we ought to behave are difficult to answer. But that doesn't mean that there is no answer for us to find, or that we can't, if we try hard enough, get closer to the truth about moral matters. What we need to do is think (and talk and discuss and argue) as sensitively and rigorously as we can about our moral problems, to help us understand their nature, and to see what it is we should really do. In this process of reflective thought and argument about morality, we can expect to resolve at least some of our moral disagreements, because we'll be getting closer to the moral truth. But because moral matters are complex, that truth won't be easy to come by, so we'll have good reason to listen to and tolerate the views of those who disagree with us, because we're likely to be able to learn from them, since they may have seen aspects of the truth which we have not.

Once we embark on this reflective practice, there are some very general questions which inevitably arise, and in trying to answer them, we quickly find that what we're doing is really what can be regarded as moral theory. We want to know what is the right thing to do, and some general questions that rapidly arise in discussion about this include: 'What is it about an action that makes it the right thing to do? Why is it usually right to struggle as hard as we can to save a patient's life, but also right in some circumstances to stop aggressive treatment and let the patient die? What do these very different right actions have in common which make them right?' This is really a request for a moral theory, since moral theories set out to tell us, at a general level, what it is about right actions that make them right. Finding this out would be interesting for its own sake, but it would also be enormously useful, since if we knew what makes right actions right we could use that knowledge to help resolve our moral dilemmas and disagreements. If we knew what feature of right actions makes them right, then we could look for that feature in our problematic moral situations, and once we found the action which possessed it, we'd know we'd found the right thing to do.

So a good moral theory would be a very useful thing to have. There are in fact several different moral theories setting out to tell us what the nature of right actions is, each with its own strengths and weaknesses. One of the most powerful ones, which has been extremely influential since it received its classic formulation in the nineteenth century, has focused on the fact that producing good consequences seems to be an important aspect of acting morally. We often think that it's morally right to do whatever will produce the best outcomes. If we develop this thought into a general account of right action, we'll get a theory which says that the right action is the one which produces the best consequences. The feature which all right actions have in common, according to this theory, is that they produce the best available outcomes. This theory, known (unsurprisingly) as consequentialism, is in many ways a very attractive theory. It tells us that it's *always* right to try to make the world a better place (since producing the best available consequences is just making the world a better place), and that sounds morally very convincing. The more we look at all the suffering there is in the world, the more we're inclined to think that it must be right to try to remove that suffering.

Of course, we may disagree about what counts as good consequences – people differ about what's good just as much as they do about what's right. The question of what things (and hence what consequences) are really good is another topic for moral theory, just as important as the question of what actions are right. What consequentialism says, however, is that whatever conclusion we come to about what things are good, the right action will be the one that produces the greatest amount of that good as possible. One very famous and influential form of consequentialism claims that what's ultimately good is human happiness or welfare, and so the right thing to do is to maximise human happiness. According to this theory (known as utilitarianism) the right action will always be the one which tends to produce the greatest happiness (or welfare) of the greatest number of people. And since there's a great deal of unhappiness in the world, the view that morality tells us always to try to reduce that unhappiness seems a very plausible one.

There are, however, several objections to this moral theory. First, it tells us that so long as we're producing the best consequences, it doesn't matter what kind of things we do ('the end justifies the means' is a very consequentialist thought). So if we can make most people's lives go better by treating a few people badly – by exploiting them, for example – then that's what we should do. If we can keep patients happy by lying to them about their illness, then that's the right thing to do (so long as there are no other bad consequences). Even if an action is an absolutely horrific one, if it would produce the best outcomes then according to consequentialism that's what we should do – so if we could save a large number of people's lives by torturing an innocent person, then that would be the right thing to do. Many people feel that this aspect of consequentialism is morally unacceptable.[3]

A second objection to consequentialism is that it provides us with a very impersonal view of morality: it tells us to do what's best for everyone, and not to give any special attention to the people we're closest to. 'Everyone counts for one, and no one for more than one' is a very consequentialist view, and it leaves no room for special obligations to our family or to our own patients or students or clients. In some circumstances this seems right, since it prevents favouritism, but many people feel that we do have special duties to those who are especially close to us, and consequentialism doesn't seem to have any room for that kind of thought.

A third objection to consequentialism is that it's an enormously demanding moral theory: it tells us that the right thing to do is to produce the best consequences (sometimes referred to as 'maximising the good'), and if we're not maximising the good, then we're doing the wrong thing. But most of the things we do in our lives don't maximise the good, and if we tried to maximise the good all the time we'd never have any time to conduct a normal satisfactory life – we'd be too busy making things better for other people all the time. Maybe this is a life that saints can lead, but most of us can't manage to be saints, and morality, according to this objection, shouldn't demand of us something that most people just can't do. We need a moral theory that shows that we can live moral lives in a way that is bearable for most of us, that isn't so overwhelmingly demanding as consequentialism seems to be.

An alternative view of morality is provided by deontology, a theory which says that though producing good consequences is indeed morally important, it isn't the only thing which matters, morally speaking. According to deontology, sometimes the right action is the one which maximises the good, but sometimes it isn't. For example, if you've borrowed some money from a rich friend, then when the time comes to return it, you ought to pay it back to him, even if you could do more good by donating the money to charity. If you've promised a patient not to tell her family about her illness, then you should keep that promise, even if it might do more good for you to reveal the truth. Deontologists think that there are certain kinds of actions which we just shouldn't do (lying, stealing, and killing the innocent are typical deontological prohibitions) and other kinds of actions which we definitely ought to do (such as looking after our own children, keeping our promises, paying our debts, protecting the innocent). So whereas consequentialists have one overarching moral principle ('act so as to produce the best consequences'), deontologists think that there are a range of different moral principles, prohibiting some actions and requiring others. As long as we conform to those moral principles or rules, then we'll be doing the right thing. (And many of the actions we might want to do – such as going to a football match, or a walk in the country, or taking up a new hobby – won't appear on either list, so we can do them or not, as we please.)

Deontology is much closer to common sense morality than consequentialism: so long as we stick to the rules, we're free to do as we please, so it's a much less demanding theory of morality than conseqeuntialism. And the rules generally include ones about special duties to our nearest and dearest (a typical deontological principle of this kind will say that we have a special duty to look after our own children, for example – though this doesn't rule out the possibility that we have some, less demanding, duties towards all children too.) And most importantly, deontology won't endorse any horrific actions, since such actions will be prohibited by deontological rules, which means that they'll be wrong even if doing them would produce good consequences.

But deontology has problems of its own. Because there are several moral rules in this theory, there is the possibility of the rules coming into conflict. Many actions are ones which fall under more than one rule – for example, if a young patient tells me in confidence that a relative is abusing him, keeping his confidence will involve failing to report a case of child abuse. But it's reasonable to think that there's a moral principle telling us to keep confidences, and another moral principle telling us to take action against child abuse. What happens when we can only obey one rule by breaking another?

The problem arises here because we tend to think of moral rules and principles as being absolute – that is, as having no exceptions. We're inclined to feel that taking morality seriously involves treating moral principles as having no exceptions at all. But absolute, exceptionless rules leave us with nowhere to go when they come into conflict (which they often do) – in those situations, it looks as if whatever we do will be wrong. And a moral theory whose output leaves us in the position where anything we can do will be wrong is not a very helpful moral theory!

One way in which deontologists can deal with this problem of conflict of duty is to interpret moral principles in a different way – to think of them not as absolute, but as capturing moral tendencies.[4] On this understanding of moral rules, they specify features of actions which tend to make them right or wrong. So the moral principle which tells us that we shouldn't lie is, in this view, telling us that if an action involves lying, that tends to make it wrong. And the moral principle which tells us to try to save lives means that if an action involves saving a life, that tends to make it right. And if we can only save a life by telling a lie, then that action will have two different moral tendencies – the fact that it's a lie will tend to make it wrong, but the fact that it saves a life will tend to make it right. Which tendency wins out will, on this account of morality, vary from case to case – perhaps in most cases the fact that the action would save a life is more important than the fact that it would involve telling a lie, so that means it's the right thing to do. But there might be some circumstances in which telling the truth is more important than anything else – perhaps when it's the only way to clear an innocent person from a criminal charge – and even if it means that someone else's life is put at risk, that might have to come second.

This form of deontology has many attractions as a moral theory. In particular, it ensures that our moral judgements are very sensitive to context, since it tells us to be aware of all the moral principles (that is, all the tendencies to be right or wrong) which may be present in each situation, and to take all these tendencies into account before deciding what's the right way to act in that situation. And because moral principles aren't understood as being absolute, we don't have the insoluble conflicts of duty which are such a problem for absolutist deontology. This theory (unlike consequentialism) doesn't offer a simple rule for deciding what's the right thing to do, what the right action is. There's no simple shortcut to that: there's no substitute for using our judgement about moral matters. But what we can learn from our moral principles is what kind of consideration will be relevant to that final judgement, what tendencies to look for in any situation in which we're wondering what is the right thing to do. Because there are principles prohibiting lying and stealing, we know that these things tend to make actions wrong; because there are principles telling us to keep our promises and to try to help others we know that these features of an action will tend to make it right. But which actions are *actually* right or wrong will depend on all the details of each unique situation, on all the tendencies that are present in it.

This form of deontology, with its interpretation of moral principles as specifying right-making or wrong-making features of action, has recently been very influential in medical ethics (and increasingly in other kinds of professional ethics too). A version of it, deriving from the work of Ross, has been developed by the ethicists Tom Beauchamp and James Childress (2001), who suggest that there are four moral principles which capture the core of our ethical thinking in the domain of health care. The principles which Beauchamp and Childress propose as central to health care are the principles of beneficence, non-maleficence, respect for autonomy, and justice, and each of them has widespread implications for our health care practice. These principles are deontological ones – they include considerations which aren't exclusively about good consequences – but they're not absolute, exceptionless principles, and each one is constrained by the presence of the others. No principle is always the most important one – which one matters most varies from case to case, and always depends on the specific features of the context in which health care professionals (and others) are acting.

The principle of *beneficence* tells us to do good to our patients. Implications of this principle are that we should protect others from harm; defend their rights; prevent harm from occurring to others; remove conditions that will cause harm to others; help persons with disabilities; rescue persons in danger.

The principle of *non-maleficence* tells us not to harm the patient. Implications of this principle are that we shouldn't kill; we shouldn't cause pain or suffering; we shouldn't incapacitate; we shouldn't cause offence; we shouldn't deprive others of the goods of life, whatever they are.

(It's worth noting that these two principles – beneficence and non-maleficence – can be accepted by any consequentialist. This reflects the fact that all moral theories acknowledge that producing good consequences is morally significant: the core distinction between consequentialism and deontology is that the latter, but not the former, thinks that other things are morally significant too.)

The principle of *respect for autonomy* tells us to respect the autonomy of the patient – that is, we shouldn't prevent (autonomous) patients from making and acting upon their own autonomous decisions. (Autonomous decisions are ones which are made by competent agents who understand the situations in which they're acting and who aren't subject to controlling influences.) Implications of this principle include the requirements that we should tell people the truth and refrain from deceiving them; respect the privacy of others; protect confidential information; obtain consent for interventions with patients; when asked, help others make important decisions.

The principle of *justice* tells us to treat people fairly, and so it tells us to ensure that the costs and benefits of treatment are fairly distributed between patients. What this amounts to is sometimes summed up in the dictum 'Equals must be treated equally, and unequals must be treated unequally', but this abstract requirement needs to be filled out by an account of which equalities and inequalities are the important ones in the health care context. A particularly significant one is often thought to be medical need, so that we should give equal treatment to people with equal levels of medical need.

This 'four principles' approach, as it is sometimes known, to health care ethics tells us which features are likely to be most important for our ethical decision making. But these moral principles are not absolute ones – each one can be overridden in some circumstances by one or more of the others. They don't provide a formula for deciding what's right to do, and they don't remove the need for sensitive moral judgement. The principles tell us what is morally important; but only careful and sensitive attention to the context will tell us what's most important *here*, in each specific situation, and hence what it's right to do.

Morality is a very complex matter, and studying ethics helps us to understand not only our own moral views and concerns, but also those of others, including people who disagree with us. We can come to see that their views may be driven by a moral theory which, though we may not agree with it ourselves, has strengths that are evident to us, even if we don't endorse it. Morality is not like physics, and we're unlikely to find the single best moral theory any time soon. Studying the range of moral theories on offer makes us better able to work out what actions are most justifiable, and also to see and often respect why others sometimes come to differing views.

Notes

1   The word 'ethics' can be used to mean two somewhat different things. Sometimes it means 'the study of morality', sometimes it's used just to mean 'morality' itself. In this chapter I'm using it in the former sense.
2   Sophisticated forms of relativism have been developed to meet this kind of objection, but there isn't room to deal with them adequately here.
3   The consequentialist can reply to this objection by saying that the only time his/her theory tells us to commit horrific actions is when the alternative is even more horrific.
4   This form of deontology derives from the work of the philosopher W.D. Ross, who suggested that moral principles be thought of as stating what he called prima facie duties – that is, features of actions which tend to make them right or wrong.

References

Beauchamp, T. and Childress, J. (2001) *Principles of Biomedical Ethics*. Fifth edition. Oxford: Oxford University Press.

16

The Role of the Family in Patient Care

Anne-Marie Slowther

> The family is the natural and fundamental group unit of society and is entitled to protection by society and the State. Universal Declaration of Human Rights Article 16.3

The paradigm relationship, both clinical and moral, in health care is that between the clinician and the patient. However, this relationship does not exist in a vacuum. Other relationships impact in a variety of ways on the central interaction between a health professional and her patient, and often the most important of these are relationships with the patient's family. In some cultures decisions about health care are seen as a familial rather than individual responsibility,[1] but even in cultures where a more individualistic model of health care is the norm, such as the UK, consideration of a patient's family is often integral to clinical decisions. Such situations include treatment of children where parents are the proxy decision-makers, treatment of adults who lack capacity where families contribute to the decision-making process, and cases where decisions about patient treatment or investigation have an impact on other family members, for example genetic testing.

Relationships with patients' families are often a source of ethical discomfort for clinicians, raising questions about how much weight to give to family members' views, how to balance interests of family members with patients' interests, or simply what to say to a family and when. These difficulties can be compounded when more than one family member is a patient of the same doctor, as is often the case in primary care. Studies of referrals to clinical ethics committees or requests for ethics case consultation frequently cite conflicts between patients' families and clinicians among the most frequent reasons for referral.[2, 3] In 2005, Canadian bioethicists were asked to identify the top ten health care ethics challenges facing the public. The top ranked challenge was disagreements between patients/families and health care professionals about treatment decisions.[4] What are the ethical considerations that should guide clinicians in their relationships with patients' families, and how can ethical conflicts be resolved?

Family as decision-maker

Families have responsibilities as decision-makers in a range of situations in health care, and in relation to both living and dead patients. Under the Human Tissue Act, which came

'The role of the family in patient care' by A.-M. Slowther, *Clinical Ethics*, 2006; 1(4): 191–3. Reproduced by permission of The Royal Society of Medicine Press, London.

into force on 1 September 2006, family members may be required to give proxy consent for use of organs or tissue after a person has died. However, any consent or refusal given by the patient before death cannot be over-ridden by the family.[5] As a general rule, parents have the responsibility of making decisions on behalf of their children, at least until the child has reached sufficient maturity to make an autonomous decision for herself. When an adult lacks capacity to make treatment decisions for herself, the person with decision-making responsibility can vary. In some countries, for example, the USA, the next of kin is proxy decision-maker. The current situation in England is that [...] under the Mental Capacity Act [...] it will be possible for an adult to appoint someone to make health care decisions on her behalf should she lose capacity at some future date.[6]

The ethical (and legal) principle governing proxy decision-making can also vary in different situations. Thus, in the USA proxy decision-makers for adults who lack capacity are expected to make a decision based on what the patient would have wanted for herself (a substituted judgement).[7] The underlying ethical principle here is that of respect for autonomy. In contrast, in the UK, the ethical principle underlying proxy decision-making is that of beneficence, or acting in the person's best interests. This is articulated in law in both the Children Act[8] and the Mental Capacity Act.[9] However, while the prime principle for proxy decision-making in the UK may be beneficence, respect for autonomy is still important. Any judgement about what is in someone's best interests must take into account (in so far as it is possible to know) what that person would want if he or she could say.

In many cases, involving both adults and children, the patient may lack capacity to actually make the decision, but still be able to participate in a discussion about the decision or indicate a preference for one course of action or another. Respect for autonomy would require that clinicians and proxy decision-makers involve the patient in the decision as much as possible. For example, the guidance on withdrawing and withholding life sustaining treatment in children by the Royal College of Paediatrics and Child Health recognizes different levels of involvement by the child in the decision-making process:

1   Informing children;
2   Listening to them;
3   Taking account of their views so that they can influence decisions;
4   Respecting the competent child as the main decider about proposed health care interventions.[10]

When conflict arises between clinicians and family members (whether or not the family member is the proxy decision-maker) about what is the appropriate treatment for a patient who lacks capacity to decide for themselves, it can be difficult to find common ground. A first step can be to agree on the underlying principle of acting in the patient's best interests. Deciding what is in the patient's best interests is a complex judgement which requires input from both clinicians and families.

Family as provider of information

Close family members are likely to know the patient as a person much better than will the clinicians caring for them, although this is not always the case. This knowledge is important when deciding what course of action is in the patient's best interests. An assessment of best interests clearly includes a judgement on the relative benefits and risks of treatment, but it also includes psychological, social and spiritual factors that are specific to the individual patient. Family members may be able to provide insight into these factors. Recognizing and respecting the contribution of family members to these often difficult treatment decisions benefits both patient and family. While clinicians may not owe a direct duty of care to family members, good clinical practice would include providing support and minimizing their distress. Involving them in the decision-making process may help to achieve this.

Conflicts of interests between patients and families

Ethical difficulties often arise for clinicians when diagnosis or management of their patients' condition is inextricably linked to other family members. Clinical geneticists may be faced with a patient (A) whose positive test for the BRCA 1 gene has implications for her sister's (B's) risk of developing breast cancer, and who specifically states that she doesn't want B to have this information. Disclosing this information would breach A's confidentiality, but not informing B denies her the opportunity to make important decisions about her own health. The principle of respect for the patient's autonomy, underpinning a duty of confidentiality, may then conflict with the principle of avoiding harm, or, indeed, with respect for another family member's autonomy. Resolution of the conflict involves balancing the competing principles and likely harmful consequences of different courses of action. In general the duty of confidentiality to a patient takes precedence, but if there was a high risk of serious harm to another family member a breach of confidentiality might be justified (see five minute focus in issue 2[11]). There has been some discussion in the ethics literature about whether genetic information is different from other patient information and should be regarded as owned by the family rather than the individual.[12] Conflicts of values between patients and their families can be particularly problematic when dealing with adolescents with health problems.

Another common area of conflict of interest within families that can lead to ethical difficulties for clinicians is when a patient is being cared for by a partner or other family member, and the burden of care is causing physical or psychological harm to the carer.[13] Various ethical conflicts may arise and consideration needs to be given to the autonomy and best interests of both patient and carer. In these situations it may not be possible, or desirable, to completely dissociate the interests of the patient from the carer. Having a carer who is physically or psychologically unwell will not be in the interests of the patient who relies on them. Caring for a patient in the social context of their family can create ethical difficulties that are not readily resolvable by reliance on principles alone. Other ethical approaches such as an ethic of care, which places more emphasis on relationships and responsibilities, or casuistry, which focuses on the particularities of the specific case, may provide alternative perspectives, shifting the emphasis from conflict to negotiation.

Most of us do not live as isolated individuals and for many people relationships with family are a key part of their lives, particularly during times of illness. Clinicians caring for patients need to consider what role, if any, the patients' family is playing in the context of their treatment or care. The clinical and moral focus is on the individual patient, but appropriate involvement of the patients' family can enhance patient care.

Summary points

- Patients' families often have a significant role to play in patient care.
- Conflict between clinicians and families, and between family members, can be a source of ethical concern.
- When family members are proxy decision-makers, the guiding principle for their decisions is the best interests of the patient.
- Family members can contribute key non-clinical knowledge about a patient's preferences and values when determining what is in the best interests of a patient who lacks capacity to decide for herself.
- The interests of patients and other members of their family can conflict. Clinicians may need to assess and balance competing interests, and to ethically justify their decision.

Further reading

Nelson HL, Nelson JL. *The Patient in the Family: An Ethics of Medicine and Families*. New York: Routledge, 1995

McHaffie HE, Liang IA, Parker M, McMillan J. Deciding for imperilled newborns: medical authority or parental autonomy? *J Med Ethics* 2001; 27: 104–9

References

1. Jafarey AM, Faroqui A. Informed consent in the Pakistani milieu: the physician's perspective. *J Med Ethics* 2005; 31: 93–6
2. DaVal G, Sartorius L, Clarridge B, Gensler G, Fanis M. What triggers requests for ethics consultations? *J Med Ethics* 2001; 27: 24–9
3. Hurst S, Hull S, CDuVal G, Danis M. How physicians face ethical difficulties: a qualitative analysis. *J Med Ethics* 2005; 31: 7–14
4. Breslin J, MacRae SK, Bell J, et al. Top 10 health care ethics challenges facing the public: views of Toronto bioethicists. *BMC Med Ethics* 2005; 6: 5
5. Brazier M, Fovargue S. A brief guide to the Human Tissue Act. *Clin Ethics* 2006; 1: 26–32
6. Mental Capacity Act 2005, Section 9. Available at www.opsi.gov.uk/acts/acts2005/50009--b.htm#9
7. Lang Forrest, Quill T. Making decisions with families at the end of life. *Am Fam Phys* 2004; 70: 719–23

8. Children Act 1989, Section 1 Available at www.opsi.gov.uk/acts/acts1989/Ukpga_19890041_en_2. htm#mdiv1
9. Mental Capacity Act 2005, Section 1(5). Available at www.opsi.gov.uk/acts/acts2005/ 50009–b.htm# 4
10. Royal College of Paediatrics and Child Health. Withholding or with drawing life sustaining treatment in children: A framework for practice. London: RCP, 2004: s2.6.1. Available at www. repch.ac.uk/publications/recent_publications/Withholding.pdf
11. Slowther A. Sharing information in health care: the nature and limits of confidentiality. *Clin Ethics* 2006; 1: 82–4
12. Parker M, Lucassen A. Concern for families and individuals in clinical genetics. *J Med Ethics* 2003; 29: 70–73
13. Rosin AJ, Van Dijk Y. Subtle ethical dilemmas in geriatric management and clinical research. *J Med Ethics* 2005; 31: 355–9

17

Should Children's Autonomy be Respected by Telling Them of Their Imminent Death?

T. Vince and A. Petros

A 14 year old boy was admitted to the paediatric intensive care unit (PICU) with acute on chronic respiratory failure and was mechanically ventilated. He was known to have obliterative bronchiolitis secondary to an episode of Stevens-Johnson syndrome. He also had a past history of IgG2 subclass deficiency and phenylketonuria but was developmentally normal. He had severely impaired lung function with both forced expiratory volume (FEVI) and forced vital capacity (FVC) at around 20% of that predicted for his age and was receiving home oxygen. He was being considered for lung transplantation.

Throughout the admission he was difficult to ventilate but five days after admission he was extubated. He was, however, unable to maintain adequate spontaneous ventilation and rapidly deteriorated, requiring reintubation under sedation and reventilation. It soon became apparent that, rather than just an acute deterioration of respiratory function following a chest infection, this was the presentation of terminal respiratory failure. A multidisciplinary discussion involving the respiratory, transplant, and intensive care teams and the boy's parents took place to review the management options. The lung disease was felt to be irreversible and of such severity and progression as to be rapidly terminal. It was agreed by all that lung transplantation was not a viable option as transplantation in children ill enough to need mechanical ventilation had previously been uniformly unsuccessful. It was also unanimously agreed that to continue aggressive intensive therapy, including tracheotomy and short term chronic ventilation, was futile in the face of deteriorating lung function and inadequate gas exchange. There was uniform consensus that withdrawal of therapy was the only option.

Having achieved unanimous agreement on this point, intense discussion took place regarding how best to proceed. One view was that as the boy had been able to communicate and show understanding immediately prior to this admission, sedation should be stopped, he should be woken up fully, and given the opportunity to be aware of his terminal condition. Awakening him would also allow him to express and exercise his choices around his death, in particular, the chance to say goodbye to his family, and make his last wishes known. An opposing view felt, however, that it was wrong to wake him up just to tell him he was going to die. There were also concerns about how competent the decision making of an adolescent with respiratory failure and hypercapnia could be. The deciding factor was the boy's parents, who felt strongly that it would be too distressing for their son to wake him and discuss his inevitable death. A multidisciplinary ethical meeting was held to discuss the dilemma. It was ultimately agreed that the parent's wishes should be respected. The boy was not woken up, all infusions were maintained and he was extubated. He died comfortably in his sleep in the company of his family.

Discussion

This case provoked considerable debate amongst those caring for the child. Our patient was felt to have no chance of recovery. He had severe lung disease and it was agreed that life sustaining treatment would only "delay death without significant alleviation of suffer-ing", thereby fulfilling category four of the guidelines from the Royal College of Paediatrics and Child Health on withholding or withdrawing life saving treatment in children.[1] All those looking after the child were agreed on this point. There were, however, two differing viewpoints on how to proceed and manage the child's death. One felt the young boy should be fully awoken from his sedation and informed of his imminent death because he had the right to know and that not to do so would deprive him of his autonomy and his right to be involved in discussions surrounding his imminent death. The contrast-ing view was that he should be kept comfortable and adequately sedated and have treat-ment withdrawn; to wake up the child and inform him of his death would be cruel and unnecessary. This was recognised as a paternalistic approach but felt to be in the child's best interests and was the viewpoint supported by the parents.

It was argued that if the child was deemed competent and capable of understanding his terminal situation, the medical team had an ethical duty to inform him of their discussions and decisions and to involve him in the process of his own death. By not doing so were the team violating his personhood, autonomy, and human rights? An individuals has "person-hood" if he is able to value his own existence and has hopes and desires for his future life.[2] An individual's right to life emanates from that personhood rather than his innate biolog-ical form.[3] With personhood comes the benefit of autonomy, in that we place a high moral value on the ability and freedom to make choices consistent with our hopes and desires.[2] In fact, many would argue that respect for autonomy is the highest moral principle because it embodies the essence of being a person.[2,4] In acknowledging personhood, we are duty bound to respect autonomy and the right to self determination. Thus, recognition of the child's personhood was integral to respect for his life. Clearly, before his admission the boy was functioning normally at school and, for all purposes, was a person. By ensuring the boy remained comfortable and allowing him to die peacefully, without the stress of being awoken only to discuss his imminent death, the team was exercising an extreme degree of paternalism, which denied his autonomy and his right to self determination.

Before this admission, the boy had been living a normal but restricted life and on PICU, while intubated and mechanically ventilated but with sedation lifted, he had demonstrated good non-verbal communications. As such, there was no reason to believe that he would not have been able to understand the gravity of his condition. Nonetheless, it was suggested that be was too young to cope with the knowledge of his death. Yet it is well recognised that children with chronic illness as young as 10 years old, can be aware they are dying and can benefit from participating in decisions surrounding death such as funeral arrangements.[5] In retrospect, this case highlights the need for early and ongoing discussions about death with children with chronic illnesses. In this case, the child was aware of the chronic nature of his condition and the probable need for lung transplantation in the future. Discussions about death had not been previously broached with him, however, as they had not seemed pertinent to his primary physicians. Furthermore, on this admission, his acute deterioration was more rapid and severe than expected and it was unclear how he would have coped with this type of discussion in his current condition. Nevertheless, some members of the team felt he should be allowed the option. Indeed, if the outcome of withdrawal of therapy is the death of a person who is able to understand then should not consent be sought irrespective of age? Allmark would argue that this paternalistic approach to withdrawal of treatment, for fear of causing distress, denies a child his personhood and is unacceptable.[6]

During the boy's admission, and while ventilated, the advice of the specialist teams was that if he was unable to breathe spontaneously and was dependent upon mechanical support, his chances of successful lung transplantation were extremely poor. The PICU team relayed this opinion to the family, but until the child required reintubation this was merely a probability rather than fact. Thus the future management plans were dependent upon how the child responded. Moreover, the speed of his respiratory deterioration further precluded discussions of death and dying during the admission to PICU including prior to the trial of extubation. It is standard practice to anaesthetise children for intubation and then sedate them while ventilated, not least to avoid the physical consequences of fear and discomfort, and the child agreed to this. By the time child was reintubated, the multidisciplinary meeting with his parents had not occurred. When it did take place, the medical teams, and in particular the transplant team, confirmed the child was not suitable for lung transplantation while dependent on mechanical ventilation. Consequently, the child remained entirely unaware of the ultimate significance of resedation and reintubation.

All parties agreed that the child was clearly not capable of consent whilst sedated. Subsequent discussions focused on whether the sedation should be lifted while maintaining the child on mechanical ventilation to allow him to be involved in decisions around his death with minimal impact on his respiratory status. Perhaps the real ethical dilemma centres, however, on the purpose of awakening the child. Was it to obtain his consent for withdrawal of treatment, or was it to inform him of his imminent death so that he could "put his affairs in order"? Some members of the team were concerned that the boy's respiratory failure and subsequent hypercapnia might have compromised his level of consciousness and competence, thereby affecting his ability to consent. An individual's competence arises from his experiences and values, not his chronological age.[7,8] Moreover, competence has differing ethical and legal definitions. A person is deemed competent if he is able to assimilate information, apply it personally, and thereafter make an informed decision. In medicolegal terms, a competent person may consent to or refuse a treatment as long as he or she is fully informed, including being cognisant of the consequences. It is an ethical and statutory requirement to seek consent prior to treatment of a competent person and to respect his choice to refuse treatment even if it not in his best interests.[2,5] The situation is different for children. The Gillick ruling in 1985 stated that a child deemed competent could consent to treatment[9] but later judgments ruled that although competent children could consent to treatment, they could not refuse it, and could be overruled by parents or doctors.[10] In ethical terms, maintaining a distinction between accepting and declining treatment have different moral values attached to them when in fact they are exactly equal but opposite. More importantly, the legal standpoint questions the value of consent of children in paediatric critical care in general. If the child remains sedated, he is incapable of consent and is the passive recipient of the discussions and actions of others. In contrast, awakening the child might enable him to consent, but is this truly possible? Consent is the voluntary, uncoerced agreement to a proposal and is made by a competent, autonomous person in the full knowledge of the consequences.[11] In this case, the doctors would continue to act in the patient's best interests by laying down the facts of his condition before him. They may even recommend a course of action, including withdrawal of intensive care support. By adopting a paternalistic attitude and using persuasive arguments, the medical staff assume an authority that directly impacts on the child's ability to concur freely and without coercion. As a result, the child is not truly autonomous and what we obtain from his is not consent but acquiescence[2]: thus the issue of this competent child's autonomy has been, as it were, overlooked. If this argument is continued, awakening the child, in effect to obtain his acquiescence, may actually be unethical because his right to autonomy remains denied and the process may cause him distress and harm.

The alternative reason to awaken him, to allow him to "put his affairs in order," bears consideration. As the outcome is inevitable, it may be postulated that the child had no real choices except in controlling some elements of the manner of his death. The opportunity to say goodbye may be vital for the child and may prove helpful for the family at the time of their son's death and afterwards. Perhaps, for these reasons alone, awakening the child may be beneficial.

[…]

In the end, the team decided to withdraw intensive care support without informing the child. It was felt that the manner in which the child died would be much more significant for the family than for the various sections of the medical team. The parents were adamant that they did not want to risk any chance that their son might be distressed if awoken. By acquiescing with the parents' wishes, the medical team allowed them some control in their son's death. The actions of the healthcare team and the parents may be described as paternalistic, but based on the ethical principle of non-maleficence, the healthcare team acted in what they perceived to be the best interests of the child. In doing so, they prioritised their own and the parents' non-maleficent decisions over the patient's right to autonomy. This may well have been the right thing to do. It may also be argued that the nature and acute circumstances of his illness never truly allowed the child to determine his future. The question remains, however, whether an individual's best interests can truly be respected if he is denied the opportunity to exercise his autonomy.

References

1   Royal college of Paediatrics and Child Health. *Withholding or withdrawing life saving treatment in children: a framework for practice.* London: RCPCH,1997.
2   Harris J. Consent and end of life decisions. *J Med Ethics* 2003;29:10–15.

3　Tooley M. Decision to terminate life and the concept of person. In: Beauchamp T, Perlin S, eds. *Ethical issues relating to life & death*. New York: Oxford University Press, 1979:64–5.

4　Gillon R. Ethics needs principles–four can encompass the rest–and respect for autonomy should be "first among equals". *J Med Ethics* 2003;29:307–12.

5　Himelstein BP, Hilden JM, Morslad Boldt A, *et al.* Pediatric palliative care. *N Eng J Med* 2004;350:1752–62.

6　Allmark P. Death with dignity. *J Med Ethics* 2002;28:255–7.

7　Sensky T. Withdrawal of life sustaining treatement. *BMJ*, 2002;325:175–96.

8　Street K, Ashcroft R, Henderson J, *et al.* The decision making process regarding the withdrawal or withholding of potential life saving treatments in a children's hospital. *J Med Ethics* 2000;26:346–52.

9　Gillick v West Norfolk and Wisbech Area Health Authority [1985] 3 All ER 402 (HL).

10　Re J [1991] fom 33.

11　Habiba MA. Examining consent within the patient doctor relationship. *J Med Ethics* 2000;26:183–7.

18

Critical Moments: Death and Dying in Intensive Care

Jane E. Seymour

Social action surrounding critically ill people in intensive care is, in many ways, on 'fast forward'. In a time span covering only a few days or weeks, people are admitted, diagnosed, investigated, discussed and cared for until their death or recovery. During this time, inter-professional activity can be frenetic and fast moving. Clinical knowledge must be produced about the ill person; relationships formed and sustained among healthcare staff, patients and patients' companions. Further, the technological environment of intensive care and its relationship to the highly segmented hospital organization allows some conclusions to be drawn about the impact of the 'hyper-specialization' of contemporary healthcare on the management of ill and dying people.

[...]

The situation in which intensive care becomes responsible for the disentanglement of end-of-life problems causes acute difficulties for medical and nursing staff as they attempt to care for dying people in a humane and appropriate way. It also engenders potential confusion in their relationships with the ill patient's companions. Companions have varying responses depending on their perception of the situation. For example, they may believe that 'intensive care' is a particular sort of modern day saviour, only to feel let down, angry and grief stricken when their husband, wife, partner or child eventually dies, especially if intensive care has been withdrawn and the death of that person occurs elsewhere in the hospital. They may feel disempowered because of a sudden, inexplicable, input of 'technology' when they believed that an expected death was imminent. Of course, such experiences of loss and bereavement are not exclusive to those who have contact with intensive care, they are a feature of 'normal' patterns of grieving following deaths in other situations. However, they are a central and recurring feature of life in intensive care: problems that have to be faced and resolved on an almost daily basis.

The way in which healthcare delivery is currently structured is, it may be argued, at the root of such problems. The 'acute care culture' [...] depends on a hospital organization structured around finding solutions to *immediate*, short-term health problems. This is done primarily by means of gathering a series of 'specialist' opinions, each of which focuses on a particular aspect of 'the patient'. Decisions are then made on the basis of information that becomes progressively narrower and less contextual in nature, and the threat of death is contained, postponed and deconstructed into a series of potentially soluble puzzles (Illich 1976; Bauman 1992; Moller 1996). What occurs is a cascade of decisions (Slomka 1992); in which there are a myriad of contributors, each of whom believes that their version of 'the patient' is the most cogent. The clinical ownership of patients by particular 'firms' directs the gathering of specialist opinions; the value of which are adjudicated according to judgements that are presented as purely technical. Accordingly, the wider social and human issues are often either ignored, alluded to only in passing, or seen as introducing murky irrationality into the whole medical enterprise. [...] In the extract below, Moller refers to what he later describes as the 'roller coaster journey' of the patient who is eventually designated as dying:

> the technical care of dying patients enables physicians and other medical staff to treat the dying patient with the same set of expectations and responses applied to other medical patients. It is for this reason that dying patients with a lingering trajectory are often cast in the sick role, and attention is focused primarily on the management of physical symptoms. By focusing on the manageability of symptoms, the unmanageability of dying is superseded and deferred. As a result the process of dying is prolonged in such a way that it is often filled with uncertainty and ambivalence. (Moller 1996: 68)

[...]

Intensive care units, then, grapple increasingly with the legacy of the failure of that wider system to come to terms with the changing face of illness and death in modern societies. [...]

Enabling continuity of care

[...] [T]he issue of 'continuity' of care across the healthcare system is revealed as problematic. This has significant effects on both the development of treatment plans for individual patients first admitted into intensive care from other areas of the hospital and on the perceptions of their companions regarding the purpose, direction and quality of care. One aspect to this [...] is the limited, immediate availability of comprehensive information regarding the patient's health history and quality of life. This constrains the ability of clinicians to develop treatment plans and, in the cases examined, leads to an apparent over-use of intensive therapies in patients who are reaching the end of a course of chronic illness. The attempt to compile a profile of the health history and quality of life of each patient is shown as an ongoing feature of clinical work in intensive care, but one that features particularly strongly in the preliminary assessment of patients. This study suggests that such information is crucial in determining not only the extent of treatment given to an individual but, more fundamentally, the initial placement of patients in intensive care. [...]

The other aspect to the problem of continuity concerns the organization of medical and nursing work across the hospital site; and the way in which care is planned and co-ordinated predominantly *within* individual wards and intensive care units, rather than *across* those organizational boundaries. [...]

[The] transfer of patients from intensive care to a general ward highlights a particular problem. In some cases patients were clearly going to die in the short term, while in other cases patients had been designated as not likely to benefit from further intensive therapy, i.e. as likely to die in the medium or long term. When this occurred it was often because of limited bed availability, but it led to an exacerbation of confusion and regret over the delivery of care expressed by patient's companions. While companions understood the need for transfer, they expressed regret at losing the attentive nursing care that intensive care could provide to the dying person, and the emotional support they had gained from the formation of close relationships with the nurses primarily responsible for the patient.

Models of practice are available, which could be adapted to address these problems. In the SUPPORT study, for example, an intervention was designed by researchers to improve the level of information available to physicians about the prognoses of patients. The intervention had three components. First, a brief written report regarding a patient's probability of surviving for a six-month period, likelihood of being severely functionally impaired at two months, and probability of surviving cardiopulmonary resuscitation. Second, a written report was provided regarding the patient's views on cardiopulmonary resuscitation, treatment preferences, and perceived prognosis. These reports were prepared by the researchers. Third, specially trained nurse facilitators were given responsibility for initiating and maintaining communication among patients, their companions and the healthcare staff.

Such initiatives could be helpful in informing decision making particularly in the case of those patients whose referral for admission to intensive care follows a period of treatment elsewhere in the hospital organization. It may also be possible to incorporate some aspects of the first two stages of the intervention into the information recorded about elderly and chronically ill patients in the primary care setting, although this presumes that such patients have had regular, close contact with their general practice prior to the onset of an acute exacerbation of their condition. That this is not necessarily the case is an indicator of the extent of the information gap that needs to be addressed. Enhancing the quality and range of information from primary care would, however, be a necessary component in informing the very rapid process of decision making that takes place around critically ill patients admitted from home to hospital via a general practitioner referral.

[...]

One example will be given here of an innovation in care that focuses specifically on the management of patients designated as dying within intensive and acute care settings. Reporting on experience of a 10-year 'end of life' service in a University hospital in Detroit, US, Campbell and Frank (1997) describe the establishment of a nurse-led palliative care service, which has served the acute care providers. This service shares some features with hospital palliative care services in this country. However, rather than being predominantly advisory and concerned with patients suffering mainly from malignancy, Campbell and Frank assume responsibility for the direction and planning of the care of all patients referred to them. They exercise this responsibility by conducting shared 'rounds' and by liaising closely with other medical and nursing staff responsible for implementing care. Patient referrals come largely from the medical intensive care unit, from the accident and emergency department, or from the acute medical and surgical departments. Where patients are referred from intensive care, Campbell and Frank become involved in, and facilitate, withdrawal of treatment discussions held with patients' companions and with intensive care staff. Further, they assume responsibility for the transfer and placement of patients to suitable non-intensive care areas. Once transfer has been completed, an inter-disciplinary 'therapeutic plan' is instituted for each patient, in which nursing and medical goals are coalesced. Campbell and Frank report that the service has been a viable 'triage' option for the medical intensive care unit in the management of dying patients: allowing intensive care beds to be vacated and significant cost savings, but at the same time, ensuring high quality nursing and medical care to those who are dying and their companions.

[...]

Re-examining the involvement of companions during care decision making

[...] [C]ommunication between intensive care staff and patients' companions is predicated on a perceived need to 'warn' of the likelihood of death. Emphasis was placed on the role of the medical staff in delivering a formal presentation to companions regarding the condition of patients. In this formal presentation, efforts are made to stress the pessimistic aspects of an individual's prognosis. Nurses regard themselves as playing an important role in 'preparing' companions for this presentation and for the eventual death of a patient. Considerable energies are invested in facilitating the expression of grief and in developing a state akin to 'anticipatory grief' (Lindemann 1944) within companions. Furthermore, healthcare staff, who were interviewed, expressed the belief that families and companions should not be expected to assume responsibility for decisions regarding the continuation of care for patients. Rather, such an expectation was seen as placing an unfair burden on companions and as leading to a risk of 'abnormal' grieving in the future.

In some cases, however, this attention to the promotion of anticipatory grief, and to the removal of responsibility for care decisions from companions, may be misplaced. What has been seen [...] is first, a variable tension between vulnerability and control within companions (Lupton 1996); and second, a very individual response to the prospect of death. Cray (1989) gives an example of how room for such individual variation might be addressed in a description of a family intervention programme in a medical intensive care unit. In this programme, special attention was given to the balancing of structured, routine approaches to the information needs of families and their individual circumstances. In this model, a clinical nurse specialist acted as a facilitator; in much the same way as reported by Campbell and Frank (1997) and Ritter et al. (1992) cited above. While this may be seen as an infringement of the role of the primary nurse, it would alleviate some of the problems reported by nurses in this study, where they described being 'torn' between the needs of their patient and the often very considerable demands and needs of that patient's companions for information and support. Further, it would ensure that specialist education could be targeted at the key individuals undertaking these roles. These individuals could then assume a counselling role directed at facilitating mutual understanding in a way that nurses at the bedside may not be able, or willing, to undertake. Such an individual could act as a supportive resource for companions and families both during the experience of critical illness and afterwards. Bereavement and critical illness follow-up could then be carried out with companions/families in a way that may not be practicable or desirable for patient-focused nurses (Jackson 1996). Such an intervention could be targeted to identify those most in need of follow up, following an approach identified by Kissane *et al.* (1996). This model creates an opportunity to move beyond a narrow definition of 'needs' encouraged both by the understandable tendency for staff under stress to follow 'routine' procedures and the continued reliance on research findings based on a 'tick-box' inventory of people's feelings.

These three suggestions are not intended as simple recipes for action. Rather they are 'food for thought' for those involved in the stressful and demanding processes of delivering care to critically ill and dying people. Further research will be required to elucidate and evaluate the most appropriate approaches to the care of such patients and their companions. This study has, it is hoped, made some contribution to that process. The primary motive behind this research has not been criticism, but rather the development of knowledge and understanding to help practitioners to alleviate the suffering that remains part and parcel of the modern healthcare environment. I hope that I have also added a small further force of leverage on the gradually opening sociological 'window' on death, dying and end-of-life decision making.

References

Bauman, Z. (1992) *Mortality, Immortality and Other Life Strategies*. Oxford: Polity.

Campbell, M.L. and Frank, R.R. (1997) Experience with end of life practice at a university hospital. *Critical Care Medicine*, 25: 197–202.

Cray, L. (1989) A collaborative project: initiating a family intervention program in a medical intensive care unit. *Focus on Critical Care*, 16: 212–18.

Illich, I. (1976) *Limits to Medicine/Medical Nemesis: The Expropriation of Health*. London: Penguin Books.

Jackson, I. (1996) Critical care nurses' perceptions of a bereavement follow up service. *Intensive and Critical Care Nursing*, 12: 2–11.

Kissane, D.W., Bloch, S., Onghena, P., *et al.* (1996) The Melbourne Family Grief Study I. Psychosocial morbidity and grief in bereaved families. *American Journal of Psychiatry*, 153(3): 659–66.

Lindemann, E. (1944) Symptomatology and the management of acute grief. *American Journal of Phychiatry*, 101: 141–8.

Lupton, D. (1996) Your life in their hands: trust in the medical encounter, in V. James and J. Gabe (eds) *Health and the Sociology of Emotions*. Oxford: Blackwell.

Moller, D.W. (1996) *Confronting Death: Values, Institutions and Human Mortality*. New York, Oxford: Oxford University Press.

Principal Investigators for the SUPPORT Project (1995) A controlled trial to improve care for seriously ill hospitalized patients: the study to understand prognoses and preferences for outcomes and risks of treatment (SUPPORT). *Journal of the American Medical Association*, 174: 1591–8.

Ritter, J., Fralic, M.F., Tonges, M.C., *et al.* (1992) Redesigned nursing practice: a case management model for critical care. *Nursing Clinics of North America*, 27: 119–28.

Slomka, J. (1992) The negotiation of death: clinical decision making at the end of life. *Social Science and Medicine*, 35: 251–9.

19

Brain Death: A Sociological View

Allan Kellehear

Determining death by employing brain death criteria has been and continues to be controversial. Apart from technical and philosophical objections to brain death criteria there are several fundamental sociological problems. Without a balanced understanding about death that includes both biological and social influences on people's experiences of death, brain death criteria are remote, abstract and over-medicalised ideas about the end of life. As a result, people commonly greet such criteria with suspicion and ambivalence. This chapter summarises the technical problems of brain death criteria but also provides observations on the sociological impoverishment of current efforts to define death in these reductionist, medical ways.

The modern determination of death

Until the 1960s, cessation of heart and breathing activity were the main signs employed to diagnose death (Waisel and Truog, 1997: 683) and these remain largely the cardinal signs even today outside hospital situations (Knudsen, 2005; Poppe and Bottinger, 2006). However, despite these longstanding signs, the interest in determining death through employment of brain death criteria has grown steadily over the last few years.

In 1968, a combination of developments in intensive care technology and the rapid rise and interest in human organ transplant surgery prompted the Harvard Medical School to convene an Ad Hoc Committee to develop a new criteria for death that matched the complexity and biological implications of those developments (Giacomini, 1997). Since that time there have been other legislative and professional changes that have advocated one of two definitions of brain death. In the US, the President's Commission report (1981) on *Defining Death* and the Uniform Determination of Death Act settled on a 'whole brain' definition of death (Truog and Fletcher, 1990). In the United Kingdom, the Conference of Medical Royal Colleges and their Faculties settled on a 'brain stem' definition of death (Sundin-Huard and Fahey, 2004). Over 80 countries have now adopted one or the other of these definitions of brain death (Bernat, 2005b).

The clinical pathway to determination of brain death begins with a state of coma. Depending on the cause of the coma and the extent of brain damage, patients may develop locked-in syndrome, a vegetative state, chronic coma or brain death (Laureys, Owen and

Schiff, 2004). Brain damage begins a few minutes after cessation of cerebral blood flow (see Bernat 2004: 163) with global destruction of brain cells after 20–30 minutes. Brain cell death leads to diffuse cerebral oedema with a resultant increase in intracranial volume (and therefore pressure). As pressure builds in the rigid skull vault, intracranial pressure exceeds the pressure of blood flowing to the brain and circulation ceases. The contents of the brain then start to partially herniate into the brain stem.

During these physiological changes further changes at the cellular and molecular level occur (in the rostral ventrolateral medulla) that create a deteriorating conflict between 'pro-life' and 'pro-death' neural programmes, with 'pro-death' programmes becoming dominant (Chan, Chang and Chan, 2005). These processes in their turn accelerate a programmed cell death both as a response to interruption of vital metabolic nutrients and vicariously from stress (Vaux and Korsmeyer, 1999; Vaux, 2002). 'Whole brain' death originally included the cerebral hemispheres, brain stem, cerebellum and spinal cord, but the spinal cord was dropped from the definition when it was discovered that most 'dead' people retained or regained reflexes from this area after a short time (Truog and Fletcher, 1990: 204).

Determining whole brain death or brain stem death follows the same clinical principles: assessment of state of coma, establishment of sustained apnea, and assessment of brain stem reflexes (Plum, 1999). Confirmatory tests are also helpful. These tests include EEG (electroencephalograph), cerebral angiography, transcranial Doppler ultrasonography, somatosensory-evoked potentials and scintigraphy (nuclear imaging) (Sundin-Huard and Fahey, 2004). The general criteria for death is irreversible cessation of circulation and respiration or irreversible brain function (whole brain, that is, cerebral hemispheres and brain stem; or brain stem alone). These criteria are not reliable in the newborn period (Diamond, 1998).

There has been significant debate about why brain death was chosen as the main criteria for death itself. These reasons include: a desire to relieve financial costs to families (Schlotzhauer and Liang, 2002), the social pressure to bring psychological relief to families of the sick, freeing up beds or respirators in intensive care units (ICU) (Pernick, 1999), and removing grounds for objections to organ harvesting (Karakatsanis and Tsanakas 2002). The increasing demand for organs has been regularly implicated in discussions about motives for brain-based determinations of death (Truog, 1997; Doig and Rocker, 2003; Bos, 2005). Against this view, Diamond (1998) rejects any suggestion that support for concepts of brain death are a result of a conspiracy of 'body-snatchers', 'grave robbers' and transplant lobbies. However Giacomini (1997), in an extended document analysis of the 1968 files of the Harvard Ad Hoc Committee, has persuasively demonstrated the powerful influence exerted by the transplant lobbies within the medical community at that time.

Summary of the clinical, philosophical and sociological objections

During the 40 years or so since the deliberations of the Harvard Committee, there has been a mounting litany of objections to the concept of brain death with no recent indication of a slow down of these doubts and criticisms (see Youngner, Arnold and Schapiro, 1999; Machado and Shewmon, 2004). Some authors have argued that organic definitions of brain death will never replace cultural and social definitions of death (Gervais, 1989; Sass, 1992; Gareth-Jones, 1998), and besides, consciousness cannot be checked by any medical test so the diagnosis of brain death remains an unproved hypothesis (Karakatsanis and Tsanakas, 2002: 140). Creating a sharp division between life and death has also been argued to be artificial since no such distinction actually exists in nature itself (Halevy and Brody, 1993).

Bernat (2004) and Laureys (2005) assert their distaste for the phrase 'brain death' on the grounds that it implies that there are other kinds of death or that it is only the brain that is dead in these cases. Bernat (2004: 370) further asserts that death is 'fundamentally' a biological phenomenon, all other uses being merely 'metaphorical'. People 'must be' dead or alive because no one can reside in both. Their assertions fly in the face of a diversity of findings about both biological and social understandings about death.

For example, many authors have questioned the veracity of brain death even when the criteria have all been met. The question, 'Is the brain really dead?', seems to have plenty of evidence for a decisive 'no' (Truog, 1997; Waisel and Truog, 1997; Karakatsanis and Tsanakas, 2002; Banasiak and Lister, 2003; Zamperetti et al., 2004). The work of Vaux and Korsmeyer (1999) and Vaux (2002) ably demonstrates the coexistence of both live and dead and living and dying cells in all multi-cell organisms including humans. Furthermore, Waisel and Truog (1997: 684) point out that many so-called brain-dead patients are capable of reproduction, a criterion that many biologists would regard as the '*sine qua non* of life'.

Several researchers have observed how both health care workers and families hold ideas about life and death in coexistent and situationally contingent ways (Lock, 1996; Sundin-Huard and Fahey, 2004; Kaufman, 2005, Veatch, 2005). This complements the very long-standing work by medical and social science colleagues, outside the determination of death field, that death and dying are viewed as *social* and not simply biological experiences (see Hartland, 1954; Blauner, 1966; Kalish, 1968; Vernon, 1970; Vollman et al., 1971; Cassell, 1974; Michalowski, 1976; Leming, Vernon and Gray, 1977; Charmaz, 1980). Kalish (1968), for example, has argued that concepts of organic, clinical, and social perceptions of death are commonly fluid ideas and may coexist and change for carers and the dying person. Cassell (1974) has argued that both death and dying – for clinical staff and families – are not simply viewed as bodily processes alone but are personal and social experiences. Categories of 'death' or 'dying' are not so simply characterised in real-life situations as 'living' or 'dead' or as 'metaphorical'.

Other objections include the tendency for the absence of evidence about consciousness to be construed as evidence of absence of consciousness (Diamond, 1998); the tendency for brain shock (ischaemia penumbria) to mimic brain death and obscure possible recovery (Sundin-Huard and Fahey, 2004); and vague and imprecise use of the concept overall (Shewmon et al., 1989; Truog and Fletcher, 1990). Many others have also questioned the problem with phrases and terms such as 'futility of treatment' or 'irreversibility' of brain function. These have been questioned conceptually (Cole, 1992; Cohen-Almagor, 2000; Bernat, 2005a) and clinically and statistically (Shewmon, 1987).

Finally, there has been widespread concern about how well understood the concept is among clinicians, including those who work in transplantation and intensive care (Winkler and Weisbard, 1989; Youngner et al., 1989; Conrad and Sinha, 2003), not to mention that many places do not have experienced neurologists available to help with any of this uncertainty (Bernat, 2005b). In some developing countries the number of neurologists per capita of population is estimated at one in three million people (Baumgartner and Gerstenbrand, 2002). There are further concerns, in more affluent countries, about the wide variation in experience and qualifications of doctors involved in brain-death determination (Sundin-Huard and Fahey, 2004: 69).

And the problems don't stop here. Although according to Gervais (1989: 9) we 'normally' proceed from theory to criteria to tests, not only have we got this process out of order by beginning with criteria but the tests themselves are not entirely compatible with those criteria (Waisel and Truog, 1997). Tests for brain death have been subject to equal criticism and scepticism. As Bernat (2004) reminds us, making the claim of irreversibility of brain death is one thing but proving it is quite another. The tests for brain death are about as good as the operators in charge of the tests and the people interpreting them (Conrad and Sinha, 2003; Young and Lee, 2004).

Tests in cerebral angiography are invasive and technically difficult to perform (Young and Lee, 2004: 503) and may have deleterious impacts on other clinical signs (Sundin-Huard and Fahey, 2004: 69). Sonography and CT scans also have major problems with false positives, and MRIs are insufficient tests on their own (Young and Lee, 2004: 503). EEGs cannot diagnose brain death though they may help confirm it (Moshe, 1989; Schneider, 1989) and anyway do not supply information about brain-stem function (Facco and Machado, 2004). Scintigraphy – the use of a nuclear tracer chemical to assess blood flow – is apparently an excellent test, but much depends on how well the test is actually performed. Therefore, given this rather common problem, even this test can only provide conditional support rather than replace clinical assessment (Conrad and Sinha, 2003: 313; Laureys, Owen and Schiff, 2004: 537; 543). This is an ironic, final observation given that the tests are frequently looked for as confirmatory of the clinical assessments and not the reverse.

In concluding this summary it should also be observed that the regular reviews of the recent debate about the determination of death in general, and brain death in particular, has been singularly self-referential. In other words, most of the deliberations about brain death are conversations between a small circle of disciplines particularly medicine, philosophy and law. Comparatively speaking, the presence of the social sciences is seldom seen. How the determination of death by the medical or legal profession is itself a social and cultural activity is rarely acknowledged. Important social studies of dying have not been consulted to understand congruence or dissonance between biomedical and social ideas of death and dying. Why such definitions are resisted or supported by wider communities has witnessed few attempts (see Veatch and Tai, 1980, Pernick 1996; 1999, for important exceptions) to check and examine the parallel history of how understandings of death have changed or evolved in human cultures in general.

Some authors have argued that the early Harvard Committee and President's Commission displayed a distrust of non-medical, outside opinion about determination of death, especially suspicion of those from law, philosophy and 'thanatology' (Pernick, 1999: 13–18). However, it is also true that seminal histories about our changing understandings of death by the French Historian Philippe Ariès (1974; 1975; 1981) were too early for the Harvard Ad Hoc Committee (1968) (but not for the 1981 President's Commission). On the other hand, other important related work did exist at that time, and was ignored, and unfortunately these did have important historical bearings for that committee's work (for examples, Freud, 1915; Moore, 1946; Borkenau, 1965; Williams, 1966; Sudnow, 1967; Toynbee, 1968; van Gennep, 1969).

Williams (1966), for example, surveyed 30 years of psychological abstracts to assess changing attitudes to death during this period, primarily in the US. Sudnow (1967) studied 200 hospital deaths, most of them comatose before their death, and made careful observations of staff reactions. He argued that social meanings of death are drawn from particular professional practices of a situation. Van Gennep (1969) is a classic anthropological work that provides important insights into how dying and death is commonly divided up by onlookers into social stages of transition. This process rarely results in an idea of death as annihilation but rather transformation – a crucial insight in explaining why modern peoples might not easily go along with a definition of death divorced from matters of identity and social relations. Had even the most basic findings and insights of these early works been highlighted or incorporated into deliberations about brain death in the late 1960s, both observations of staff and family behaviour and/or the policy recommendations might have looked substantially different. Observations of staff or family behaviour would not have been commonly described, as they often are, as ignorant or inappropriate. Policy deliberations would probably have included the general public and other health care staff if they had known exactly how resistant staff or communities could subsequently be to formulations that do not have social factors built into their policy and practice recommendations.

Further underlying sociological problems

Although the concept of brain death has suffered a litany of technical objections these objections themselves are founded on a broader, and arguably more important set of sociological problems. Definitions of brain death have ignored the historical and sociological basis of human understanding of death itself. This promotes a medicalisation of death that privileges remote and technical understandings of death over social understandings of death founded and supported by communities themselves.

The literature on the determination of death has ignored, and continues to ignore, the social sciences and its empirical studies and theoretical insights into how communities understand death, dying, loss and care. There are few sociologists or anthropologists cited in the determination of death literature. There are few social studies of dying consulted by the determination of death literature. The conceptual emphases and priorities of sociological disciplines – particularly context, culture and community, comparative methods, or the social nature of identity – are seldom mentioned by the determination of death literature, and yet such ideas are crucial to understanding family and community responses to their dying and dead.

Ignoring social science studies of dying conduct ensures that the tradition of research into how communities act in matters to do with death are summarily ignored. Indeed, many studies of how 'communities understand death' are in fact studies of how poorly communities seem to understand (or not) the medical criteria for death (see the review by Siminoff and Bloch, 1999). There is no doubt that determination of death, or the termination of artificial life support, are topics discussed with most families. But it is not clear how much of that discussion is actively led and shaped by the authority of the medical ideas about brain death promoted in those settings, rather than a by desire to encourage and support any alternative ideas that families may hold. We simply do not have the studies that would illuminate these kinds of questions.

An antipathy towards sociological questions also promotes the uncritical acceptance of a biologically reductionist view of death. The idea that death may equal brain death makes no more social sense than a genetically driven view of health. To most people, 'death' is a conclusion they derive from an assessment about the integrity and sustainability of a relationship. Physical factors are a necessary, but not always sufficient, decider in that assessment. Not to understand or appreciate this long-standing observation about how communities and families respond to their ill and dying is both sociologically and historically naïve.

Finally, not to explore the sociological basis of current interest in brain-death determination with respect to people in comas is to ignore or minimise the extraneous influences on, not only the whole policy push in this area, but also the policy pursuit of certainty. There is little doubt that the accelerated and recent interest in brain-death determination has behind it several sociological pressures: the demand for organ donation, the desire to free up expensive respirators and other life-support equipment, the desire to cut costs especially (but not only) for families, the desire to minimise trauma to families, the need to determine legal settlements around matters to do with inheritance, marriage, health, work or insurance entitlements. No reading of academic or policy pronouncements about the so-called 'certainty' of brain-death criteria, or of the tests claimed to confirm these criteria, can be divorced from an appreciation of how these factors may act as important political pressures on promoting so-called 'certainty'.

These pressures encourage policy claims and clinical pronouncements to appear more confident, unambiguous or certain than the science may warrant or the general public can believe. Explaining the reluctance of particular communities or families to embrace brain-death criteria by attributing this to their medical ignorance is to sell short their understanding of death as a wider social matter for them. But it downplays community suspicion that haste or confidence in the determination of death may not always be what it seems – as these are represented to them by hospital or medical interests. Until these and other sociological questions are taken seriously and addressed – by attention from research teams that are truly interdisciplinary, or by the incorporation of insights from the long tradition of social studies of dying – resistance to brain-death criteria and their proponents will continue, indefinitely and with considerable justification.

References

Ad Hoc Committee of the Harvard Medical School to examine the definition of brain death, (1968) 'A definition of irreversible coma', *Journal of the American Medical Association,* 205 (6): 337–40.

Ariès, P. (1974) *Western Attitudes Toward Death.* Baltimore, MA: Johns Hopkins University Press.

Ariès, P. (1975) 'The reversal of death: changes in attitudes toward death in Western societies', in D. Stannard (ed.), *Death in America.* Philadelphia: University of Pennsylvania Press. pp. 134–58.

Ariès, P. (1981) *The Hour of Our Death*. London: Allen Lane.

Banasiak, K.J. and Lister, G. (2003) 'Brain death in children', *Current Opinion in Pediatrics,* 15: 288–93.

Baumgartner, H. and Gerstenbrand, F. (2002) 'Diagnosing brain death without a neurologist: simple criteria and training are needed for the non-neurologist in many countries', *British Medical Journal,* 324: 1471–72.

Bernat, J.L. (2004) 'On irreversibility as a pre-requisite for brain death determination', in C. Machado and A. Shewmon (eds), *Brain Death and Disorders of Consciousness*. New York: Kluwer Academic Publishers. pp. 161–7.

Bernat, J.L. (2005a) 'Medical futility: definition, determination and disputes in critical care', *Neurocritical Care,* 2: 198–205.

Bernat, J.L. (2005b) 'The concept and practice of brain death', *Progress in Brain Death,* 150: 369–79.

Blauner, R. (1966) 'Death and social structure', *Psychiatry,* 29: 378–94.

Borkenau, F. (1965) 'The concept of death', in R. Fulton (ed.), *Death and Identity*. New York: John Wiley and Sons. Pp. 42–56.

Bos, M.A. (2005) 'Ethical and legal issues in non-heart beating organ donation', *Transplantation,* 79 (9): 1143–7.

Cassell, E.J. (1974) 'Being and becoming dead', in A. Mack (ed.), *Death in American Experience*. New York: Schocken. Pp. 162–76.

Chan, J.Y.H., Chang, A.Y.W. and Chan, S.H.H. (2005) 'New insights on brainstem death: from bedside to bench', *Progress in Neurobiology,* 77: 396–425.

Charmaz, K. (1980) *The Social Reality of Death*. Boston, MA: Addison-Wesley.

Cohen-Almagor, R. (2000) 'Language and reality at the end of life', *Journal of Medicine and Ethics,* 28 (3): 267–79.

Cole, D.J. (1992) 'The reversibility of death', *Journal of Medical Ethics,* 18: 26–30.

Conrad, G.R. and Sinha, P. (2003) 'Scintigraphy as a confirmatory test of brain death', *Seminars in Nuclear Medicine,* 33 (4): 312–23.

Diamond, E.F. (1998) 'Brain-based determination of death revisited', *Linacre Quarterly,* 65 (4): 71–80.

Doig, C.J. and Rocker, G. (2003) 'Retrieving organs from non-heart beating organ donors: a review of medical and ethical issues', *Canadian Journal of Anesthesia,* 50 (10): 1069–76.

Facco, E. and Machado, C. (2004) 'Evoked potentials in the diagnosis of brain death', in C. Machado and A. Shewmon (eds), *Brain Death and Disorders of Consciousness*. New York: Kluwer. Pp. 175–87.

Freud, S. (1915) 'Thoughts for the times on war and death', in J. Strachey (ed.), *Standard Edition of the Complete Works of Sigmund Freud*. London: Hogarth Press. Pp. 275–300.

Gareth-Jones, D. (1998) 'The problematic symmetry between brain birth and brain death', *Journal of Medical Ethics,* 24: 237–42.

Gervais, K.G. (1989) 'Advancing the definition of death: a philosophical essay', *Medical Humanities Review,* 3 (2): 7–19.

Giacomini, M. (1997) 'A change of heart and a change of mind? Technology and the redefinition of death in 1968', *Social Sciences & Medicine,* 44 (10): 1465–82.

Halevy, A. and Brody, B. (1993) 'Brain death: reconciling definitions, criteria and tests', *Annals of Internal Medicine,* 119: 519–25.

Hartland, E.S. (1954) 'Death and disposal of the dead', in J. Hastings (ed.) (with assistance of J.A. Selbie), *Encyclopedia of Religion and Ethics*, Volume 4. New York: Charles Scribner and Sons. Pp. 411–44.

Kalish, R.A. (1968) 'Life and death: "dividing the indivisible"', *Social Science & Medicine,* 2: 249–59.

Karakatsanis, K.G. and Tsanakas, J.N. (2002) 'A critique on the concept of "brain death"', *Issues in Law and Medicine,* 18 (2): 127–41.

Kaufman, S.R. (2005) *And a Time to Die: How American Hospitals Shape the End of Life*. Chicago: University of Chicago Press.

Knudsen, S.K. (2005) 'A review of the criteria used to assess insensibility and death in hunted whales compared to other species', *The Veterinary Journal*, 169: 42–59.

Laureys, S. (2005) 'Death, unconsciousness and the brain', *Nature Reviews Neuroscience*, 6: 899–909.

Laureys, S., Owen, A.M. and Schiff, N.D. (2004) 'Brain function in coma, vegetative state and related disorders', *Lancet Neurology*, 3: 537–46.

Leming, M.R., Vernon, G.M. and Gray, R.M. (1977) 'The dying patient: a symbolic analysis', *International Journal of Symbology*, 8 (2): 77–86.

Lock, M. (1996) 'Death in technological time: locating the end of a meaningful life', *Medical Anthropology Quarterly*, 10 (4): 575–600.

Machado, C. and Shewmon, D.A. (eds) (2004) *Brain Death and Disorders of Consciousness*. New York: Kluwer.

Michalowski Jr, R.J. (1976) 'The social meanings of violent death', *Omega*, 7 (1): 83–93.

Moore, V. (1946) *Ho for Heaven! Man's Changing Attitude Toward Dying*. New York: EP Dutton and Co.

Moshe, S.L. (1989) 'Usefulness of EEG in the evaluation of brain death in children: the pros', *Electroencephalography and Clinical Neurology*, 73: 272–5.

Pernick, M.S. (1996) *The Black Stork*. New York: Oxford University Press.

Pernick, M.S. (1999) 'Brain death in a cultural context: the reconstruction of death, 1967–1981', in S.J. Youngner, R.M. Arnold and R. Schapiro (eds), *The Definition of Death: Contemporary Controversies*. Baltimore, MA: Johns Hopkins University Press. Pp. 3–33.

Plum, F. (1999) 'Clinical standards and technological confirmatory tests in diagnosing brain death', in S.J. Youngner, R.M. Arnold and R. Schapiro (eds), *The Definition of Death: Contemporary Controversies*. Baltimore, MA: Johns Hopkins University Press. Pp. 34–65.

Poppe, E. and Bottinger, B.W. (2006) 'Cerebral resuscitation: state of the art, experimental approaches and clinical perspectives', *Neurology Clinics*, 24: 73–87.

President's Commission for the study of ethical problems in medicine and biomedical and behavioural research (1981) *Defining Death: Medical, Legal and Ethical Issues in the Determination of Death*. Washington DC: Government Printing Office.

Sass, H.M. (1992) 'Criteria for death: self-determination and public policy', *Journal of Medicine and Philosophy*, 17: 445–54.

Schewmon, D.A. (1987) 'The probability of inevitability: the inherent impossibility of validating criteria for brain death or "irreversibility" through clinical studies', *Statistics in Medicine*, 6: 535–53.

Schewmon, A. Capron, A.M. Peacokk, W.J. and Schulman, B.L. (1989) 'The use of anencephalic infants as organ sources: a critique', *Journal of the American Medical Association*, 261 (12): 1773–81.

Schlotzhauer, A.V. and Liang, B.A. (2002) 'Definitions and implications of death', *Hematology/Oncology Clinics of North America*', 16: 1397–1413.

Schneider, S. (1989) 'Usefulness of EEG in the evaluation of brain death in children: the cons', *Electroencephalography and Clinical Neurology*, 73: 276–8.

Siminoff, L.A. and Bloch, A. (1999) 'American attitudes and beliefs about brain death: the empirical literature', in S.J. Youngner, R.M. Arnold and R. Schapiro (eds), *The Definition of Death: Contemporary Controversies*. Baltimore, MA: Johns Hopkins University Press. Pp. 183–93.

Sudnow, D. (1967) *Passing On: The Social Organization of Dying*. Englewood Cliffs, NJ: Prentice-Hall.

Sundin-Huard, D. and Fahey, K. (2004) 'The problems with the validity of the diagnosis of brain death', *Nursing in Critical Care*, 9 (2): 64–70.

Toynbee, A. (1968) *Man's Concern with Death*. London: Hodder and Stoughton.

Truog, R.D. (1997) 'Is it time to abandon brain death?', *Hastings Center Report,* 27 (1): 29–37.

Truog, R.D. and Fletcher, J.C. (1990) 'Brain death and the anencephalic newborn', *Bioethics,* 4 (3): 199–215.

van Gennep, A. (1969) *The Rites of Passage.* Chicago, IL: University of Chicago Press.

Vaux, D.L. (2002) 'Apoptosis timeline', *Cell Death and Differentiation,* 9: 349–54.

Vaux, D.L. and Korsmeyer, S.J. (1999) 'Cell death in development', *Cell,* 96: 245–54.

Veatch, R.M. (2005) 'The death of whole-brain death: the plague of disaggregators, somaticists, and mentalists', *Journal of Medicine and Philosophy,* 30: 353–78.

Veatch, R.M. and Tai, E. (1980) 'Talking about death: patterns of lay and professional change', *Annals of the American Academy of Political and Social Sciences,* 447: 29–45.

Vernon, G.M. (1970) *Sociology of Death.* New York: Ronald Press.

Vollman, R.R., Ganzert, A., Picher, L. and Williams, W.V. (1971) 'The reaction of family systems to sudden and unexpected deaths', *Omega,* 2: 101–6.

Waisel, D.B. and Truog, R.D. (1997) 'The end-of-life sequence', *Anesthesiology,* 87 (3): 676–86.

Williams, M. (1966) 'Changing attitudes to death: a survey of contributions in psychological abstracts over a thirty-year period', *Human Relations,* 19 (4): 405–23.

Winkler, D. and Weisbard, A.J. (1989) 'Appropriate confusion over "brain death"', *Journal of the American Medical Association,* 261 (15): 2246.

Young, G.B. and Lee, D. (2004) 'A critique of ancillary tests for brain death', *Neurocritcal Care,* 1 (4): 499–508.

Youngner, S.J. Arnold, R.M. and Schapiro, R. (eds) (1999) *The Definition of Death: Contemporary Controversies.* Baltimore, MA: Johns Hopkins University Press.

Youngner, S.J., Landfield, C.S., Coulton, C.J., Juknialis, B.W. and Leary, M. (1989) 'Brain death and organ retrieval: a cross-sectional survey of knowledge and concepts among health professionals', *Journal of the American Medical Association,* 261 (15): 2205–10.

Zamperetti, N., Bellomo, R., Defanti, C.A. and Latronico, N. (2004) 'Irreversible apnoeic coma 35 years later: towards a more rigorous definition of brain death?', *Intensive Care Medicine,* 30: 1715–22.

20
Palliative Care and the Doctrine of Double Effect

Stephen Wilkinson

What is the doctrine of double effect?

Although frequently criticized by moral philosophers and others, the doctrine of double effect is widely accepted by health care professionals and by various religious groups (most notably, the Catholic Church) and many (though not all) academic lawyers believe that it is part of UK law (Beauchamp and Childress, 1994: 206–11; Brazier, 1992: 447; Gillon, 1986: 133–9; Glover, 1977: 86–91; Harris, 1985: 43–5; McHale et al., 1997:822–3; Mackie, 1977: 160–8; McMahan, 1994: 201–12; Randall and Downie, 1996: 71–3). The main idea behind the doctrine is that, provided certain conditions are met, one is not fully responsible for *all* the effects of one's actions, but only for those which are *intended*. It is normally applied therefore to cases in which an action (for example, administering a drug) has both a good effect (for example, pain relief) and a bad effect (for example, adverse side-effects, including perhaps shortening life).

What the doctrine of double effect says about such cases is roughly the following. Provided that the good effect is what was intended and the bad effect is a *foreseen but unintended* side-effect, then the action is ethically acceptable. Although most commonly discussed in the health care setting, the doctrine is meant to capture a general ethical truth (i.e. one which is applicable to everyone, not just health care workers) and, as such, has been used, for example, in attempts to differentiate the 'strategic bombing' of military targets (which is supposed to be acceptable – at least sometimes – because the civilian deaths involved are foreseen but unintended side-effects) from the 'terrorist bombing' of non-combatants (which is supposed to be morally indefensible because the civilian deaths involved are the *intended* means of achieving political or other objectives).

Here is a more precise account of the doctrine: an action is morally acceptable provided that all of the following conditions are met (Beauchamp and Childress, 1994: 207).

'Palliative care and the doctrine of double effect' by Stephen Wilkinson in Dickenson, Johnson, Samson Katz (eds), *Death, Dying and Bereavement*, 2nd edn. SAGE, 2000, pp. 299–302. Reprinted by kind permission of the publisher and author.

a The action is not *intrinsically* wrong (i.e. wrong considered apart from its effects).
b The person acting is aiming to do something good (for example, to relieve pain).
c The bad effects are *not* aimed at and are *not* means of achieving the good effects.
d The good effects are sufficiently good to outweigh the bad effects. (This is some-times referred to as the 'proportionality criterion'.)

Why is the doctrine of double effect relevant to palliative care?

The doctrine of double effect is often illustrated by reference to the use of diamorphine. Take the case of a weak, terminally-ill patient who is in pain. In order to alleviate the pain, a doctor administers diamorphine, which (in the case in question) causes depressed respiration and hastens the patient's death. Why isn't this (either morally or legally) a case of murder? The short answer is that the doctor didn't have the relevant intention, since (let's assume) her intention was to relieve the patient's pain, not to kill her.

A fuller answer can be provided using the doctrine of double effect. Assuming that the administration of diamorphine is not intrinsically wrong (wrong independently of its effects) we need to ask three questions, corresponding to parts (b)–(d) of the doctrine in order to see whether it would classify the action as permissible.

First, was the intended end (pain relief) good? Almost certainly 'yes': relieving pain seems uncontroversially to be a good thing. Second, was the bad effect (hastened death) aimed at and was it a means of achieving the good effect (pain relief)? Again, almost certainly 'no' (to both parts of the question). The doctor did not intend death (on the contrary, she would probably prefer the patient to survive) and death was not the means of causing pain relief. Rather, death and pain relief were both effects of the same cause: the administration of diamorphine. Finally, is the good effect (pain relief) sufficiently good to outweigh the bad effect (hastened death)?

This last question is much harder and the answer will vary depending on the details of the case. To take one extreme, if the pain in question was minor and the patient lost 10 years of life, then many of us would say that the 'proportionality criterion' clearly had *not* been met. In other words, the patient would be better off keeping both the pain and the extra 10 years, rather than losing both. At the other extreme, if the pain was intolerable and the patient only lost a few minutes of life then many of us would say that the patient had benefited overall from the administration of diamorphine – in spite of its hastening her death. In between these two extremes there is, unfortunately, an enormous grey area in which 'quality of life' must be weighed against 'quantity of life'. And to complicate matters still further there may also be cases in which the patient is judged to have a *negative* quality of life: cases in which, because quality of life is so poor, death is seen as benefiting (or at least as not harming) her.

It may seem as if the doctrine of double effect sanctions some forms of euthanasia, since I have started to talk in terms of patients benefiting from having their lives shortened. However, it should be stressed that the doctrine is *not* supposed to be a way of justifying euthanasia. It is rather an attempt to establish that there is a morally significant difference between those cases where death is a foreseen but unintended side-effect of an intervention, and those in which it is intended, either as an end in itself, or as a means of achieving pain relief. Only cases like the latter can be cases of euthanasia, since *euthanasia is the intentional killing of a patient*, performed by someone who believes death to be in the patient's best interests. Euthanasia, therefore, is not sanctioned by the doctrine, since it (by definition) involves intentional killing.

Before moving on to consider briefly some of the problems with the doctrine, one further point of clarification needs to be made. Some health professionals argue that effective pain management never, or at least hardly ever, requires us to give life-shortening doses. Twycross (1999: 639) for example, suggests that 'when correctly used, morphine and other strong opioids are safe – safer than non-steroidal anti-inflammatory drugs, which are prescribed with impunity'. Whether this is actually true is not something that can be considered here. What *can* be considered here though is this question: what ethical implications would there be *if* it were true?

The main implication is that the idea of 'double effect' would become almost totally irrelevant as far as palliative care is concerned. For, if life-shortening interventions are never required, what reason could there be for a person to give patients drugs which shorten life? There are two main possibilities. Either she does so because she *wants* to cause death – in which case we have a case of *intentional* killing and the doctrine of double effect doesn't apply. Or she does so accidentally and/or negligently and does not foresee the lethal side-effect – in which case the doctrine again doesn't apply because death isn't even a foreseen side-effect (since it's not foreseen). (Of course, we may, in certain circumstances, wish to condemn the doctor in such a case for being negligent and incompetent but that is another matter.) For these reasons, then, the doctrine only has relevance to palliative care if it is true that good palliative care sometimes necessarily involves interventions with life-shortening side-effects.

A problem with the doctrine of double effect

When applying the doctrine, we need often to make very difficult judgements about which effects are intended and which are not. But (and this is the main problem) *how do we know* what is intended and what is not? This question can arise from two different perspectives. First, from the 'first person' perspective, if a doctor administers diamorphine to relieve pain, but at the same time would be glad if the patient's death was hastened (perhaps because she believes that the patient would be 'better off dead') she may not be sure herself which effects she intends and which she doesn't. Second, from the 'third person' perspective, how are other professionals, relatives and the public to know what was going on 'in the doctor's head' when she administered the drug? How are they to know what she intends? This problem may render the doctrine unworkable in practice. Furthermore, it also opens up the possibility of health carers abusing the doctrine and using it as a way of 'smuggling in euthanasia by the back door'. In other words, the acceptance of the doctrine might make it possible to kill patients intentionally while *pretending* that their death is an unintended side-effect.

Conclusions

The doctrine of double effect is a potentially useful tool for distinguishing *intentional* killings (such as euthanasia) from cases in which hastened death is only an *unintended* side-effect. Practitioners, however, should remain aware that there are both practical and theoretical problems (including several that have not been discussed here) with the doctrine and that it should not be accepted or applied uncritically.

References

Beauchamp, T. and Childress, J. (1994) *Principles of Biomedical Ethics*, 4th edn. Oxford: Oxford University Press.

Brazier, M. (1992) *Medicine, Patients and the Law*, 2nd edn. Harmondsworth: Penguin.

Gillon, R. (1986) *Philosophical Medical Ethics*. Chichester: John Wiley and Sons.

Glover, J. (1977) *Causing Death and Saving Lives*. Harmondsworth: Penguin.

Harris, J. (1985) *The Value of Life*. London: Routledge.

McHale, J., Fox, M. and Murphy, J. (1997) *Health Care Law*. London: Sweet and Maxwell.

Mackie, J. (1977) *Ethics*. Harmondsworth: Penguin.

McMahan, J. (1994) 'Revising the doctrine of doubt effect'. *Journal of Applied Philosophy*, 11(2): 201–12.

Randall, F. and Downie, R. (1996) *Palliative Care Ethics: A Good Companion*. Oxford: Oxford University Press.

Twycross, R. (1999) 'Palliative care physicians always have their patients' best interests in mind', *British Medical Journal*, 319 (4 September 1999). www.bmj.com/cgi/content/full/319/7210/63.

Part IV

Exploring Grief and Ritual After Death

Introduction

Sarah Earle

Part IV focuses on exploring what happens after death and seeks to understand the changing landscape of grief and ritual. The readings illustrate that there is no one model or approach to understanding how people grieve, and highlight the importance of understanding the diverse needs of different groups of people. In this part of the book, attention is given to issues of disposal, bereavement and memorialisation as well as exploring some of the theoretical ideas which underpin practice in this area.

This part of the book begins with Reading 21 by Neil Small which offers a critical review of theories of grief. In this reading, Small briefly outlines the development of a theoretical system of grief beginning with a brief overview of the work of Sigmund Freud and other psychoanalysts. Small then moves on to describe the attachment theory of grief, developed by John Bowlby; a theory which challenged and revised psychoanalytic approaches and has been enormously influential in the field of grief and loss. In the final part of this reading, Small critiques approaches to grief and loss which include stage theories, notions of 'letting go', or of continuing bonds, and argues for a better understanding of the sociality and historicity of death.

Reading 22, by Leonie Kellaher, David Prendergast and Jenny Hockey, discusses the modern disposal practice of cremation. Drawing on a qualitative study of the destination of ashes, the authors explore the ways in which such practice is informed by the more traditional practice of whole-body burial. In this reading Kellaher, Prendergast and Hockey note that while cremation is now the most common form of disposal in the UK, a new trend is emerging whereby innovative ways of disposing of ashes are becoming commonplace.

The next three readings focus on bereavement. In Reading 23, Miri Nehari, Dorit Grebler and Amos Toren turn their attention to the issue of grandparents' bereavement. They argue that when discussing bereavement, the needs of grandparents are either not considered or they are simply not seen to be part of the bereaved family. Drawing on research carried out with a support group for bereaved grandparents in Israel, the authors explore how there is often no 'place' for grandparents to express their grief. Furthermore, while grandparents are often grieving for their grandchildren, as well as wanting to help their own bereaved children, Nehari, Grebler and Toren argue that their grief often goes unacknowledged both within the family and by wider society.

Reading 24, by Liz Rolls, also focuses on the subject of bereavement but here the focus is specifically on children's bereavement (see also Reading 1). In this reading, Rolls draws on a UK study of childhood bereavement services exploring their role in supporting bereaved children and families through ritual. Rolls describes the role that childhood bereavement services undertake working with children and families both directly and indirectly, individually and through group activities, discussing – in particular – the ritual performance of candle-lighting and balloon-releasing events. The author concludes by arguing that childhood bereavement services support children through ritualised performance by placing them (actually and symbolically) into groups of other bereaved children.

In the third reading to focus on bereavement, Reading 25 explores the facilitation of bereavement for the victims of genocide. Focusing specifically on the aftermath of the 1994 genocide in Rwanda, and based on her work at the Kigali Institute of Science and Technology Counselling Centre, Eugénie Mukanoheli recounts the trauma experienced by the survivors of this atrocity. Mukanoheli highlights the significance of traditional death rituals and the absence of these following the genocide. She outlines the way in which Rwandan society has sought to facilitate bereavement and points to the work yet to be done.

The final two readings in this part of the book focus on the issue of memorialisation. In the first of these, Reading 26 discusses the making of roadside memorials. Here, Jennifer Clark and Majella Franzmann, who draw principally on an analysis of roadside memorials across Australia and New Zealand, argue that the making of these memorials – together with accounts of their construction – demonstrate an increasing desire for individual expressions of grief. The authors argue that the making of roadside memorials – which is an increasingly international phenomenon – 'turns a public place into a sacred space', and is one which challenges both civil and religious authorities.

In the final reading in Part IV, Kylie Veale explores the growing practice of online memorialisation. Veale argues that cyberspace provides an alternative space for remembering the dead which offers some advantages compared to traditional (physical) memorialisation practices. In particular, she argues that online memorialisation is timely, accessible and cost-efficient as well as offering a range of opportunities for creativity and expression. This reading also explores what motivates individuals to memorialise online and examines some of the key features of online memorialisation.

21

Theories of Grief: A Critical Review

Neil Small

[…]

Psychoanalysis

Freud saw grief as something that would free the ego from attachment to the deceased and, in so doing, allow new attachments to be formed. Silverman and Klass (1996) claim that this is a formulation that Freud arrived at via the selective use of the data available to him. In effect they argue that there was a difference between Freud's theories and his own experience of grief. Silverman and Klass (1996: 7) read into those of Freud's letters that describe his own bereavement experiences a realization that he could not cut old attachments and form new ones.

[…]

Klass and Silverman, and other critics of the Freudian prescription of cutting the bond with the deceased so that new attachments can be formed, underemphasize the sense of the positive associated with the Freudian model. This includes the process of overcoming denial of the loss and hence enriching the self. To summarize, simply to talk about letting go and moving on, which is the way the critics of Freud précis his position, does not do justice to the idea of resolution presented by the Freud and then developed by others from within the psychoanalytic school.

[…]

Steiner (1993: 35–6) offers the example of Melanie Klein's Writings … as illustrative of this post-Freudian position. In 1940 she published an article, which included a case summary of Mrs A, whose son had died. Mrs A's early reactions were of feeling numb and closed up, wishing to deny the reality of her loss. Subsequently a dream allowed her to both see her true feelings but also to disentangle this loss from the death in childhood of her own brother. A further dream helped her understand how her son's death had made her fearful of her own. But she realised she could, and would, go on living and this meant that she could accept the event of the death free of the entanglements of her own fears and fantasies (Klein 1940). Hence, what one is freed of is not the person who has died but the projective identification we have lodged in them, that is the parts of our self we have allowed them to act out for us. We have to re-own those parts so we can properly relate to the person who has died.

[...]

Attachment theory

The attachment theory of grief, developed by John Bowlby, was central to his attempts to revise psychoanalytic theory and has been hugely influential in developing understanding of grief and loss. Bowlby, working both in the Tavistock Institute in London and as a consultant to the World Health Organization on the needs of homeless children, based much of his work on the observation of children. This was a different approach to the Freudian or Kleinian perspectives, which engaged with psychic trauma in the internal world. Much of his theory developed from observation of children's separation, in stressful circumstances, from their mothers. James Robertson had observed children in short- and long-term residential nurseries and in hospital children's wards. His resulting stage theory saw children responding with protest, despair and then denial (also called detachment) (see, for example, Robertson 1958). Bowlby's attachment theory replicated these stages and linked them with the central problems of psychoanalytic theory. That is, protest can be linked to separation anxiety, despair to grief and mourning and detachment to defence (Bowlby 1973: 27). Essentially Bowlby's theory of bereavement is an extension of his theory of separation anxiety. He saw the psychological response to the trauma of separation as something biologically programmed, just as we physiologically respond to trauma. For example:

> Following Darwin, Bowlby sees the facial expressions and crying of the bereaved as a resultant of the tendency to scream in the hope of awakening the attention of the negligent care-giver. … This is then an evolutionary view (not the teleological view of Freud in which the survivor detaches memories and hopes from dead). (Holmes 1993: 91)

> Bowlby categorizes four phases of mourning: numbness; yearning, searching and anger; disorganization and despair; and, reorganization. These stages are seen as occurring successively and, as such, they suggest a possible blueprint for those who wish to offer help to the bereaved. A model of the 'work of grief' was developing.

[...]

By 1979 Bowlby was considering whether the term mourning should be replaced by grieving (Bowlby 1979: 91). In part this was an attempt to create some distance from the specific analytic understanding of mourning – to overcome some of the confusion created when analytic terms were transposed into popular usage. In part the shift in terminology was also designed to emphasize the internal world of grief as opposed to the social manifestation of mourning.

The capacity for healthy grieving, according to Bowlby, was shaped by childhood experience. Specifically, it was shaped by the extent to which attachment behaviour had been regarded sympathetically as opposed to it being something to be grown out of as quickly as possible. Indeed the experience of a positive attachment experience allows the necessary first expressions of feelings. Bowlby believed that one should encourage the bereaved, in Shakespeare's words, to 'give sorrow words'. In the process it is:

> Both unnecessary and unhelpful to cast ourselves in the role of a [representative of reality] ... our role should be that of companion and supporter, prepared to explore in our discussions all the hopes and wishes and dim unlikely possibilities that he still cherishes, together with all the reproaches and the disappointments that inflict him ... Yearning for the impossible, intemperate anger, impotent weeping, horror at the prospect of loneliness, pitiful pleading for sympathy and support – these are the feelings that a bereaved person needs to express, and sometimes first to discover, if he is to make progress. (Bowlby 1979: 94–6)

[...]

Modernity and sequential time

The quintessential modernist construct is that of time – metanarrative and sequential organizing epitomized. The ability to have popularly accepted the idea of present work for future gain, and the compartmentalization of the day into defined work/non-work sections was essential to the triumph of the industrial revolution and, in particular, the factory system. That the gain could be on earth or in heaven was at the heart of Protestantism, as one lived one's life with an eye to the future judgement that would be brought to bear on it. This can be contrasted with the cyclical and less differentiated agrarian community that preceded the industrial/modern.

Models of bereavement and grief, described above, all draw on models of sequential time and time-defined lives. But, it may be argued that bereavement fractures the sequential experience of time and that any model of grief and mourning that relies on a straightforward passage of time construct is inappropriate. Myerhoff offers the idea of 'simultaneity' where 'a sense of oneness with all that has been one's history is achieved' (Myerhoff 1982: 110). At this point the sequential arrangement of events across time is temporarily undone. As applied to mourning such an approach critiques Freud in much the same way as does the Klass *et al.* critique presented in *Continuing Bonds*.

> Freud ... suggests that the completion of the mourning process requires that those left behind develop a new reality which no longer includes what has been lost. But ... it must be added that full recovery from mourning may restore what has been lost, maintaining it through incorporation into the present. Full recollection and retention may be as vital to recovery and wellbeing as forfeiting memories. (Myerhoff 1982: 110).

However, it is not just the Freudian view that can be critiqued if one abandons the idea of time-defined lives and time-framed experiences. Any approach that includes stage theories, any sense of letting go, or of continuing bonds, is also constrained by linear time assumptions.

In effect the modernist understanding of time, like the modernist constructions of order and control, does not survive the impact of extreme experiences like bereavement. The modern exists as a layer on top of other ways of making sense of experiences; for example, fate, faith and so on. Once fissures appear in the veneer of the modern we are allowed glimpses of the underlying residual belief systems, many of which are pre-modern. The coming together of the dying person or the bereaved, within this complex of beliefs, and the professional trying to cling to the structures of the modern creates the sorts of dissonance that can make for problematic encounters with bereavement services.

There are many examples in literature of ways we move beyond the contingency of linear time. Ralph Waldo Emerson wrote that 'Sorrow makes us all children again'. Psychoanalyst Adam Phillips (1999) has observed that nobody grows up in relation to death. That is, we are always the same age in relation to it. He is suggesting that we can travel one of two routes; either accept that we live in nature and that one of its basic conditions is that we might die at any time, or live our lives without an awareness of our mortality. It is not then how old we are but how we engage with the physicality of our existence that defines our relationship to death. Novelist Jim Crace argues that death reminds us that we are not future leaning but essentially live our lives retrospectively. In his story *Being Dead*, the narrative begins with the deaths of his central characters and then looks back on their lives – an interlude between the formlessness of how they began and the formlessness of what they will become (Crace 1999). But it is not just in relation to our personal histories that linear time is displaced; there is also the domain of the social and its history.

Rethinking historicity and the science of the indefinite

In a challenging book about the historicity of both AIDS and nuclear terror, Havers (1996) brings a different sort of language to the Freudian discourse on mourning and melancholia. He describes Freud's world of mourning as, 'a process by which the dead are rendered radically other by means of a process of dissociation or separation' (Havers 1996: 57). They are objectified as an abject object in the work of mourning, which historicizes the dead. In so doing the wounded ego is restored to an integration it seeks. If that wounded ego is not restored and there remains a (narcissistic) identification of the ego with the abandoned object (Freud 1917: 246); then melancholia results. (This condition, Havers suggests, is represented by the vampires and ghosts in our literature.)

However, Havers goes on to argue that this construction misses out the sociality that is 'the very existentiality of historicity' (Havers 1996: 60). It is in, and through, our exposure to death that we can appreciate the contingency of our intersubjectivities, of our relationship with our friends and with our 'cultural consolations'. If we relegate the dead 'other' to a historicism that we separate ourselves from, we do not see mourning as central to the cultural world of society and to our own sociality. While Havers's subject is mourning we can see that if we can redirect his concerns towards grief and bereavement we can re-emphasize the social and the relational, rather than that which is located in the internal world.

That interface between the social and the internal worlds is negotiated via the medium of language, which constructs, and gives expression to, concepts of the self and the emotions. The emotional self is a dynamic project existing at the intersection of the past, the present, the personal and the social. Some of it exists at an unconscious level. But, while language constructs and gives expression to this self, there is also a sense that the emotional experience has an embodied dimension (Lupton 1998). Seale (1998) uses the experience of dying to illuminate embodiment in social life and presents an 'imagined community' in which dying and bereaved people can live and where they can draw on various cultural scripts as well as their own narrative biography.

Against logic, for the sociality of our existence

Irigaray has argued 'the West has been slow to develop a science that can measure and model patterns of the indefinite and of fluidity' (see Battersby 1993: 35). 'We need to think individuality differently; allowing the potentiality of otherness to exist within it, as well as alongside it; we need to theorise agency in terms of patterns of potentiality and flow' (Battersby 1993: 38).

Thinking about individuality and agency in new ways allows us to move beyond modernity. One route is to look to the small narratives and contingent meanings that characterize the postmodern (see Mannion and Small 1999). The death of someone close to us takes us, as individuals, to a place that exists at the brink of the crisis of modernity. We are not in control, we do not understand. Our sense of self, our relations with others, even the way we experience time is challenged. Those whom we meet at this place can stay with us or they can try and pull us back. The modernist discourse of grief and bereavement risks the charge of hubris because it offers a route map to impose a meaning that is form there not here, that is theirs not yours. That many of those we encounter at this point do not seek to impose their meaning is a tribute to their recognition of the poetics of loss rather than the logic of theories of loss. They accept that they do not understand your loss but do appreciate the sociality of all our lives and deaths.

References

Battersby, C. (1993) Her body/her boundaries, in A. Benjamin (ed.) The Body. *Journal of Philosophy and the Visual Arts:* 31–9.
Bowlby, J. (1973) *Loss: Sadness and depression.* Newyork: Basic Books.
Bowlby, J. (1979) *The Making and Breaking of Affectional Bonds.* London: Tavistock.
Crace, J. (1999) *Being Dead.* London: Viking.

Freud, S. (1917) Mourning and melancholia, in J. Strachey (ed.) *The Standard Edition of the Complete Psychological Works of Sigmund Freud,* Vol. 14. London: Hogarth Press and Institute of Psycho-Analysis.

Havers, W. (1996) *The Body of this Death.* Stanford University Press.

Hertz, R. ([1907] 1960) *Death and the Right Hand.* New York: Free Press.

Holmes, J. (1993) *John Bowlby and Attachment Theory.* London: Routledge.

Klass, D., Silverman, P.R. and Nickman, S. (1996) *Continuing Bonds, New Understandings of Grief.* Washington, DC: Taylor & Francis.

Klein, M. (1940) Mourning and its relation to manic-depressive states. *International Journal of Psycho-Analysis,* 21: 125–53.

Lupton, D. (1998) *The Emotional Self.* London: Sage.

Mannion, R. and Small, N. (1999) Postmodern Health Economics. *Health Care Analysis,* 7: 255–72.

Myerhoff, B. (1982) Life history among the elderly: performance, visibility and remembering, in J. Ruby (ed.) *A Crack in the Mirror: Reflexive Perspectives on Anthropology.* Philadelphia, PA: University of Pennsylvania Press.

Phillips, A. (1999) *Darwin's Worms.* London: Faber.

Robertson, J. (1958) *Young Children in Hospital.* London: Tavistock Publications.

Seale, C. (1998) *Constructing Death.* Cambridge: Cambridge University Press.

Silverman, P.R. and Klass, D. (1996) Introdution: what's the problem?, in D. Klass, P.R. Silverman and S.L. Nickman (eds) *Continuing Bonds. New Understandings of Grief.* Bristol, PA: Taylor & Francis.

Steiner, J. (1993) *Psychic Retreats.* London: Routledge.

Steiner, J. (1996) The aim of psychoanalysis in theory and practice. *International Journal of psycho-Analysis,* 77(6): 1073–83.

22

In the Shadow of the Traditional Grave

Leonie Kellaher, David Prendergast and Jenny Hockey

This [reading] draws on data from a qualitative study of the destinations of ashes now being removed in increasing numbers from crematoria, the practice of cremation, and particularly the private disposal of ashes outside crematoria. It explores the case that such disposals may frequently be informed by the recollection, or awareness, of practices surrounding whole body burial. These include notions of bodily integrity, the creation and preservation of a clear, bounded space for the deceased, and expectations and negotiations about grave visiting and upkeep. The [reading] therefore seeks to determine whether new ritual practice is being developed, or instead, whether a reformulation of traditional beliefs and between burial and cremation practice or a serious intention to stand clear of the shadow of the traditional grave. In addition we discuss a smaller body of material which reveals more ambiguous approaches that do not support either argument. By examining data within these categories, the article explores the varying degrees of alignment between traditional burial and cremation practices and asks whether cremation provides scope for a return to positively perceived aspects of burial, while side-stepping its less welcome aspects, such as slow bodily deterioration.

[…]

Cremation in the ascendant

Cremation is now the most common form of disposal in the UK. A comparatively new practice, it was only legalized in 1884 following an intense period of campaigning by its supporters, including the Cremation Society of Great Britain. (Cremation Society of Great Britain, 1974; Jupp, 2005; White, 2002). Despite the public promotion of cremation towards the end of the nineteenth century, it did not become a popular alternative for disposal until after the Second World War. Indeed, cremation only surpassed full body burial as the most common preference in the late 1960s. Since the early 1970s, however, two

'In the shadow of the traditional grave' by Leonie Kellaher, David Prendergast and Jenny Hockey, *Mortality*, 10(4), 2005, Taylor & Francis Ltd. Reprinted by kind permission of the publisher and Leonie Kellaher (www.informaworld.com).

thirds of all annual disposals have been cremations, rising to an average of 71.54% since 2000 (*Pharos International,* 2004, p.20), making this the customary choice in the UK.

While cremation has now achieved ascendancy over burial, another significant change has been occurring in recent decades as ever more family members and friends choose not to leave cremated remains in the hands of crematoria staff to be interred or scattered within the garden of remembrance. In the 1970s, only around one in 10 sets of ashes were taken away for private disposal; by 2004 this proportion had risen nationally to over 56%, with considerable local variation. This equates to almost a quarter of a million sets of ashes removed annually. Intriguingly, there are only limited statistics, official or otherwise, tracing the eventual fate of most of these ashes, aside from those very few sets that are recorded as openly returned to gardens of remembrance for one or other form of placement, or to cemeteries for ash burial. Even where some official information can be obtained, the picture remains unclear. For instance, applications for burials by the Council in Sunderland show that, between 1999 and 2004, approximately 8% of ashes taken away from its crematorium were placed in family graves in the cemetery. What these statistics do not show however, are the numbers of ashes that were buried or scattered on graves illicitly. This may be in an attempt to avoid paying the costly fees involved; or from ignorance or even distaste that permission is required in the first place. [...] We might argue that such covert practices indicate the paucity of choices on the part of providers, who appear to have offered limited forms of memorialization, such as wall plaques and inscription in the book of remembrance, until, relatively recently. At the same time, we could acknowledge this as one facet of the effort to keep costs associated with cremation low, in contrast to what has always been understood as more expensive burial options.

[...]

Strong parallels between burial and cremation practice

[...]

Vignette of Doris Penny

Doris had created a small plot for the ashes of three family members who died at intervals over the previous 15 years: her father, mother, and an aunt. The father died first. In his will he requested cremation, for as Doris said, he had always 'been a bit against burial'. However, as in many other cases, he did not specify what he wanted doing with the ashes. In contrast, Doris had always considered herself to be somewhat 'anti-cremation' because she felt that 'you are just burned and there is nothing there and there is nowhere to visit'. This perception of cremation arose from the belief that, as in the 1970s and 1980s, there were few options available for the disposal of ashes. Speaking of her abhorrence of the placelessness which she felt accompanied the dispersal of ashes, she commented:

Where would I go talk to them? Where would I relate to them? He would I know who I was talking to? My husband's dad died and was scattered in the crematorium garden of remembrance and Tony said 'I have nowhere to relate to'. I think it would have been better for him had he been able to. My mother always said 'I don't want to be buried as they forget you and then there's no flowers on the grave'. Well that may be true, but there might be another generation who wants to come and visit you and see where your last resting place was.

For Doris Penny, like many other interviewees, the availability of a 'focus' seemed essential; a permanent place to visit where she felt that her parents somehow lingered, their presence symbolized by the ashes. When asked if she had considered splitting the ashes and disposing of them in several locations, she reacted with horror, declaring 'I wouldn't chop my dad in half would I? He's whole isn't he … it would be like chopping his legs off'. When asked if she had mingled her parents' ashes together in one container, she replied that she preferred to keep the sets of ashes separated. Her own husband had recently suggested the possibility of mixing their own ashes after their deaths but, though she humoured his romantic inclination, she secretly disliked the idea.

It was not until after her father's death in 1990 that Doris Penny discovered to her surprise that it was possible to bury ashes. As a result, the family discussed how they felt about it. None of them knew much about the practice and so they approached a funeral director to find out more. They were shown a cemetery and told they could buy a plot which would hold three caskets. The potential for reuniting family members through sharing grave space decided the matter, particularly for Doris Penny's disabled mother who changed her views as result and said 'Yes let's do it, as I'd like to be with Dad when something happens to me'. It was agreed at the same meeting that her father's sister, who for many years had lived with her brother and his wife in the capacity as carer, would take the third space in the plot once the time came. For Doris, this ashes' plot had taken on the significance of a family grave. The urns of her father and mother were now buried together at the centre of the plot, and those of the aunt were placed at one side. Her mother had reportedly been quite pleased to think that when she died, her family would be able to visit them all together.

Doris Penny's view on visiting match very closely with the views of informants who contributed to *The secret cemetery* by Francis, Kellaher and Neophytou (2005), where the focus is the grave established for whole body burial. Family members, or others who were close in life, frequently expressed wishes to be buried in the same grave, the same section, or at least in the same cemetery. This emerged as significant for people with a range of ideas about reunion in an afterlife. Proximity was as urgent for those with secular views as for those with either firm or uncertain beliefs about a form of resurrection. Comfort appeared to be drawn from the prospect of 'company', when faced with the dissolution of death, as did a notion of security in numbers, not least for those from immigrant groups such as Greek Cypriot Orthodox, more recent Bangladeshi Muslims, or longer established Irish catholic families and communities. The possibility of family and community remembrance was also seen as more likely where the dead had been placed in close proximity.

The reaction of the Penny family seems to reflect these more widely held preferences for a grave or area where visiting and tending a plot allows for meaningful engagement, including conversation. For instance, Doris Penny visited regularly, particularly on anniversaries. Initially she had found herself drawn to the grave at surprising times of the day. This intense compulsion had lessened by the time of the interview, but she still could not ignore the urge to visit. At the site of ash interment, Doris Penny talked to her deceased family about her daily life and brought them flowers, because that is what she had done when they were alive. She hated to see dead flowers on a grave, or items such as plastic flowers, figurines, or wind chimes, arguing that it was a question of respect. In her view cemeteries were 'sacred places, though I'm not a believer. And that one has to resist making them like a decorated house outside at Christmas with glitter and lights on off, on off, on off'. The only exceptions she made to this were children's graves. Photographs, she believed, should be kept away from the public arena of the cemetery as they were too intimate, even though she had many images around her house that often brought her warmth, a sense of closeness, memories, and, at times, sanity. She felt these were very personal and should be kept private. The fresh flowers she took to the plot, however, were important as gifts which demonstrated that she remembered. She felt that her habits or rituals of visiting had helped with her grieving process by giving her a defined space that in turn both offered and demanded a time to think. In her refusal of the placelessness of scattered ashes, Doris Penny therefore turned to more traditional ritual practices, and her dislike of the newer practice of extending the domestic sphere into the site of disposal through fairy lights and photographs also indicates that for her the removal of ashes from the crematoria was not viewed as an opportunity to innovate.

[...]

Other strong parallels between burial practice and decisions surrounding the disposal of ashes were repeatedly voiced by our interviewees. One informant, Maria Warburton, spoke repeatedly of here mother's ashes being 'laid to rest'. Describing her repatriation of the ashes to Ireland, she recalled; 'People said "You've brought her home". It was very important that she should come home, to be laid out in her own house in Ireland'. Maria recounted how she had placed the ashes on the windowsill the night before a ceremony which involved scattering them on the sea nearby. This echoes an Irish wake with a candle in the window and people visiting. Traditionally, repatriation to Ireland would be of the body for burial, and the appearance of a container with ashes would not generally be expected in a country where the cremation rate is still around 2%. Maria, however, constructed an account that fits with bodily repatriation and all its beneficial possibilities for remembrance fixed in time and place. Indeed she argued that burial per se had a problematic finality: 'A funeral is over, but if you are so inclined you can visit (the grave). With cremation it is not (a case of) "the lid's closed and that's that"'. In carrying out this process of ritualization, Maria has overcome reservations about cremation which were expressed by some of the people we interviewed in their 'professional' capacity. For example, a representative of the Compassionate Friends in Glasgow said that whereas people whose children have been buried 'go up once a week, but people that have scattered ashes don't have that, and they all regret it, most of them do'. With regard to her own son whose body was buried rather than cremated, she said 'I just feel he's still there, there's part of him still there, if I'd got him cremated I think it'd have been, that would have been finished if you know what I mean'. Similarly a Nottingham outreach nurse said 'when people are cremated it's almost as if they're wiped off the face of the earth, I mean I, know they are anyway when they die but it's more of a really, more as if they never existed than if you've got a grave to visit'. Maria, however, had ensured that her mother's expressed wish to be cremated and then repatriated for scattering on the sea still provided opportunities for memorialization at a pace that she herself could set, and which, in her view, greatly eased her feelings of grief. At the same time, and more publicly, the idiom of burial was brought into play.

[…]

In each of these instances, the placing of cremated remains in a public place, or, in the case of Maria Warburton, arranging for a series of traditional, public and religious ceremonies, may be the link that connects ash disposal with the grave and burial. The insistence on not splitting ashes, indeed on portraying the practice as a form of desecration, also seems to reflect the law and custom about not disturbing human remains. Though there are some ambiguities in such cases, these bereaved people acted and thought within frames that seem to lie deep in the shadow of traditional burial not least because the disposal of the ashes entailed strong elements of placement in a public arena. In the next section we examine several cases where, by contrast, the intention has been to ensure that the final destinations of the ashes are clear of the public domain, as represented by the cemetery or the crematorium garden of remembrance.

Of wind and tide: resisting the shadow of the traditional grave

During many of our interviews, it immediately became clear that the choice of cremation was heavily influenced by a dislike of the idea of burial in the earth. As an interviewee with a terminal illness said, just 3 days before his death, he had decided on the 'oven' instead of the grave because it would be 'bloody freezing down there'. Other frequent comments reflect those gathered in Davies and Shaw's (1995) study in revealing the desire to avoid slow decay, the fear of being 'buried alive' or 'being eaten by worms', or simply a concern to eliminate the effort and trouble descendants would incur in attending to a grave. It is noteworthy that these views are commonly cited as the wishes of the deceased, or articulated by those contemplating their own deaths; among those attempting to plan a relative's disposal without instructions, they are far less evident. The inter-related themes of confinement and release are particularly significant here. As indicated in the previous section, for many of those seeking the focus and protection of a carefully defined, bounded, and permanent burial or scattering place, the notion of keeping the ashes together, or at least distributed within a readily identifiable area, such as around the base of a favourite tree, was important. What then of people who chose to scatter to the winds or to the tides, often citing the aim of 'freeing' the deceased? Do their choices reflect a desire to escape the shadow of the grave?

   This was certainly the case for Daniel McGough, a plasterer from Glasgow. He argued that the grave is 'confinement to you as a person cos you're there for all time, or until the council wants to build houses then relocate you … confining to the people who only think they're with you when they go to your grave'. For himself, Daniel claimed: 'if they just take my ashes up the hill and let them blow away in the wind, I'll be quite happy. I like the idea of the freedom'.

A significant number of other interviewees would agree. Bill Oswald, a 90-year-old inter-viewee, still had his wife's ashes on his bedside table, despite having been a widower for a decade. He had plans for their mingled ash-remains to be scattered, by friends from their rambling club, from the top of a favourite peak in Derbyshire, a place of fond memory. For him this would signify an ending, but one which embraced his wife, in a non-confined and starkly beautiful place with fine views. Asked about cemetery interment he replied:

> Well, I think cemeteries are depressing places. I have the deeds for the grave where my mother and father are buried, but I think all this remembrance and crosses and these things are not necessary. I mean, I was religious when I was young – 'til I was around 14 and then I thought 'I've started to think for myself'. I won't say that I'm an atheist but I did not – well I didn't have a service for the cremation, because I do not believe in using the church just for marriages, deaths, and christenings.

His intentions were clear but, in the meantime, his wife's ashes had been 'disposed of' in a way which is private and intimate. Every night before he went to sleep, he sat in bed talking to the ashes of his wife, telling her about his day. He said he could only talk to the ashes as these alone were the material remains of his wife; for him a photograph was no substitute (see Gibson, 2004).

[...]

It is evident, therefore, that even in cases which appear to demonstrate an escape from the shadow of the grave, rituals and meanings associated with burials can continue to exert a powerful influence. Our final group of interviewees were more ambivalent towards the ideas of a public grave, regulated by municipal or ecclesiastic institutions. In these instances, the placing of ashes tends to take place away from public areas, usually in more private and personally meaningful sites. While we might here include the media-attractive strategies of rocket despatch and transformation into gems (diamonds especially), our informants described more modest domestic and familial approaches. While less dramatic, these may be no less challenging to tradition and to institutions that have hitherto deter-mined and controlled the manner of disposal after death.

Ambiguous or liminal? The interim and the domestic

Alice Robson's mother had died several years previously and, at the insistence of her sister, the ashes had been divided. Some were taken to New Zealand, a place that had been a favourite holiday destination, and the rest had been kept at the sister's house. Alice did not think it right that the ashes had been split, so had nothing to do with the remaining ashes. She believed that her mother was not at peace because of this division. Last year, Fred, Alice's husband, also died and was cremated. When it came to choosing a final destination for his ashes, her decision was informed by both her dislike of how her mother had been treated and her observations of other ashes being left at impersonal, distant and unwelcoming gardens of remembrance. After a discussion with her son and his wife, they decided to keep the ashes close by, burying them in the son's garden in a Chinese vase which Fred had always been fond of. He had loved the son's garden and spent much of his retirement sitting there, so felt this was a safe and suitable location. Being so close also meant that Alice did not have to get three buses to the cemetery, and they could always feel Fred was with them.

They buried him in the garden in a post-funeral ceremony for family and close friends, marking the spot by placing a birdbath over the ashes, and surrounding it with his favourite flowers. A small brass plaque bearing Fred's name was attached to the birdbath. This arrangement can be seen as a compromise between a range of choices. The ashes were buried underground with a formal monument marking them. Though not countenanced by the current regulations about exhumation, these ashes were considered portable by the family, should they ever move house. This can be seen to reflect their location (fixed within the private domain by the family) and not officially recognized or recorded within the public domain. The potential informal removal of interred ashes is of course much more problematic within a cemetery, a space where official regulations about exhumation can more easily be enforced.

Another interviewee, Carole Devon, who buried her father's ashes in a family garden, echoed many of these explanations and rationales. Of a neighbour who had left her husband's ashes to be scattered at the crematorium, she said that it was a disgrace that so little regard had been shown for him, even the neighbour's dog's ashes had been placed on the mantelpiece. Carole Devon, like Alice Robson, stressed the pressures associated with cemetery visiting and added that she wanted to avoid passing such a responsibility to her children. Instead, by having the father's ashes buried in her daughter's garden, she felt they were safe and well looked after, in a pleasant, lively garden with children running around.

In general, keeping ashes within the garden, whether irretrievably scattered or buried whole in a polytainer, is usually seen as a more final destination than those kept inside the house. Retention in the house usually seems to be chosen as an interim holding strategy, even if for a prolonged period. In such cases, interviewees described a planned reunion when they themselves died. For some this entailed placing the ashes in their coffins, prior to burial; for others the ashes were to be mingled, for joint burial or scattering. Others had requested that their ash containers be buried side by side, or perhaps placed together in an above ground sanctum. Cremated remains can also be kept in commercially produced containers, ranging from coloured glass dolphin statuettes to carved hard-wood boxes that one widow said reminded her of a coffin. This diversity is matched by the variety of locations in which ashes are placed within the household. Frequently taking up initial residence to the forefront of social life, perhaps on the mantelpiece or under the television set, they often retreat over time, migrating to 'back-stage' regions, such as under the stairs, in the garage, or the attic, or indeed into very private space such as the bedroom. Here the permanency of the grave or indeed of dispersal, of a *final* decision, is often fended off as unwelcome. At this point, the ashes can be seen as liminal, imbued with a social life and identity, yet reserved in a cupboard.

[…]

Note

1   To ensure confidentiality, all proper names used are pseudonyms.

References

Cremation Society of Great Britain (1974). *History of modern cremation in Great Britain from 1874: The first hundred years.* Retrieved September 12, 2005, from http://www.srgw.demon.co.uk/CremSoc/History/HistSocy.html

Davies, D., and Shaw, A. (1995). *Reusing old graves: A report on popular British attitudes.* Kent: Shaw & Sons.

Francis, D., Kellaher, D., and Neophytou, G. (2005). *The secret cemetery.* Oxford: Berg.

Gibson, M. (2004). Melancholy objects. *Mortality,* 9, 285–299.

Jupp, P. C. (2005). *From dust to ashes: Cremation and the British Way of Death.* Basingstoke: Palgrave Macmillan.

Pharos International (2004). Disposition of cremated remains in Great Britain. *Pharos International,* 70, 20.

White, S. (2002). A burial ahead of its time? The Crookenden burial case and the sanctioning of cremation in England and Wales. *Mortality,* 7, 171–190.

23

A Voice Unheard: Grandparents' Grief Over Children Who Died of Cancer

Miri Nehari, Dorit Grebler and Amos Toren

Introduction

Research on families who have suffered the death of a child has given us a great deal of information on responses, processes, and ways of coping with bereavement of parents, siblings, orphans, and spouses. However, there are few published accounts regarding the grief process of the grandparents or psychological work with them (Gerner, 1990; Ponzetti & Johnson, 1991; Ponzetti, 1992; Fry, 1997; Rothman, 1999; Reed, 2000; Dent & Stewart, 2004). Indeed, when discussing bereavement, grandparents are not usually considered part of the 'bereaved family.'

Nevertheless, evidence seems to suggest that grandparents have an important function in the bereaved family and that their grief has some unique characteristics. Reed (2000) writes about the 'double pain' of bereaved grandparents. They experience the pain of the loss of their grandchild and also the pain of their own child's bereavement. Ponzetti (1992) writes about the 'triple pain' of grandparents who are mourning for their dead grandchild, their grieving wounded child, and themselves. Rothman (1999) writes about the grandchild's role to ensure eternity for the grandparents', which is lost by his/her death.

A support group for bereaved grandparents was conducted at Beit Wiesel palliative care unit for children with cancer in Safra Children's Hospital [Israel]. A bereaved grandparents' group is a pioneer effort, and in our literature search we were unable to find any detailed report about such a group. This is somewhat surprising, since we witnessed in Beit Wiesel that grandparents are often very much involved in taking care of the sick child, as a result of practical needs of the family having to deal with long and difficult treatments and hospitalizations. The physical involvement heightens the emotional and intimate ties, both with the sick grandchild and with the family as a whole.

During discussions in the grandparents' group, significant topics were raised and a door was opened into an important area that has been only slightly touched by research. The unique aspect of this information has to do with the tasks grandparents are asked to perform during a long and difficult illness of a grandchild, as well as their special position

Excerpts from 'A voice unheard: Grandparents' grief over children who died of cancer' by Miri Nehari, Dorit Grebler and Amos Toren, *Mortality*, 12(1): 66–78, 2007, Taylor & Francis Ltd, reprinted by kind permission of the publisher and Miri Nehari (Taylor & Francis Ltd., www.informaworld.com).

in the complex family dynamic developed during the time of the child's long illness. The purpose of this article is to describe grandparent's dealing with bereavement and the dynamics of three generations of a bereaved family through an analysis of the group work.

[…]

The grandparents' group

Grandparents of children who died in Beit Wiasel in the past 2 years and were known to the staff were invited to join a grandparents' bereavement group. Of the 15 couples invited, six joined the group. Seven couples expressed their wish to come but could not do so because of poor health or death of a spouse. Two couples said they did not need such a group. The group was heterogeneous: the age of participants ranged from early 50s to late 70s; some participants were employed and others fully retired. There were grandparents whose children had left home and others who still had children living with them (two couples). […]

Here follows a description of the six grandchildren: four males, two females. Two aged 0–5, three aged 6–10, and one aged 16–20. Length of illness for five children was 6–12 months, with one being ill over 12 months. Lapse of time between death and beginning of the group: four children, 3–12 months; two children, 13–20 months.

Despite differences in age, background, and education, the cohesion of the group was established quickly, and attendance was almost complete. A senior clinical psychologist and a head nurse, both trained in group work, led the group.

The sessions

[…]

Group meetings included problem solving, as well as emotional focused support (Thoits, 1986). Problem solving focused support relates to providing tools to understand what is happening in the grief process, to developing abilities to cope with problems, to developing alternative ways of seeing reality, and to coping in the behavioural sphere. Emotion-focused support relates to an opportunity to share emotions, provide empathetic listening, deal with emotions of loneliness and isolations, sorrow, pain, or anger, by allowing each group member to share their stories repeatedly, and to experience acceptance from the group.

Two topics were planned to be introduced in the discussions in a structured way. The first subject was the relationship of the grandparents with their own children, the parents of their late grandchild. We planned to investigate emotions, behaviours, and family dynamics from the grandparents' point of view, that is, the intergenerational level. The second subject was the relationship of the grandparents with the deceased grandchild, which was approached through a model developed by Byock (1997) to be used with families of dying adult patients. Byock's model consists of five phrases which the patient and his family members should talk about. The phrases are presented as beginnings of sentences to be completed as specifically and as fully as possible. The phrases are:

I forgive you for…
I ask your forgiveness for…
I thank you for…
I love you for…
I say goodbye in parting from you…

[…]

Results: content raised during meetings

During the course of the group meetings, different subjects were raised, set aside, and raised again. Group members shared their stories and listened to each other's narratives while processing their own loss and pain. The content of the discussions was recorded verbatim and analysed by methods influenced by Strauss and Corbin (1990). Five main themes* emerged, here follows those themes presented with quotations from the participants:

A 'place' for mourning of grandparents

The REAL mourning is that of our children [the parents]. Who are we? Just grandparents.

I wanted a copy of the video [of the deceased grandchild] and my daughter-in-law asked me, what for?

Strong expressions of feelings that there is no 'place' for grandparents' mourning were expressed. Members of the group debated whether or not their pain was legitimate compared to the pain of the parents of their deceased grandchildren. In addition to the strong experience of meeting other people in a similar situation, participants expressed the importance of the group experience validating their grief, which emphasized the lack of acceptance of their mourning in the general culture:

There is nowhere else that I can speak of my grief over the death of my grandson.

I can speak to you [another grandfather in the group], I can't speak about this to anyone else, a grandfather is different.

In our estimation, the quick, deep bonding of the group is evidence not only of the experience of support but also of the significant lack of a place for grandparents to mourn in our society. The group created a place by legitimizing the grandparents' grief, by creating a physical place where grandparents' grief can formally be expressed, and by having a stage where grandparents' grief is acknowledged. Therefore, problems related to this social identity could be raised and discussed.

[…]

---

*Only four of the five themes are discussed here.

Parting from the grandchild: pain, loss, and memory

There were a lot of discussions about the grandchildren, the pain, and the memories. In the beginning, participants were hesitant, it was difficult to express in words, to share. As the meetings continued, it was difficult to staunch the verbal flow of pain, yearning, and memories. What to do with the possessions of the grandchild, things they used to do together. The group focused on the range of emotions and provided for expression of pain, emptiness, sharing, and support. Group members debated, advised each other, and reported developments between meetings on practical problems: where to place the grandchild's pictures in their home; parents' wishes regarding the grandchild's possessions; caring for other grandchildren; what to do with the toys and clothing; when to visit the grave; to speak about the deceased grandchild or not; to tell others about him/her; how to find a space for the deceased grandchild while leaving a space for surviving ones; to find a space for their children, especially the one who is the parent of the deceased grandchild. They struggled with the issue of how to go with the flow of different family members' needs and their own needs, without hurting or being hurt.

Following stories about how wonderful the dead child was, and the size of the vacuum he left in their lives, the grandparents were presented with the Byock model. They were asked to write letters to the late grandchild, based on the model. The meetings, when each participant read out his/her letter to the grandchild, were exceptionally difficult to bear:

My daughter said: 'Let him go!' but I could not until the very last moment.

My son said: 'Mom, release him. Almost 2 years have passed!' But I still can't let him go.

What can I forgive him for, he was so little and he had no time to do anything bad.

The group swung from pain, emptiness, and loss to memories of happy moments and joy with the grandchild.

The bereaved family: grandparents' point of view

The group discussed, at length, the dynamics of the bereaved extended family and the special role of grandparents in this dynamic. The different ways of mourning of family members, the difficulty of bridging these differences, and the desperate need to do so were also discussed. The difficulty of the emotional relationship to surviving grandchildren came up. For example:

I am afraid to love [sibling of the deceased grandchild]. I am not attached to him the way I was to [deceased grandchild].

There were discussions about other grandchildren: whether or not to speak with them about the deceased grandchild, whether it was okay to give other grandchildren the toys or clothing of the deceased child. The participants discussed the questions, shared and consulted, suggesting ways of coping with the situation. Many questions were raised regarding children that still lived with the grandparents (aunts or uncles of the deceased grandchild). Situations were raised where grandparents become mediators for their children. For example: one grandmother found herself caught between her daughter (mother of the deceased grandchild) whose marriage is crumbling, the grandfather (her husband) whose life has stopped as he has lost himself in the depths of grief, and her son (16 years old, the uncle of the deceased child) who acts as if death had not visited the family at all.

The grandparents discussed how to find their place in the multigenerational bereaved family. Many hurt feelings, much anger and pain were expressed concerning the parents of the late grandchild. The group spoke of the distance between the generations:

The children don't come for holidays.

They are moving to a new apartment far away.

The spoke of the silence:

They won't talk with us about the pain.

A planned meeting was suggested by the grandparents between our group and a group of bereaved parents. A bereaved parents group was conducted by two social workers during the same period in Beit Wiesel. Many of the participants in the parents group were children of the participants in the grandparents group. The issue of communication between the two bereaved generations was so intense emotionally that the parents group deliberated over it for a few sessions. They feared too much hurt would come out of such meeting. They decided, instead, to send a representative, a bereaved mother that was not the daughter of any of the grandparents in our group. The joint meeting was highly emotional, and unusually honest and open:

When we [parents] want to distance ourselves from you [grandparents] it's not that we have anything against you, this is our way of dealing with our pain. I understand that this is perceived as hurtful to you, but this is not our intent.

We [parents] have a hard time with your [grandparents] pain, we can barely manage our own pain and that of our other children. We decided to do what is best for us and put you out of the picture.

You [grandparents], it's like you are stealing our grief. You came before us to the grave and you lit the first memorial candle [the role of the primary grievers].

The mother told the group that according to the parents the relationships between them and the grandparents are dynamic and could have three meanings:

1 The parents distance themselves from the grandparents with no hard feelings, only because they have no energy to reach out to them, being too involved in their own grief.
2 The parents distance themselves because the grandparents' grief is a burden they could not or would not carry.
3 There is a situation where the parents actually feel some kind of struggle over who has the primary role in the grief or who takes decisions about family issues related to the dead child.

I suffer doubly for my daughter and my grandson. I have a great vacuum in my heart. When my daughter smiles, I am happy. When she is down, my world falls apart.

In the beginning the illness brought us together. Now we have stopped talking about it and it's frightening. It's impossible to talk about it with my daughter. There is too much [emotional] distance.

I [grandparent] used to be the head of the family [before the death]. I am no longer the head. Now I just get in the way.

Another thing is difficult for me. I am growing old; I didn't want her [my daughter] to move far away [geographically]. I may need her help but they are moving to another city.

The grandparents talk of their double pain over their child and their grandchild, about the emotional distance which makes it impossible for them to support their child or be supported by him/her or even get practical help as they grow old.

Return to living

I was at a meeting in my senior citizens club, it was nice and I laughed, when suddenly I said to myself, 'How can you laugh? Your grandchild is dead!' And I got up and left.

The group talked about returning to living, giving permission to laugh, to enjoy. They advised each other about how to return to family celebrations that, until then, they had not attended. They deliberated whether or not to return to hobbies, to go on outings that they so loved, encouraging each other to do so. They advised each other on how to deal with the sudden burst of tears that well up in public places and how to cope with the pain that surprises you as you pass near the toy store that the grandson so loved.

Perhaps it is harder for retired people like ourselves. When people are not busy, it is harder.

The question was raised:

Should we plan extended family meetings when these cause so much pain, both for us and for our children?

The hope was expressed that the grandparents' isolation and distance from their own children would pass in time:

I have begun to understand my daughter. I thought that I am the mother and she must come to me for help, but she distanced herself from me. Now I understand that she needed her space as I needed mine.

I understand their pain [the parents]. They are trying to cope and we sometimes interfere. I am less angry and hurt by this now.

The group also found itself smiling. Together, they were able to allow themselves to share some of the good things that had happened to them since their last meeting. They could also discuss other things besides their grief, to plan their return to hobbies, and even sometimes to argue about politics.

Subjects that arose during the course of the meetings will continue to occupy the participants long after the group is over. There will continue to be fluctuation between pain and yearning and the good memories:

> Time heals, I believe this saying. But it says with you all your life. You continue living, but this wound slowly eats at your heart.

The group sadly parted but with a feeling of achievement, of openness to others who shared their fate, and the feeling that the group helped with their own families. The feeling that the group was the place that shared, listened, understood, and enabled them to continue their own journey.

Discussion

The goal of this article was to touch on the grieving process of bereaved grandparents through a description of a group's work. This is a case study in an area barely touched in the professional literature. This unique group of bereaved grandparents was formed as a response to a need identified, first by the medical team serving the families and reiterated by the bereaved parents of these same deceased grandchildren. Analysis of the main themes brought up in the group showed that a special human experience occurred in the group which reflects the similarities and differences of two generations within a bereaved family.

The expression 'bereaved grandparent' is not common. This expresses, in our opinion, the cultural sociological expectation that bereavement is related almost exclusively to the nuclear family. There are bereaved parents, bereaved siblings, widows, widowers, and orphans. Grandparents are not included in this small circle of formal grievers. Their loss has no specific place in terms of conceptual or cultural frameworks. There is a culture of bereaved parents (Riches & Dawson, 1996) but not one for bereaved grandparents. Tajfel (1978) claims that the overall social tasks of the individual determine his/her social identity. The roles we perform and the expectations of society determine who we are and what we expect of ourselves. It appears, therefore, that the absence of a clear social position and social role for bereaved grandparents, within the culture and the family framework, causes vagueness concerning what they are expected to be and how they should cope. The emotional response by our group participants to the reality that we recognized their grief and gave it legitimacy was, in itself very strong, bringing tearful thanks.

The isolation of the bereaved grandparent can be a very heavy burden, especially when considering the depth of the experience. Some grandparents are no longer young. Most of them have already dealt with loss of parents, spouse, siblings, or good friends. They compared those losses with the loss of a grandchild and came to the conclusion that losing a grandchild is by far the most difficult blow. Some of them are already retired, and have less to occupy their time. Some have limited social support networks. In many cases, as they age, they have lost the energy to support others while trying to hold their own heads above water. However, some grandparents are relatively young, in their 50s, and are still working, some at the height of their career. The grief can affect their ability to fulfill their daily tasks, but they are not given allowances while recuperating, as parents are.

In the family too, the place of the mourning grandparent is not clear. Meetings of the extended family for events, holidays, and in the normal course of life can be very difficult and the pain over the deceased grandchild is especially pronounced. The differences between mourning styles can affect the nature of relationships and closeness among family members. For example, when the family gathered at the Sabbath dinner table, the grandparents wanted to leave an empty chair for the dead grandchild but the parents objected and refused to stay. This caused further emotional pain, physical distance, and distress. Nadeau (2004) writes about the importance of families making sense of death to aid the coping with grief. In our group, the grandparents yearned to be part of the grieving family but did not feel so.

Isolation and alienation between bereaved parents described in the literature occurs also with grandparents. Bereaved parents cannot carry the additional weight of their own parents' grief, so they become more distant and the grandparents find it difficult to cope with the grief of their children, so they become silent. They might not be able to find a way to support each other or speak of their grandchild or of their own pain. Grandparents, additionally, experience the pain of separation, distance, isolation, and inability to help their children, which is their role as parents.

[...]

References

Byock, I. (1997). *Dying well, place and possibilities at the end of life*. New York: Riverhead Books.

Dent, A.L., and Stewart, A.J. (2004). *Sudden death in childhood: Support of bereaved family*. Elsevier: Butterworth, Heineman.

Fry, P.S. (1997). Grandparents' reactions to the death of a grandchild: An exploratory factor analytic study. *Omega*, 35, 119–140.

Gerner, M.H. (1990). *For bereaved grandparents*. Omaha, NE: The Centering Corporation.

Nadeau, J.W. (2004). *Families making sense of death*. Newbery Park, CA: Sage.

Ponzetti, J.J. (1992). Bereaved families: A comparison of parents' and grandparents' reactions to the death of a child. *Omega*, 21, 63–71.

Ponzetti, J.J., and Johnson, M.A. (1991). The forgotten grievers: Grandparents' reactions to the death of grandchildren. *Death Studies*, 15, 157–167.

Reed, M.L. (2000). *Grandparents cry twice*. Amityville, NY: Baywood Publications Co.

Riches, G., and Dawson, P. (1996). Communities of feelings: The culture of bereaved parents. *Mortality*, 1, 143–161.

Rothman, J.C. (1999). *The bereaved parent's survival guide*. New York: Continuum.

Strauss, A., and Corbin, J. (1990). *Basics of qualitative research*. Newbery Park, CA: Sage.

Tajfel, H. (1978). Social categorization, social identify and social comparison. In H. Tajfelt (ed.), *Differentiation between social groups*. London: Academic Press.

Thoits, P. (1986). Social support as coping assistance. *Journal of Consulting and Clinical Psychology*, 54, 416–423.

24

The Ritual Work of UK Childhood Bereavement Services

Liz Rolls

Introduction

Within the wider context of UK health and social care services, childhood bereavement services are a recent form of provision that support children who have lost a significant person through death (Rolls and Payne, 2003). Furthermore, there appears to be a continuing rise in the number of services being developed (Rolls, 2007). In this chapter, I consider their work as one of 'ritual performance' and argue that UK childhood bereavement services appear to be a 'ritualised activity' (Árnason, 2007) whose influence on UK society is increasing. I begin by briefly considering the loss of ritual in bereavement, and outlining the work of services with bereaved children and families. Drawing on a study of UK childhood bereavement services[1] in which I was the principal researcher, I then explore the ritual aspects of two commonly used activities, including the creative and transformative dimension that these activities provide both psychically and culturally. The study was designed to explore how providers develop and deliver their services, and what bereaved children and their families found helpful in their experience of childhood bereavement service provision. It was undertaken in two phases: a national postal survey of 91 UK childhood bereavement services (Rolls and Payne, 2003), and eight in-depth organisational case studies, selected through maximum variation sampling. These included interviews with paid and unpaid service providers (n = 60) and stakeholders (n = 6), a postal survey of unpaid service providers (n = 74), and interviews with 14 families (24 children and 16 parents) who had used one of the case study childhood bereavement services (Rolls and Payne, 2004; 2007; 2008; Rolls and Relf, 2006). It also included my participant observation in six group interventions (three for children, one for adolescents, and two for parents). Until this study, no formalised, academic research of UK childhood bereavement services had been undertaken. However, following the tradition in services for adults who have been bereaved (for example, Hislop, 2001; Firth, 2005), service providers had made a contribution to the literature including describing the types of interventions that were used (Fleming and Balmer, 1991; Stokes and Crossley, 1996; Potts, Farrell and O'Toole, 1999; Paton, 2004; Stokes, 2004).

In the context of this chapter, the term 'parent' is used to mean biological and adoptive parents, while the term 'family' is used to mean the 'network of people in the child's immediate psychosocial field' (Carr, 1999: 3), including those who play a significant role. However, the broad use of these terms does not intend to ignore the variety of family compositions within the UK, nor the impact of the individual family constellation on a child who has been bereaved (Rolls, 2008).

The role of ritual in bereavement and consequences of its loss

Theories on the role of ritual point to a number of features. Ritual is seen as an event in which a participant emotionally, structurally, and ideologically 'makes change' and 'moves' (Turner, 1969), from one social status to another (Littlewood, 1992). This helps bring order to transition (Romonoff and Terenzio, 1998; Kobler, Limbo and Kavanaugh, 2007) by enabling participants 'to understand the world, and how individuals should operate within it, in a particular way' (Hockey, 2001: 206). It differs from ceremony which 'marks a change that has been effected elsewhere' (Hockey, 2001: 206). The key dimensions of ritual are intention, participation, and meaning-making (Kobler, Limbo and Kavanaugh, 2007), and appear to have three functions: to validate and reinforce values in the face of psychological disturbances; to reinforce group ties; and aid status change by acquainting people with their new role (Taylor, 1980). Rituals are cultural devices that make use of symbols in either a public or private performance framework, and these symbols contain meanings that are also either publicly (socially) constructed or privately emotionally charged (Romonoff and Terenzio, 1998).

Bereavement can result in a psychological disturbance in which a significant tie to an individual is broken, leading to a loss of status and the need to acquire another. Bereavement rituals appear to mediate the social and psychological transition of bereaved people from the life to death of the those who have died, and from one social status to another (Romonoff and Terenzio, 1998), at the same time as helping to maintain appropriate connection to the deceased person (Silverman and Klass, 1996). In helping to moderate the sense of self, mediate status and provide continuation of the connection with those who have died within a communal context, rituals encompass the intrapsychic, the psychosocial, and the communal (Romonoff and Terenzio, 1998).

However, within an increasingly secular society, religiously based community rituals and bereavement support have been lost. The rise in individualism (Beck, 1991; Walter, 1994; Wilkinson, 1996), and an increasing cultural anxiety about death (Mellor, 1993) has given way to the privatisation, commercialisation, and the professionalisation of death (Hockey, 1990; Walter, 1994; Illich, 1995). This has consequences for individuals as 'the absence of death from the public space makes its presence in the private space an intense and potentially threatening one' (Mellor, 1993: 21). The deconstruction of shared rituals at the time of death results in the deterioration in meaning (Romonoff and Terenzio, 1998), and ambiguities and contradictions for individuals who no longer know how to act (Mellor, 1993). Walter (1994) argues that a characteristic of the 'revival of death' is that while personal experience invades and fragments public discourse, expert discourse manipulates private experience – further distancing the personal experience of bereaved people. Winkel

(2001), however, argues that what is often called 'denial' is in reality a problem of communication and describes the 'new institutions for grief work and bereavement support … as a turning point in communication' (2001: 73). Winkel sees these organisations as part of the uninterrupted individualisation of mourning, based on a general emotionalisation and psychologisation of the self. They generate the expression of grief and channel it at the same time through a re-ritualisation of mourning. Nevertheless, while new rituals that end with the disposal of deceased people are helpful in providing immediate structure, the long-term needs of those who are bereaved may be being ignored; bereavement has arguably become an incomplete rite of passage (Hunter, 2007).

There are also important consequences for bereaved children (Dyregrov, 1991; Worden, 1996; Rolls and Payne, 2007). Alongside the cultural changes in rituals surrounding death and bereavement, there is uncertainty about their status and agency (Rolls and Payne, 2004), and the long-term impact of bereavement on them (Harrington, 1996). Children are subsumed within the privatised nuclear family, but bereaved children often feel isolated within the family (Rolls and Payne, 2007), as well as from their peers and within the school setting where they may be marked out as 'other' and be targets for bullying (Rowling, 2003; Rolls and Payne, 2007). With the loss of a set of practices and rituals that inform how adults act, the position of children has become increasingly precarious.

The work of UK childhood bereavement services

During the last decade within the UK, there has been a cultural shift in the discourse on 'children' and on 'bereavement', and this has led to a rise in the number of services being provided to meet their needs following a significant death (Rolls and Payne, 2003). However, this development is not without critics. Harrington (1996) argues that bereavement does not necessarily make children ill. In addition, the need for childhood bereavement services is contested – with some (for example, Kmietowicz, 2000) arguing for the need for more services, and others questioning their value and arguing that counselling after bereavement, however well intentioned, may be harmful to some children (Harrington and Harrison, 1999).

In my own study of childhood bereavement services (Rolls and Payne, 2007), children came from a wide range of socio-economic backgrounds, and many services provided outreach services in socially deprived areas. Nevertheless, a child's access to a service was dependent on a number of features, including the presence of a local service. In addition, services had different referral policies in terms of who had died or whether a professional referral was required, and some limited their service to a specific age group or type of death (Rolls and Payne, 2003).

Services were also offered to children in different ways: either directly in face-to-face encounters, or indirectly, for example, through a telephone helpline or the agency of another person such as a parent or teacher. Direct work with children may be on an individual basis in the form of assessment, ongoing weekly sessions, and pre- and/or post-group support, or it may take place in groups organised on an ongoing weekly basis or over a weekend period. These two forms – individual work and group work – were not mutually exclusive. Furthermore, the groups may be organised solely for children, or they may include other family members, for all the sessions or only for some of them. Where groups were organised for parents, these were run concurrently with those of their child, and an activity that brings the family members together at the end was arranged (Rolls and Payne, 2004). Most, but not all, services supported bereaved parent(s), placing particular emphasis on helping them understand more about childhood bereavement, and enabling them to parent a bereaved child.

Across all age groups, services provided a wide range of experiential activities that utilised a variety of techniques, including the use of puppetry, picture and collage-making, and the creation of 'memory boxes' and salt sculptures. These activities were purposeful in contributing to naming feelings, thinking about the person who had died, about what had happened, and how children (and their parents) could help and support themselves in the future. Underlying these activities were a set of common objectives to provide a secure place to enable participants to create memory and story through: an exploration of their experience of bereavement; accessing their unspoken and unconscious feelings; and helping them make sense of what had happened and how they felt. Services also helped children manage these feelings, improve communication between family members, reduce feelings of isolation, and hold the possibility of hope for their future (Rolls and Payne 2004; Rolls, 2008).

Two ritual performances

There are two commonly used activities in group-based UK childhood bereavement services, each of which constitutes a ritual performance. The first is a 'candle-lighting' event and the second is a 'balloon-releasing' event. During my study, I participated in both children's and parents' candle-lighting events. In some services, the candle-lighting event takes place during the programme series, while in others it forms part of the ending of the programme of events. In either case, it is held after a period of group activities designed to create an environment of trust. Thus, by the time the candle-lighting event begins, the participants have been able to get to know each other and the staff members, and have begun to speak about the person who has died and about their grief. In the children's group programme I attended, children and staff sat on the floor in a circle. Music was played 'to set a reflective tone' (Stokes, 2004: 112) and all participants – children, staff and, in this instance, myself as participant observer – were invited, each in turn, to light our candle and to say who we had come to remember and anything else we would like to say about them. For example, I said I had come to remember my brother John; I lit my candle for him and said that I was sad that he no longer walked the Earth, but that when I looked at the stars and moon (he had been an astronomer), I thought of him. Children did not have to speak or they could use a staff member to speak on their behalf. Nevertheless, they participated in the circle, lighting their own candle. Once the circle of candles was complete, more music was played and the group remained quiet for a time. Some of the children and staff members cried and were offered comfort by another. Once the music stopped, and after a further brief period of silence, the facilitator drew it to a close. Participants were asked to blow out their candles one at a time around the circle in the order in which they had been lit. Participants were also encouraged to keep their candle for another occasion. The candle-lighting event in the parent group mirrored that of their child's; it followed a similar pattern, although adults were invited to create their own circle and to sit on chairs. A poem was also read. During participant observation, it seemed as if many parents found it hard to speak, and I noticed that some parents also found it very difficult to blow out their candle at the end. Both events were, for all participants including staff and myself, an emotional experience.

The balloon-releasing event is a commonly used activity among UK childhood bereavement services. It takes place at the end of a group session and, unlike the candle-lighting activity, it involves both children and their parent(s) together as a family group. However, preparations usually occur independently beforehand during one of their last separate sessions. In their own group, children and their parent(s) will have been asked to write a message to their deceased relative. Once families are reunited, they are given a balloons upon which each family member ties their message. In the activity in which I participated, a staff member stood in front of the group holding his balloon. Silence descended for a moment before he released it, and this acted as a signal to us to release our balloon, watching them take our messages and thoughts with them. I released mine, and watched the wind catch hold of it and lift it up high. It was very moving for me to write a message to my long-dead brother, and I noticed how hard I found it to release the balloon. I felt captivated by its movement and its stoic effort to rise up and away, and felt fear that it would not. I was standing close to a man whose partner had died, and with whom I had shared an earlier activity. He said the whole thing had been a wonderful experience: 'almost spiritual'.

Ritualised performances in UK childhood bereavement services

Stokes (2004) describes the candle-lighting event as 'a simple ritual, which allows participants the opportunity to remember the person who has died and to connect with some of the feelings of deep sadness that may have rarely surfaced outside the group environment' (2004: 112). In the candle-lighting events that I observed, they appeared to include the three common themes described by parents in a candle-lighting event for those bereaved of a child, each of which equate to dimensions of ritual. These included the importance of the spiritual nature of the service; a bond with others who were sharing the same bereavement/occasion through hearing the names of others; and a continuing relationship to those who have died by remembering one's own (Hislop, 2001).

The activity contained a number of symbols or symbolic activities. Candles have personal, cultural, and religious meaning; they are used to celebrate 'life' ('birth' day), and bring 'light' – illuminating dark corners. In a religious context, they represent prayer, a contemplative, reflective activity on the meaning, joys and trials of life. Blowing out a candle, rather than leaving it behind as a sign of one's 'prayer', is a decisive act that may symbolise 'ending', 'being snuffed out', or 'allowing the dark to return'. Retaining the candle may provide a sense of continuity by becoming an artefact of remembrance, not only of the person who has died, but also of the event of remembrance itself. Circles also have symbolic meaning. It is a symbol used across cultures and 'expresses the totality of the psyche in all its aspects ... it points to the single most vital aspect of life – its ultimate wholeness' (Jung, 1964: 240). In the circle, we were 'levelled' – made equal – in the face of death; we were also symbolically created as 'one' in a never-ending circle. The use of music and poetry enhanced the ritual mood in which we could express intense feeling as we named, remembered, and reflected upon those who had died.

Balloons carry less cross-cultural meaning than candles and circles, and in the UK they are symbolic artefacts of 'party' and 'celebration'. However, their use in this context differed. The balloon-releasing activity reunited families. The balloon becomes a symbol of this; the individual message of each family member is actually and symbolically tied together and a message (even one unsent) unites sender and receiver. But the balloon-releasing activity also marked the end of the group sessions. Release of something 'into the unknown', to be taken 'up and away', to go 'who knows where', is a potent symbol of the uncertainty families, and others, feel about what happens after death, and of the uncertainty of what will happen to families on their return home to 'normal' life. For some children, balloon-releasing holds the prospect that the message will reach the dead person (Stokes, 2004), thus keeping open the possibility of a connection to their dead relative, while for some parents, there is a need to metaphorically 'let go' of their grief and construct a different family life (Stokes, 2004).

UK childhood bereavement services: creating 'symbolic communitas'

Nwoye (2005) argues that bereaved people in Africa are never left in the dark about what is expected of them or what to expect from the culture, and that healing comes to those who have been bereaved where these expectations are fulfilled. African grief rituals are designed to heal the memory components of people who have been bereaved, including the *fact,* the *behavioural,* the *event* and the *prospective* memories. Mourning rituals such as cutting hair, ritual bathing and formal removing and disposal of the mourning dress are intended to symbolise for bereaved people the idea of formal leave-taking; they are rituals that signify 'the exit of the old order and opening of space for the inauguration of a new one' (Nwoye, 2005: 152).

Both of these ritual performances commonly used by UK childhood bereavement services centred on powerful organising images, which brought together the psychological/emotional and abstract/conceptual domains (Hockey, 2001). They connected the participants to the dead person at the same time as they symbolically relinquished or 'let go' of them; symbolising and facilitating an understanding of the ambiguity that often surrounds people who have been bereaved (Littlewood, 1992). These are examples of postmodern death rituals in which 'we can most clearly see the reanimation of ritual forms from other societies or from our own pasts' (Hockey, 2001: 206, drawing on Walter, 1996), although Winkel (2001) constructs these as an extension of modernity – 'a form of 'cultural continuity based on recourse to religious knowledge' (2001:74).

One consequence of the sequestration of death is the loss of *public* recognition for the feelings of personal mourning (Wouters, 2002). Ribbens McCarthy (2006) has argued that a special social context may need to be sought for dealing with private emotions that feel impossible to display in public settings, while Hunter (2007) has argued that people who have been bereaved could be helped by the construction of a ritual of remembrance and meaning-making, after time has allowed them to move along in meaning reconstruction processes of making sense, finding benefits, and identity change (Hunter, 2007). Both of the ritual performances described here were public performances, even if they are sequestered into the 'professional' world of a childhood bereavement service.

A central aim of ritual is 'symbolic communitas', a term used by Turner (1969) to describe generating a feeling of connectedness to a larger symbolic community. This has a double function of socially and psychically offering ways to regulate intense feeling, providing respite and communality in transition (Valentine, 2006). Mortuary ritual is viewed as the human adaptive response to death, and ritual language – the way in which individuals gain sense of self-consciousness – is its crucial form of response; giving sense of power that motivates an ongoing life (Davies, 2002). In the absence of a shared culture and ritual around death and bereavement, children do not have – and are not always given – a language with which to verbalise their experience, to ask questions, to describe their experience or to give names to their feelings. UK childhood bereavement services as 'ritualised activity' (Árnason, 2007) take children out of the privatised nuclear family and place them, actually or symbolically, into groups of other bereaved children. They explore the impact of bereavement on them from their perspective, helping them through experiential activities and through ritualised performances such as those described here. They provide a 'community' for bereaved children in which they are the chief 'scriptwriter' speaking to their memory, writing their own messages (Hockey, 2001). And while they may not change children's status in contemporary society by the provision of a more public ritual, they contribute to changing the child's view of him/herself and of their own status. Through these rituals children can assert membership of a larger symbolic community (Wouters, 2002). By introducing them to another status group; the community of 'bereaved children', children are more able to situate themselves in society. They have an account (a status) for themselves.

Note

1   The study was funded by the Clara Burgess Charity and this support is gratefully acknowledged.

References

Árnason, A. (2007) '"Fall apart and put yourself together again" the anthropology of death and bereavement counselling in Britain', *Mortality*, 12 (1): 48–65.
Beck, U. (1991) *Risk Society*. London: Sage.
Carr, A. (1999) *The Handbook of Child and Adolescence: Clinical Psychology*. London: Routledge.
Davies, D.K. (2002) *Death, Ritual and Belief: The Rhetoric of Funerary Rites*. Second edition. London: Continuum.

Dyregrov, A. (1991) *Grief in Children: A Handbook for Adults*. London: Jessica Kingsley.

Firth, P. (2005) 'Groupwork in palliative care', in P. Firth, G. Luff and D. Oliviere (eds), *Loss, Change and Bereavement in Palliative Care*. Maidenhead: Open University Press. pp: 167–84.

Fleming, S. and Balmer, L. (1991) 'Group intervention with bereaved children', in D. Papadatou and C. Papadatou (eds), *Children and Death*. New York: Hemisphere, pp. 105–24.

Harrington, R. (1996) 'Bereavement is painful but does not necessarily make children ill', *British Medical Journal*, 313, (7060): 822.

Harrington, R. and Harrison, L. (1999) 'Unproven assumptions about the impact of bereavement on children', *Journal of the Royal Society of Medicine*, 92, (May): 230–2.

Hislop, J. (2001) 'A place for my child: the evolution of a Candle service', in J. Hockey, J. Katz and N. Small (eds), *Grief, Mourning and the Death Ritual*. Buckingham: Open University Press. pp. 174–81.

Hockey, J. (1990) *Experiences of Death: An Anthropological Account*. Edinburgh: Edinburgh University Press.

Hockey, J. (2001) 'Changing death rituals', in J. Hockey, J. Katz and N. Small (eds), *Grief, Mourning and the Death Ritual*. Buckingham: Open University Press. pp. 185–211.

Hunter, J. (2007) 'Bereavement: an incomplete rite of passage', *Omega*, 56 (2): 153–73.

Illich, I. (1995) 'Death undefeated', *British Medical Journal*, 311: 1652–3.

Jung, C. (1964) *Man and His Symbols*. London: Arkana/Penguin.

Kmietowicz, Z. (2000) 'More services needed for bereaved children', *British Medical Journal*, 320, (1 April): 893.

Kobler, K., Limbo, R. and Kavanaugh, K. (2007) 'Meaningful moments: the use of ritual in perinatal and pediatric death', *American Journal of Maternal Child Nursing*, 32 (5): 288–97.

Littlewood, J. (1992) *Aspects of Grief: Bereavement in Adult Life*. London: Routledge.

Mellor, P.A. (1993) 'Death in high modernity: the contemporary presence and absence of death', in D. Clark (ed.), *The Sociology of Death*. Oxford: Blackwell. pp. 11–30.

Nwoye, A. (2005) 'Memory healing processes and community intervention in grief work in Africa', *Australian and New Zealand Journal of Family Therapy*, 26 (3): 147–54.

Paton, N. (2004) 'Dreamcatcher: supporting bereaved children', *Nursing Times*, 100, (40): 24–5.

Potts, S., Farrell, M. and O'Toole, J. (1999) 'Treasure weekend: supporting bereaved siblings', *Palliative Medicine*, 13: 51–6.

Ribbens McCarthy, J. (2006) *Young People's Experience of Loss and Bereavement: Towards an Interdisciplinary Approach*. Maidenhead: Open University Press.

Rolls, L. (2007) *Mapping Evaluations of UK Childhood Bereavement Services: Final Report to the Funders*. Cheltenham: University of Gloucestershire.

Rolls, L (2008) 'Helping children and families facing bereavement in palliative care settings', in S. Payne, J. Seymour and C. Ingleton (eds), *Palliative Care Nursing: Principles and Evidence for Practice*. Second edition. Buckingham: Open University Press.

Rolls, L. and Payne, S. (2003) 'Childhood bereavement services: a survey of UK provision', *Palliative Medicine*, 17: 423–32.

Rolls, L. and Payne, S. (2004) 'Childhood bereavement services: issues in UK provision', *Mortality*, 9 (4): 300–28.

Rolls, L. and Payne, S. (2007) 'Children and young people's experience of UK childhood bereavement services', *Mortality*, 12 (3): 281–303.

Rolls, L. and Payne, S. (2008) 'The voluntary contribution to UK childhood bereavement services: locating the place and experiences of unpaid staff', *Mortality*, 13(3): 258–81.

Rolls, L. and Relf, M. (2006) 'Bracketing interviews: addressing methodological challenges in qualitative interviewing in palliative care and bereavement', *Mortality*, 11 (3): 286–305.

Romonoff, B.D. and Terenzio, M. (1998) 'Rituals and the grieving process', *Death Studies*, 22: 697–711.

Rowling, L. (2003) *Grief in School Communities: Effective Support Strategies*. Buckingham: Open University Press.

Silverman, P.R. and Klass, D. (1996) 'Introduction: what's the problem?', in D. Klass, P.R. Silverman and S.L. Nickman (eds), *Continuing Bonds: New Understandings of Grief*. London: Taylor and Francis. pp. 1–27.

Stokes, J. (2004) *Then, Now and Always: Supporting Children as They Journey Through Grief. A Guide for Practitioners*. Cheltenham: Winston's Wish.

Stokes, J. and Crossley, D. (1996) 'Camp Winston: a residential intervention for bereaved children', in S. Smith and M. Pennells (eds), *Interventions with Bereaved Children*. London: Jessica Kingsley. pp. 172–92.

Taylor, R.B. (1980) *Cultural Ways*. Third edition. Boston, MA: Allyn and Bacon.

Turner, V. (1969) *The Ritual Process: Structure and Anti-Structure*. London: Routledge and Kegan Paul.

Valentine, C. (2006) 'Academic constructions of bereavement', *Mortality*, 11 (1): 57–78.

Walter, T. (1994) *The Revival of Death*. London: Routledge.

Walter, T. (1996) 'A new model of grief? Bereavement and biography', *Mortality*, 1 (1): 7–235.

Wilkinson, R.G. (1996) *Unhealthy Societies: The Afflictions of Inequality*. London: Routledge.

Winkel, H. (2001) 'A post-modern culture of grief? On individualization of mourning in Germany', *Mortality*, 6 (1): 65–79.

Worden, J. (1996) *Children and Grief: When a Parent Dies*. New York: Guildford.

Wouters, C. (2002) 'The quest for new rituals in dying and mourning: changes in the We–I balance', *Body and Society*, 8 (1): 1–27.

25

Facilitating Bereavement Recovery and Restoring Dignity to the Genocide Victims in Rwanda

Eugénie Mukanoheli

Introduction

During the 1994 genocide in Rwanda more than a million people were tragically massacred, and the survivors were left with severe trauma which continues to affect their daily lives. Although it sounds contradictory in light of the atrocities that were committed by a large number of Rwandans against their fellow countrymen during the genocide, Rwandans generally have a great deal of respect for human life. This reverence for human life is expressed by the ceremonies and rituals accompanying birth and death. A child's birth symbolises a social event in the family and a special day is set aside to name the child and celebrate this great event. Relatives, friends, neighbours, and especially children are invited to these celebrations. Rwandans believe that life is 'God's gift'. This is expressed in some of the names commonly given to Rwandan children such as 'Habyarimana', 'Uwimana' meaning that 'only God can give and raise children'. Because only God can give life, He is also the only one who can take it away. Therefore, when a person dies, there is an expression in our language which says that he/she has 'responded to God's call'.

It's important to note that the concept of God in the traditional Rwandan religion (Imana) is different from the one introduced by Christianity. The 'Imana' is a supreme being, the creator and the sovereign of the universe, and most importantly the guardian of Rwanda. There is a common saying that 'God spends the day elsewhere but spends the night in Rwanda'. The idea of spending the night in Rwanda reflects the close relationship between God and the Rwandan people, since one generally sleeps at home at night.

This reading explores national and community efforts to facilitate bereavement recovery for the survivors of genocide and the family and friends of genocide victims in Rwanda. It draws on personal observations and reflections on the genocide commemoration events, as well as interviews with some of the students who survived the genocide, and who regularly visit the Kigali Institute of Science and Technology Counselling Centre. This Centre provides its students with counselling on various issues such as trauma, HIV/AIDS, and other issues related to their academic, family or social life.

Before writing about what is done to restore dignity to the genocide victims, and thus facilitating bereavement recovery for the survivors, it is important to put this into context by describing traditional Rwandan death rituals and how they have changed over the years.

Death rituals

Traditionally, a person's death was accompanied by a series of rituals and ceremonies that symbolised the value and respect accorded to human life. However, the traditional rituals relating to birth and death have been changing over time as a result of influences from various cultures, such as Christianity, which has had the greatest impact. Indeed, some of the traditional practices which were relevant and important to the Rwandan culture were lost during the Christianisation period, because they were considered to be pagan – and, therefore, nonsense. The end of the 1800s was marked by the invasion of the country, first by Germans and then by Belgians. This was the beginning a new era which was going to transform the Rwandans' way of living by introducing a new way of thinking and living. For example, when somebody died, their corpse was buried in the family compound. This was due to the traditional religious belief that a dead person's spirit stayed around watching on the living, especially if it was the father, who is considered the chief of the family. The dead could also interfere with the life of the surviving family members, so the family members would visit the tomb with gifts for the dead on a regular basis, to maintain a good relationship or to make peace with him/her. The relationship with the deceased, especially one's parents, also depended on the relationship prior to death, so people made sure that they were on good terms with their parents at the time of their death. A good relationship was a source of blessings whereas a bad one caused malediction. The belief that the dead continue to stay around and watch over the living was comforting to the survivors, especially those who were in need of protection, such as widows and orphans, even though they were generally taken care of by the extended family. Sadly, this practice no longer exists today whereby when somebody dies, their body is taken to a public cemetery.

The type of rituals performed generally depends upon the deceased person's religion, but the way of mourning the dead is generally the same. What is common, for example, is the way the community accompanies the bereaved family in their grief. There is a mourning period during which family members, friends and neighbours keep company with the bereaved family offering comfort to them and taking care of them. In the past, this period could even last for a whole year, and it was characterised by a series of rituals and prohibitions which were an expression of grief. As an instance, for a whole week, the deceased's family members stayed at his/her place offering each other mutual support. Day and night, a fire was kept burning in the yard and the people sat together around the fire. Initially, this fire was started to provide light and warmth to the mourners, but over time, it became a symbol of mourning.

The traditional mourning period was marked by a series of prohibitions, such as not having one's head shaved, not eating meat, not participating in any entertainment and avoiding strenuous labour, like working in the field. The cessation of all enjoyable activities was a way of acknowledging and processing grief, which facilitated the bereaved person's recovery. This mourning period has been shortened today, and generally lasts one week, while many prohibitions have also been omitted as a result of Christianity, Western education and a modern lifestyle. A few practices remain, such as not eating meat, remaining inside the home rather than walking visitors out, not clapping when somebody makes an address and avoiding washing one's clothes.

The end of the mourning period is characterised by a lot of cleaning, drinking, eating and celebrations which mark the resumption of normal life, and the beginning of a new life for the bereaved without the deceased. On that day, the fire torch that is kept burning during the mourning period is thrown far away from the bereaved people's homes to push death away. Also on that day, speeches are pronounced to comfort the bereaved and to encourage members of the community to continue extending moral and material support to them. It is also on that day that the deceased's successor is nominated according to his will to act as the chief of a family and this is generally a man – the deceased's son or his brother – as it is a patriarchal system.

During the 1994 genocide, however, all these mourning rituals were abdicated because people were continuously hiding and running away in an effort to ensure their survival. In addition, all the traditional taboos and mourning rituals were ignored by the perpetrators. Indeed, the respect usually paid to human life was denied to the victims who were slaughtered in a manner that would be unfit even to an animal. Their dead bodies were thrown carelessly, and tossed in mass graves, street drains and filthy latrines. In fact, in addition to the multiple losses they experienced, what upsets the genocide survivors most is the dehumanising conditions in which their loved ones died. A large number of the genocide survivors also experienced torture and abusive treatment themselves which has etched indelible scars on their minds and souls. Witnessing such horrific atrocities committed against themselves and their loved ones has taken a psychological toll on the survivors who continue to experience traumatic stress and chronic grief reactions such as flashbacks, nightmares, depression, anger, anxiety, loss of future perspective, headaches, stomach aches, and maladaptive coping mechanisms such as alcohol and other substance abuse. Indeed, the suddenness of the events coupled with the violence and mutilation, multiple deaths, and the ongoing threat to the survivors are significant factors that have contributed to the prevalence of traumatic grief symptoms among a large number of the genocide survivors. A woman survivor once said, 'I'm a living dead person' to mean that she was more dead than living, that part of her was dead despite the fact that she managed to survive. Indeed, she had no more hope, no more joy, no more meaning for life.

In order to facilitate the genocide survivors' recovery from traumatic grief, the government, jointly with the association of genocide survivors 'IBUKA' which means 'remember', has decided to designate a week for the genocide commemoration during which various activities are organised to remember the genocide victims. The genocide commemoration week, which is commonly called the 'mourning week' in Kinyarwanda (Rwanda's native language) extends from 7 to 13 April of each year. This week is marked by the lighting of a torch at Kigali genocide memorial that will keep burning for 100 days, which represents the length of time that the genocide lasted. During the commemoration week, the country is encouraged to stop and think about the genocide. Various activities are organised to acknowledge the genocide and to honour its victims: mourning wakes, visits to genocide sites, cleaning around the mass graves, public lectures on topics related to the genocide, even radio and television stations are only allowed to broadcast programmes relating to the genocide. Most importantly, the remains of the victims which are still scattered all over the country are exhumed and given a proper sepulture. Many mass graves are still being unearthed since the inception of the community participatory justice system (inspired by the traditional justice system 'Gacaca'). These remains are excavated and reburied in the presence of some perpetrators and bystanders who are encouraged to disclose their actions and/or what they witnessed. This justice system was created to expedite the trials of thousands of suspects whose jail sustenance was becoming a heavy burden on the government. However, the main purpose of the Gacaca system is to facilitate reconciliation in light of the Rwandan tradition, which dictates that all members of a family or community be involved in the mending of a broken relationship between any of its members.

Learning about the circumstances surrounding their loved ones' deaths, while publicly acknowledging the victims' deaths in the presence of the survivors, as well as burying their remains, has validated and alleviated some of the survivors' grief. They feel more satisfaction when their deceased loved ones are found, because the family can then carry out all the rituals in privacy and in a more personal way: washing the bones, taking pictures, or organising a wake at their home. Speaking about the genocide commemoration, one of the students explained:

> The genocide commemoration enables us to remember about our loved ones, to think about the good things they did for us. It also enables to vent out our emotions which have been blocked in our hearts because we were not able to express them at the time of the genocide. This is some relief for us.

Unfortunately, a large number of genocide survivors still have not found the remains of their loved ones. Indeed, due to the brutal nature of the violence, the bodies were generally thrown into mass graves, which makes it difficult to identify the individual remains more than a decade later. In addition, family members hid separately, so many of them don't really know what happened to their family members, relatives and friends. In fact, some people attend all the burials in their region in case one of their relatives might be among the victims. These survivors not only suffer from the loss of their loved ones, but also from the harsh reality that their remains may never be buried. This is considered the worst kind of loss, and the absence of a dead body prevents closure for the survivors while prolonging the grief process. One of the students expressed what she felt as follows:

> Not having been able to bury my relatives hurts and worries me a lot. I feel they judge me wherever they are because I've failed to give them back the dignity they were deprived from by their perpetrators.

Another student expressed his pain in these terms:

> I've nothing to remind me of my parents or brothers. I don't even know where they died. I suppose they lie somewhere in a mass grave. I hope so. Sometimes, I think that perhaps the bones of my loved ones are still lying on a hillside somewhere. My heart aches whenever I think of it.

Traditionally, not giving proper burial to the dead was also said to have bad repercussions on the living. However, when one of my counselling clients was asked if he felt any guilt for not having been able to find the remains of his relatives and if he was afraid it could have any impact on his life, he said there was nothing he could do about it, and further explained that those who killed them are the ones who should feel guilt for having deprived humanity to their fellow human beings. Although the majority of genocide survivors are not keen on revenge, some of them wish the perpetrators' cruel acts would bring doom to them, which is viewed as a form of natural justice being avenged by a fairer God. Others think that the justice system is too lenient on the perpetrators.

Burials are organised collectively and most members of the concerned community participate in them. Even if the genocide survivors were unable to bid a final farewell to their loved ones or mourn them at the time of their death, they feel somewhat comforted by the idea that their remains are buried with dignity and respect in a public place that is considered their final resting place. It also helps them to know that the atrocious death imposed on the victims is castigated by the Rwandan government and the larger global community. Furthermore, it is comforting to be mourning together as a country which provides a sense of solidarity and belonging, whereby one is part of a larger community that is united by shared sadness and sometimes even destiny. Although the genocide-related speeches and images evoke bad memories in the survivors' minds, who in some cases experience strong emotional crises, the commemoration activities facilitate healing overall, since it enables them to process their unresolved grief. Judging and punishing the perpetrators also gives the genocide survivors a sense of justice. However, most survivors I encounter have said that they wish the perpetrators, and all the other people involved in the genocide, would publicly confess their crime and ask for forgiveness. Alas, this wish is far from being granted! Only a small number of perpetrators have the courage to confess their criminal acts with a heartfelt sense of contrition. Unfortunately, the majority have confessed in order to reduce their prison sentence, while others continue to disseminate the genocide ideology.

Conclusion

In spite of these efforts and others (such as the Fund for Assistance to the Genocide Survivors and the work of the National Commission for Unity and Reconciliation), much still needs to be done to alleviate the psychological needs of genocide survivors. The mental health field was almost unknown in Rwanda before 1994 and became enhanced only after the genocide, but there still remains a scarcity of qualified mental health professionals. Given this human resource shortage, the majority of survivors continue to experience debilitating traumatic stress symptoms and complicated grief reactions which impair their daily lives and inhibit their capacity to contribute to society. Therefore, more policies need to be implemented to facilitate the mending of the national social fabric, and the recovery of all the components of the Rwandan society. These social policies should be community oriented, emphasising diplomatic measures as a means for resolving future civil and/or ethnic conflicts within a justice system of public accountability versus impunity for crimes committed against humanity.

26
The Making of Roadside Memorials

Jennifer Clark and Majella Franzmann

Those who make memorials for the victims of motor vehicle crashes assume an author-ity to do so that stems from three main elements of experience: the over-whelming empowerment of grief; the belief that the presence of the deceased can be felt and recognized: and the understanding that the place where life was lost is a special place for memorialization. The strength of grief, the power of presence and the importance of place allow ordinary people to assume and, therefore, challenge the authority of the church and the government as official purveyors and regulators of mourning ritual.

[...]

To this end, we have examined some 430 memorial sites across Australia and New Zealand and analyzed international newspaper accounts of the memorialization process. The aim of this paper is to suggest that memorial makers assert a self-proclaimed authority in order to perpetuate a loved-one's memory but we do not propose that this argument completely explains the emergence and growth of roadside memorials as a phenomenon. That is far more complex than our concerns here; rather, we want to argue that the memorials themselves and accounts of their construction demonstrate a willingness to express grief in individual and unprescribed ways that can constitute an assumption of, or challenge to, current authorities.

[...]

The authority of grief

The current practice of erecting roadside memorials challenges accepted ideas of the road-side as public not private space, as secular not sacred space, as somewhere that is nowhere in particular rather than a special place, and something that is passed by rather than perma-nently set aside as a place of pilgrimage, somewhere that Kennerly simply describes as 'between' (2002, p. 252). The erection of memorials can represent the explicit flouting of regulations and can also be interpreted as an implicit defiance of accepted roadside use as

Excerpts from 'Authority from grief, presence and place in the making of roadside memorials' by Jennifer Clark and Majella Franzman, *Death Studies*, 30: 584–99, 2006, Taylor & Francis, reprinted by kind permission of the publisher and Jennifer Clark (Taylor & Francis, www.informaworld.com).

well. In some cases, defiance can escalate into a dispute. In California, the father of Jennifer, a fourteen-year-old girl killed while jogging by the side of the road, was ordered to remove a large and growing memorial site or else face a fine of $1,000 and six months in jail. The County Deputy Director of Public Works, although aware of the emotional nature of the situation, explained: 'we're not in the memorial business, we're in the road business. I'm not insensitive, but I have got to enforce whatever the rules and regulations are.' Jennifer's father admitted that 'I guess they are bigger and stronger than we are,' but he could still claim the high moral ground of grief: 'I'm still grieving, but I'm still grieving for the next child to be killed' (Hughes, 2002, p. 1). He turned his attention to road safety advocacy. When Brandon Blount's father was asked by county officials to dismantle his son's memorial site, he refused, claiming he would chain himself to the memorial if necessary to prevent its removal. He subsequently began gathering signatures to pressure the state legislature to legalise roadside memorials. 'This memorial is so important to us,' explained Mrs. Blount, 'it's just not right to remove it' (Verhovek, 2000, p. 12). The implication of this and similar stories is that the mourning family has the moral authority to express their grief and that this should take precedence over government regulations and concerns.

Memorials may appear to be a popular expression in contradiction to the expectations of organized authority, but this does not mean they have complete communal endorsement. Public space may be regulated by the state but it is for the use of the wider community. The non-grieving can see memorials as an intrusion upon their space. In Ormeau in Queensland, Australia, nineteen-year-old Daniel was killed when a vehicle struck him as he walked home. His memorial was repeatedly vandalized, flowers were removed and Daniel's laminated photograph was pulled down. The vandal explained these actions in a note left at the scene: 'The community of Ormeau have endured this memorial site for one year and two months and we feel that is by far long enough' (Steele, 2001, p. 7). Daniel's parents claimed the right to grieve for as long as necessary. 'It's not always going to be there,' they explained 'but it should be up to take it down when we're ready' (Steele, 2001, p.7).

The common factor in all cases of private memorial building is grief. Grief is often described as an ordered process where emotions are encountered and worked through leading ultimately to restoration of some degree of normality achieved by accepting, managing and accommodating life after loss (Bowlby, 1980/81; Glick, Weiss, & Parkes, 1974; Pollock, 1987). Schuchter and Zisook (1993, p. 23) are less prescriptive, seeing grief expression as more varied, 'not a linear process with concrete boundaries but, rather, a composite of overlapping, fluid phrases that vary from person to person.' Still, those who experience the greatest difficulties in this process, however presented, are those whose loved ones died suddenly, unexpectedly and violently, for example, in car crashes (Hayslip, Ragow-O'Brien, 1998–99, p. 308; Stewart, 1999). Yet, they are the very ones who may take positive action and put energy and emotion into making and maintaining memorials. This positive response counters the emphasis on inability and debilitation including impaired decision making processes and increased morbidity, often associated with grief, especially (Kim and Jacobs, 1993; Middleton, Raphael, Martinek, and Misso, 1993, p. 55; Shuchter and Zisook, 1993). An overwhelming grief for someone tragically killed, for someone's life 'cut short,' appears to empower family and friends for behavior out of the ordinary, enough to overcome the usual reticence of people in the face of civil and religious authority.

Grief can equally empower and embolden in the face of unofficial criticism. Penny, the mother of Josh who died in a car crash in 2001, established a memorial for her son at the site of his death. She was distressed when a passerby criticized her for leaving flowers. 'I can still hear this woman saying to me', she wrote to the Herald Sun, '"I know this was sad, but it's not fair on me to have to look at these flowers."' 'Believe me,' wrote Penny, 'this is a lot more than "sad". How anybody feels they have the right to tell somebody not to place flowers where their child died is beyond me' (Martin, 2002). Grief can empower by possessing the mourner with higher moral knowledge. Support comes from those who know. 'I, too, lost a son in a car accident,' E. Pesch wrote to the paper in support of Josh's mother. 'I only hope the woman who complained to you never has to experience the heartache of losing a child under such circumstances' (Pesch, 2002, p. 28). This is the grief not fully assuaged by the church in a funeral or by the state in a cemetery or crematorium. This is grief empowering the mourner to find satisfying expression in individualized meaning making. 'Did this woman not stop to think,' wrote Sharon also in reply to Penny's lament 'that placing flowers at these sites is part of the grieving process these families must go through?' (Munro, 2002, p. 17). Both E. Pesch and Sharon confidently express the belief that they know something about grief that clearly 'this woman' does not—grief must be allowed to take its course and be expressed in its own way, unimpaired, unjudged and free. Mourners assume the authority to construct a memorial for private purposes in a public place for as long as they need it there. They are willing to take grief out of the confines of the cemetery and beyond the emotional and spiritual boundaries of the church, to construct for themselves a new sacred place fully recognizing that this process is open-ended and only those who grieve know when it is time to stop.

Authority of presence

The roadside is public, secular space, but memorial builders assume the authority to transfer this space into a sacred place. An empowering agent may be their own sense of spirituality informed by an eclectic knowledge of religion but not necessarily dictated by the practice or ideas of any one religion or denomination. Such eclecticism may, in fact, facilitate a more open sense of the spiritual (Saraswati, 2004). Without the dictates of any organized religion, mourners may be less restricted in their sense of what is appropriate. [...]

The sacred space of the memorial is often built upon a strong and explicit cosmology that incorporates a belief in this particular space as a kind of threshold between the world of the living and the world of the dead (Franzmann, 2004). The memorials 'are not simply remembrances along the roadside,' explained Kent Duryée, but rather they are 'signposts at intersections of the spiritual and material worlds in which we live' (Duryée, 'Shrines of the Desert'). There is material evidence at the memorial sites that communication with the deceased takes place, and that the deceased is believed to be present in some way and capable of receiving the communication. A most potent statement of the cosmology of the memorial is found in South East Queensland, Australia, where a doorknob is attached at the top of the vertical stake of the cross structure, indicating that at this spot there is a supported by an explicit text written directly under the doorknob: 'The door to heaven is now open Scotty RIP.' Scott's memorial cross is the message board and Scott both the receiver of messages and the link with the spirit world implicit in another message; 'Please say hi to nana.'

Very often memorials are signed, not unlike autograph books with little messages from family and friends. These messages may be static, in the sense they are composed at a set time, either at the time of the memorial's erection, or on a significant birthday or anniversary. 'Today would have been your thirtieth birthday our beautiful son,' wrote Brad's parents, 'Still can't believe you have left this earth.' One mother was so distraught after the death of her baby daughter that she wrote a long letter to the child apologising for her failure to 'get you home safe that night'. She wrenchingly expressed her ongoing love for the baby always referring to her in the present or future tense. She refused ot say goodbye because 'you will come back and visit me and talk to me.'

Alternatively, memorials frequently contain evidence of ongoing activity beyond their construction. New mementos may be added during visits to the memorial, so that the site grows and develops, sometimes decorated for seasonal holidays. Some mementos are left by friends, other by strangers who are simply moved by the occasion. The family may then take comfort from this ongoing display of affection (Morrison, 2005). Friends and family may visit the memorial site. Malcolm's mother regularly visits a memorial where a photo of her young son is pinned to a power pole. She takes his favourite meal there on his birthday and sits for a while just to talk to him and blow kisses (Thomas-Lester, 2000).

[...]

With the predominance of crosses at memorial sites, one might assume that these are Christian memorials, but where the crosses signify something more than a convenient structure upon which to hang flowers and cards, they are general markers of death and sacredness rather than purely Christian symbols. To characterize the sacred aspect of the roadside memorial, we are, perhaps, more correct in deeming it to be spiritual or religious in the general or broadest sense, rather than explicitly linked to any particular church or religious institution. Certainly, some who erect memorials use the cross with a clear Christian intent. When Keith erected simple white cross as a memorial to his son nine years after he was killed by a drunk driver it was specifically to make a statement of Christian forgiveness (Mickelburgh, 2000). Similarly, the memorial for Sarah-Lynee and James was erected following the practices and expectations of the Ringatu faith of New Zealand Maories. Other memorials have small Christian images hung around the neck of the cross or painted on it: another cross, a crucifix or Rosary beads. Such overt connections, however, are not common and it may be to misconstrue the general meaning of the cross to argue, as some do in the United States, that the erection of roadside crosses contravene the constitutional separation of church and state (Radford, 2001). Tom Horwood, from the Catholic Church in England and Wales, believes there is a remembered sense of the solemnity and sacredness of the cross set well apart from belief. 'Even if people have forgotten what the cross meant to Jesus,' he explained, 'we still know it is something sacred' (Rowe, 2000, p. 15). The memorial cross has become a symbol of amorphous spirituality easily detached from any particular institution. 'I put up a cross not just because I'm a Christian,' said crash survivor Jeremy Haddock, 'but because it is a universal symbol for what I feel' (Radford, 2001, p. 59). The use of the cross may, in fact, be little more than an attempt to find culturally appropriate symbols to express death and the sacred, where there is a paucity of such symbols apart from those offered by institutional religion. In any case, memorial makers under their own authority most often appropriate the

Christian symbol of the cross for their own purposes, except in Britain, where the incidence of a cross at a memorial site is low (Excell, 2005; Morrison, 2005).

Authority of place

In the memorials, the presence of the deceased is directly connected to the place where their life was lost. The actual spot becomes sacred and is imbued with ritualized meaning by the creation of a memorial marker as a focus for grief and communication. Memorial makers feel authorized to claim that place for the deceased regardless of the designated purpose of that space. 'The memorial is very bittersweet for me,' said Kendra's mother. 'It's where my daughter's life here on earth ended and her life in heaven started' (Thomas-Lester, 2000, p. COI). Many memorials explicitly focus on the paramount significance of the place of death. For example, Sheryl was 'tragically killed at this spot' or even more specifically, Mark 'died adjacent to this spot on the roadway as a result of a motor accident at 4.39 Thursday 26th March 1987.' In Sydney, Australia, a large white cross is spray painted on the asphalt of a car park on the exact place where Rodney crashed his car and was killed.[1] 'This will always be your spot' wrote 'Possum' to Conor and Adam on the banks of Kakahu River in New Zealand.

It appears that for many grieving families and friends the roadside memorial may be of greater significance than the cemetery or crematorium space where bodies or ashes reside. Perhaps this is so because burial customs have gradually lost some of their spiritual dimension and attachment to place. Before the nineteenth century the place to be buried was the churchyard within the precinct of hallowed ground, with other believers of like faith. A stranger could not be buried there, nor one who committed suicide, indicating the authority of the church over demographic and theological matters. The modern cemetery developed as an alternative burial place to accommodate those who could not meet the residency and theological requirements of the church. It was a democratized and secularized place even though, in some cases, it was divided into sections for Christian denominations or other religions. In the age of liberal capitalism anyone could ensure their burial, as a commodity to be bought, not a favor to be earned. The cemetery is a civil space, open to all, regardless of belief or unbelief. Thomas Laquer (1993, p. 190) argues that it does not 'speak of a place but of people from all places … unknown to each other in life and thrown together in a place with which they might have had only the most transitory acquaintance.'

For an increasing number of contemporary mourners the cemetery is divorced from the places and paraphernalia of personal meaning. Cemetery management may even regulate how the dead are remembered, restricting the size, structure and nature of memorialization to something that meets Council approval, so that there is little scope for individual expression. 'Everything's so orderly, so retrained,' wrote Peter Read (2003, p. 17) as he wandered through Gore Hill Cemetery at midnight, hunting spirits. In contrast, the roadside memorial is built with what Gerri Excell call 'the pagan, do-it-yourself element' (Morrison, 2005).

Memorials grow and spread, taking on a life of their own as a focus for action and contemplation. The place is the significant feature, the ground that must be claimed and ritualized in a variety of ways. Memorials contain items of personal significance including clothing or possessions belonging to the diseased. Candles are commonly found, sometimes ceremonially lit on a regular basis (Williams, 2002). It is quite common for groups of friends to gather at memorials in personal vigils to grieve together and to employ self-designed rituals in the process. Often beer or spirit bottles are left at the memorial where mourners have shared a last drink; one bottle regularly remains unopened. Poems are written and attached to the memorials. In one case in New Zealand the friends of the deceased participate in a memorial act by driving past his memorial at the same speed he was traveling when he was killed. These ritualistic acts are performed at the place where life was last known. [...]

The recent and current popularity of cremation in the West may increase the tendency to divorce death from place even further by completely disposing of the mortal remains and reducing the likelihood of a continued physical connection between the mourners and the deceased. Ariès (1974, p. 91) is sure that 'Cremation excludes a pilgrimage.' Perhaps somewhat paradoxically, the trend towards scattering ashes at a place of significance for the deceased suggests a desire to express the value of place in our lives and to honour that connection for the dead. In that sense, some cremation practices may actually facilitate the revaluation of place. While in others the memorial assumes the place of significance 'Our son was cremated,' explained Mrs. Blount when describing her feelings towards his road-side memorial. 'That's all we have left of him' (Verhovek, 2000, p. 12).

Roadside memorials bear silent witness to the importance of place. To say they only mark the scene of a fatal crash is far too rational, too bureaucratic, too realistic, too modern; rather, the relationship with place should be seen in personal and spiritual terms. The place becomes important because it is invested with the emotional energy of loss, grief and the process of remembering. Memorialization, may, in fact, be part of a fight against the depersonalizing process of modernization and urbanization. [...] [However] it is difficult for individuals to claim a significant place, partly because they are [...] marginalized in a bureaucratic society and partly because the place in question may be public space. How can an individual or a small group, such as a family or, as is often the case, a group of school friends, reclaim public, secular space as a significant place? Perhaps by demonstrating an emotional and spiritual connection with that space and marking it with the symbolic white cross so that it must draw respect. The roadside memorial can represent an act of reclamation.

Conclusion

[...]

There are, currently, poorly understood personal and institutional reasons why the roadside memorial phenomenon has emerged as a strong expression of public grieving, but what is clear from the evidence inherent in the memorials themselves and from accounts of their construction, is that memorial makers are prepared to assume their own authority to build, maintain and defend roadside memorials and that this authority taking can explicitly challenge the role of the government and bypass the church as the prime social purveyors and mediators of grief rituals. Although roadside memorials have a long history across vastly changing religious climates, what we can say is that during this period of declining religiosity personal spiritual expression can surface in a resurgence and remaking of a tradition that allows for personal and eclectic mourning. Roadside memorial builders are prepared to take the role of ritual creation and practice upon themselves. It is not so much that a roadside memorial is built as an overt spiritual expression, [...] but rather, its existence indicates a willingness to take spiritual matters out of the hands of the church and to divert spiritual energy in new directions. The memorial can then become a focus for spiritual activities and rituals, especially for young mourners.

The roadside memorial is a private expression of grief that turns a public place into sacred space; its sacred space; its sacredness directly constructed and controlled by people who would ordinarily make no claim to such civil or religious authority. The roadside memorial is an expression of our current search for meaning, an attempt to find a tangible focus for memory, to take time over mourning and to acknowledge publicly one's envelopment by grief. The transformation of the roadside into sacred space occurs because memorial makers find authority in their experience of grief, presence and place.

Note

1   We are grateful to Lindsay Varcoe for this information.

Reference

Ariès, P. (1974). *Western attitudes towards death from the middle ages to the present*. Baltimore: Johns Hopkins University Press.

Bowlby, J. (1980/81). *Attachment and Loss. Vol. 3, Loss sadness and depression*. London: Hogarth.

Duryée, K. *Shrines of the desert*. Retrieved March 20, 2003 from www.oriflamme.net/Shrines/body.index.html.

Excell, G. (September 15–17, 2005). *Contemporary deathscapes: comparing US, UK and Australian roadside memorials*. Paper delivered to The Social Context of Death, Dying and Disposal Conference, Bath, UK.

Franzmann, M. (1998). Diana in death – a new or greater goodness. *Australian Folklore, 13*, 112–123.

Glick, J.O., Weiss, R.S. and Parkes, C.M. (1974). *The first year of bereavement*. New York: Wiley.

Hayslip, B. Jr, Ragow-O'Brien, D., and Guarnaccia, C.A. (1998–1999). The Relationship of cause of death to attitudes towards funerals and bereavement adjustment. *Omega, 38*, 297–312.

Hughes, T. (April 7, 2002). Roadside tributes raise safety issue. *Los Angeles Times,* part 2, p. 1.

Kennerly, R.M. (2002). Getting Messy: In the field and at the crossroads with roadside shrines. *Text and Performance Quarterly, 22*, 229–260.

Kim, K. and Jacobs, S. (1993). Neuroendocrine changes following bereavement. In W. Stroebe & R.O. Hansson (eds), *Handbook of bereavement*. Cambridge: Cambridge University Press.

Laquer, T.W. (1993). Cemeteries, religion and the culture of capitalism. In J. Garnett & C. Matthew (eds), *Revival and religion since 1700*. London: Hambledon Press.

Martin, P. (February 25, 2002). Roadside memorials. *Herald Sun* (Melbourne), p. 17.

Mickelburgh, R. (February 13, 2000). *A public grieving*. *Sunday Mail* [Queensland, Australia p. 6.]

Middleton, W., Raphael, D. and Marunek and Misse, V. (1993) Pathological grief restrictions. In W. Stroebe and R.O. Hansen (eds), *Handbook of bereavement*. Cambridge. Cambridge University Press.

Morrison, B. (November 4, 2005). Saying it with flowers. *Guardian*, Retrieved January 10, 2005 from http://guardian.co.uk/print /0,3858,5324483-103639,00.html.

Munro, S. (February 27 2002). Lack of emotion [Letter to the editor]. *Herald Sun* (Melbourne), p. 17.

Pesch, E. (March 2, 2002). Memorials helpful [Letter to the editor]. *Herald Sun* (Melbourne), p. 28.

Pollock, G.H. (1987). The mourning-liberation process in health and disease. *Psychiatric Clients of North America, 10,* 345–354.

Radford, B. (2001). Religion on the roadside: Traffic fatality markers generate controversy. *Free Inquiry, 22*, 59.

Read, P. (2003). *Haunted Earth*. Sydney: University of New South Wales Press.

Rowe, M. (September 10, 2000). Roadside flowers and plaques for accident victims multiply as shrine culture takes hold. *The Independent* (London),p. 15.

Saraswati, A. (June 25–27, 2004). A personal journey: Multiple rituals following a roadside death. Paper delivered to the First International Symposium on Roadside Memorials, Armidale, Australia.

Shuchter, S.R. and Zisook, S. (1993). The course of normal grief. In W.Stroebe & R.O. Hansson (eds), *Handbook of bereavement: Theory, research and intervention*. Cambridge: Cambridge University Press.

Steele, S. (February 11, 2001). Hard road – vandals target memorials. *Sunday Mail* (Brisbane), p. 7.

Stewart, A.E. (1999). Complicated bereavement and posttraumatic stress disorder following fatal car crashes; Recommendations for death notification practice. *Death Studies, 23,* 289–321.

Thomas-Lester, A. (May 28, 2000). Makers of Grief; each memorial tells a story – and offers a warning. *Washington Post,* p. COI.

Verhovek, S.H. (June 23, 2000). A cross on the roadside, and a continuing grief. *The New York Times,* Section A, Column 1, p. 12.

Williams, D. (June 10, 2002). Drive-by 'salutes' worry police. *Nelson Mail* (New Zealand). Retrieved June 10, 2002 from http://www.stuff.co.nz/inl/index/0,1008,1194362a1540,FF.html.

27
Online Memorialisation

Kylie Veale

In the recent past, memorialisation is largely practised via granite, marble or bronze memorials in cemeteries, requiring physical visits that can be impeded by distance or physical ability. In a society that is increasingly fragmented where families and friends, often separated by significant distances, cannot actively participate in memorialising their deceased an alternate space to the physical needs to be provided.

Several authors claim this alternate space is cyberspace. I therefore ask: how and why do memorials exist there? Is there a link between physical and online memorialisation? What kind of memorialisatoin space is emerging online? To consider these questions, this presents findings from an investigation of online memorialisation. A unique model was created based on an analysis of the work of several authors, using their definitions of memorialisation and their discussions of the motivations and characteristics of traditional memorial practices. The resulting Memorial Attribute Model was then used to understand how the web is being used as a memorialisation space. Why memorialisation may have been adopted online is then considered. In addition, I outline possible links between the remembrance of the dead in the physical space and online.

Memorialisation practice

As a form of meaningful and personal communication, memorialisation helps those who experience the death of a loved one to fight through the stages of the grieving process, providing a means to express deeply felt emotion and to honour the deceased. Memorials provide a permanent place for those left behind to connect emotionally and spiritually with their loss. They also provide an opportunity to honour and pay tribute to a person and make a statement about the impact that person had on his or her family, community, or even the world. Moreover, Ruby (1995) explains that mourners are confronted by two very contradictory needs when someone dies: to keep the memory of the deceased alive, and, at the same time, accept the reality of death and loss.

'Online memorialisation' by Kylie Veale, *Fibreculture*, Issue 3 [extract]. Reprinted by kind permission of the author and journal.

So what can cyberspace offer memorialisation? Cyberspace lacks physicality but, as Wertheim (1999) contends, cyberspace can be a spiritual space. Several authors agree this notion extends to memorialisation practice. Hallam and Hockey (2001) note that the internet offers the ability to memorialise in a public place, where anyone can visit at any time, without imposition to others, and without interruption to themselves. While Wertheim claims therapy is a quintessentially lonely experience, the author also suggests people crave something communal; something that will link their minds to others. As a result, while working 'on one's own personal demons … many people seem to want a collective mental arena, a space they might share [and I suggest, also grieve] with other minds' (1999: 233).

Academics have proven the web can be specifically used for the practice of memorialisation. Geser's (1988) early work suggests the web 'may enlarge the scope of cultural expression to new spheres of thoughts and emotions, hitherto hidden in the privacy of individual minds or informal interpersonal relations', thus providing a more enriched environment in which to memorialise the dead. The impulse to create some form of memorial to the dead seems to be nearly universal across all cultures to Marshall (2000), who indicates he is not surprised that websites as online memorials 'have sprung into existence'. In his proposal for studying the Israeli culture of mourning and memorialisation on the Internet, Sade-Beck says that 'the Internet is a new tool for the direct expression of emotions' (2003: 9).

So as cyberspace seems conductive to memorialising the deceased, how has the practice actually manifested online? This question brings me to the first task of this paper – using a model of memorial motivation and characteristics to investigate how memorials exist in cyberspace. A number of principle were ütilised to create a unique method, the Memorial Attribute Model: firstly, an analysis of memorial definitions from several authors (see Davies, 1994; Friedman and James, 2002; Ruby, 1995); secondly, an analysis of the stages of the grieving process in foundation works such as van Gennep (1960) and Kübler-Ross (1969); and finally, the model incorporates a consideration of the aforementioned specific works of Geser, Marshall and Sade-Beck. As a result, the Memorial Attribute Model consists of a list of memorial motivations and characteristics, creating two hypotheses relating to how memorials exist in cyberspace:

1   Memorials manifest online as a result of one or more of four motivations: grief, bereavement and loss; unfinished business; living social presence; and/or historical significance.
2   Online memorials adhere to one or more memorial characteristics: invoking remembrance; a demonstrable array of kinships; and/or as a surrogate for the deceased.

Each motivation and characteristic was applied to random websites claiming to be memorials, found through Google's 'search engine' and using a set of identified search terms.[1] Memorial 'gateways' (websites providing portal-like access to a number of related websites) were also utilised to find memorial content. In exploring each feature of the Memorial Attribute Model, references to memorials in the physical world, the web's predecessor in this field, are incorporated for illustrative and comparison purposes.

How memorialisation manifests online

Memorial motivations

From my brief analysis of the works of van Gennep and Kübler-Ross, I observe in the first instance that coping with grief and loss is perhaps the main impetus for memorials online. Certainly, memorialisation 'helps the bereaved to recover from their grief by providing a pleasant "memory picture"' (Metcalf and Huntington, 1991: 54) to reflect on, and can allow others to express their sympathy and consolation through active participation in the grieving process. Online memorials created in times of grief and bereavement are found through examples of online memorial text. Just as Kübler-Ross explains the five stages of grief, websites found during my investigation adhere to one or more of these stages, supporting their usage as self-help throughout the grieving process.

Expressions of denial are found on many websites, symbolised by phrases such as 'I still can't believe you're gone' (Tracy, n.d.; Woznick, n.d.). Additionally, idioms such as 'I would do anything' feature as messages on memorial texts in the bargaining stage of grief and bereavement, and the bereaved also write about how their life cannot go on after the death event. And finally, in the last stage of acceptance, acknowledgements that the deceased is not coming back are typical: 'and now I … understand that you're not coming back … ever' (Johnson, n.d.).

Secondly, Kübler-Ross notes within some communities, those who care about the deceased may need help in completing unfinished business. Kuenning (1987) agrees that a sudden death may leave the survivor with many regrets, a sense of unfinished business, and no time for an orderly farewell. Memorialisation can therefore be an outlet for those with unfinished business with the deceased to action towards completing it. Items such as personalised epitaphs, written letters placed graveside or journals created to work through the unresolved issues, are active and physical displays of this memorialsation motivation. Similarly, in his content categorisation of the Virtual Memorial Garden, Marshall uncovers that most memorials were either light or dark in tone. Light-toned memorials were often joyful dialogues about the deceased, whereas dark-toned memorials were 'often apologies, regrets and even confessions'.

The tone of the memorial is especially important when we consider unfinished business as memorial content. Online confessions of unrequited love, last-word regrets and missed opportunities for meeting the deceased are often found, for instance.

> I remembered that day as if it were yesterday. We said a lot of words, you and I. I would love the opportunity to take a lot of them back. My greatest regret is that the last words I ever said to you was that I never wanted to see you again. (In Loving Memory of DebraAnn, n.d.)

The tone of the memorial is also important when we consider that memorials have regularly been used as opportunities for conversations with the dead. In their personalised epitaphs and graveside letters, the living speak to the dead as if they were still alive, as the memorials become a 'living' social presence for the deceased. Epitaphs are written as personal, lasting messages, and as I have already mentioned, as an outlet for those with unfinished business with the deceased.

The online memorial created for a young lady who died in 1997 serves as an example (see Amanda Joy Alstatt), to which her father and brother often leave, messages on her memorial message board. Their messages are conversional in nature, as they 'talk' to her about family news and the day-to-day goings on in their lives:

> Amanda. Yea, it is me Daddy.. I know you know about the new and wonderful news. Pretty awesome, huh! That is it for now! ...

> Hi Amanda it's me Matthew, I started highschool [*sic*] on August 11th. I'm ... now in 9th grade and I'm 14 ...

Aside from mourning, grief and bereavement, memorialisation can occur on grounds of historical significance, the model's final memorialisation motivation. The maintenance of the past as a living memory is of essential importance in the life of a group and individuals. Knowing about origins, past achievements, and mistakes, allows us to understand ourselves as links in the chain of generations (Von Eckartsberg, 1988). In this way, the concept of deliberate memorialisation (see Cosslett, 2002; Searl, 2000) lends itself to historical motives, that is, dedicating a special place to the memory of someone and, in turn, strengthening the fragile bonds of memory that link the generations. This type of memorialisation can occur immediately after a death, though as Cosslett suggests, it often involves 'deliberate attempts to recapture lost memory' (2002: 252), years beyond when the actual person died.

The web is also used to memorialise everyday people from history. In the case of the historical section of The Officer Down Memorial Page www.odmp.org, memorials serve as reminders of the everyday risks facing law-enforcement officers, by establishing a sense of past in the duties still completed today. Consider Deputy Keeper James B. Lippincott (The Officer Down Memorial Page Inc, 2003), who was killed by gunfire Friday, March 2, 1894. He has been memorialised online since 2003, despite his death occurring nearly 110 years ago.

In summary, and while they are not proven to be exhaustive, online memorialisations are found to be created as a consequence of one or more motivations; grief, bereavement and loss; unfinished business; living social presence; and/or historical significance. To further investigate how memorialisation exists on the web, I present the second hypothesis of the Memorial Attribute Model, in terms of investigating three physical memorial characteristics in cyberspace.

Memorial characteristics

In the first instance, from my analysis of the work of van Gennep and Kübler-Ross, a memorial should be a catalyst for invoking memory and remembrance, due to its past or present proximity to the deceased. Property that used to belong to the deceased may invoke memories of them. The very act of visiting a grave places the deceased immediately into the memory of the visitor, due to the proximity of the deceased to the memorial. Though what of the Internet? What of a space that lacks physicality?

Similar to photo albums depicting the life of the deceased at funerals, I find online memorials mitigating their lack of proximity to the deceased by providing a vast array of textual and visual remembrances. A montage of photos, sounds and video reflects the personal values of the deceased, and hence bring into play perhaps more remembrance than a static physical memorial.

Every memorial website I visited contained at least one picture of the deceased, though many also included photos of family, and images depicting the deceased in a positive light, allowing family and friends to relive their experiences and reflect. MIDI and WAV files play songs favoured by the deceased when memorial pages open in the browser, and visitors are given the opportunity to view home videos of the person, uploaded by family and friends from personal video cameras. Similarly, technology has also enabled an everlasting reminder of the exact time the person died, beyond the static death date on most physical memorials. Using time-counters to display the exact time elapsed since the event of their death, a link between the virtual and physical space occurs, complete with second-by-second adjustments as life in the physical space continues. For example:

> 1653 days, 14 hours, 28 minutes, and 12 seconds have passed since Robbie went to heaven. (Smith, n.d.)

Perhaps the most significant memorial characteristic is that memorials are generally surrogates for the dead. Certainly in previous research (Veale, 2003), headstones are found as representations, markers or substitutes for the dead, containing one or more descriptors as information about the deceased. These surrogate descriptors, or inscriptions in the context of general memorialisation, are often crucial in establishing relationships between the memory object and the subject to be remembered. In any case, I suggest surrogate form, content and context has a profound effect upon the ways in which a memorial works as a surrogate.

Examples of memorials as surrogates for the deceased abound on the web, and the presence of this characteristic is perhaps the largest evidence of how memorialisation exists in that space. At a minimum, memorial websites contain the name and/or photo of the deceased, along with their birth and death date. However, websites are also found to contain biographies; some even chronicling the deceased's whole life from birth (see Conaway-Cameron, 2003).

Continuing the concept of memorial as surrogate, outward displays of kinship are a generally a part of traditional memorials. In a time where privacy laws and identity protection are paramount, I expected this particular memorial characteristic to be invisible on the web and thus be specifically inferior to physical memorials. Demonstrable kinships on online memorials however are similar, if not superior, to traditional memorials in this instance, due the increased space available for memorial text. They are also similar in that they contain a mix of detailed kinships. For example, in terms of specifically named relationships:

> He was the fourth child and third son of Samuel L. Diggle and Marie Louise Cobb. (Diggle (1914–1993))

And, generalised kinships:

> This page is dedicated to the memories of my beautiful granddaughter. (Stempien, n.d.)

In the same way, some online memorials (see Dube, 2002) contain links to the memorials of other deceased family members on the web, thereby stating familial relationships in the form of hyperlinks.

To summarise the above findings, websites are found to portray one or more of the Memorial Attribute Model's three characteristics – remembrance; a demonstrable array of kinships; and/or as a surrogate for the deceased. These findings however, in addition to the aforementioned five memorial motivations, raise additional questions. Why is cyberspace used for memorialisation? Are there links between the physical and virtual space? Does the existence of online memorialsation change traditional memorialisation practice? The following section attempts to explore these questions.

Why memorialisation manifests online

In a world where physical memorials can cost hundreds or thousands of dollars (Ryle, 2002), require physical attendance, and are subject to degradation and desecration, the web can be considered an additional or alternate space to memorialise the dead. To explain, I propose timeliness, cost, accessibility, and creativity as advantages of memorialising online.

Perhaps the most prevailing advantage of cyberspace for memorialisation is that the Internet, as a space, allows quick if not instant content creation, unlimited editing and updating, and a lifespan that is not subject to the degradation of the physical world.[3] Unlike physical memorials, which are erected at one point of time and generally remain unchanged, the interactive and communicative nature of the Internet allows online content be amended and added to, in subsequent periods of memorialisation.

After the initial creation of an online memorial during times of grief and bereavement, additional reflection and content is often added to create an enduring and expanding space for the deceased. For example, a memorial to SIDS infant Jordan Joseph Miller (see Miller, n.d.) contains messages authored on the anniversary of his death, over some four years since he died in 1994. Not only are memorials fluctuating and adaptive online, they are also a timely intermediary until a physical memorial is erected. As one bereaved person said in response to the World Trade Center site becoming inaccessible after the September 11 terrorist attacks: 'What are we supposed to do between now and when the actual physical memorial is there?' (Frangos, 2004). I contend that cyberspace allows memorial websites to be created more quickly than physical memorials. Within three months of the terrorist attacks, a large number of websites were erected as online memorials. Thus, in times quicker than physical memorials could be erected, the web was utilised to quickly and easily create memorialisation spaces. Similarly, online memorials do not cost as much as the physical to erect.

Furthermore, perhaps in part to the aforesaid time and cost considerations and the increasing number of people accessing to the Internet, the web as a memorialisation space is also more open and available to a diverse group of people than physical memorials. As Marshall explains, online 'memorials are often created by people unable to attend funerals [and] who live far away from the burial place'.

As a result, funerary web-casting has become popular online, as a way to participate in memorialisation practice virtually. Made available via Internet technology, funerary web-casting enables a funeral service to be watched live through the use of webcams, as downloadable files in an online or at a later date from a recording of the service. They are often supplementary material to online websites, archive of the memorial service. In fact, Karen Kasel made a funeral webcast available for the family of her deceased mother, because:

> It cost[s] money to drop everything and come to a funeral. It's difficult in this day and age of everyone living so far away. I think it's just wonderful that [the family] were seeing this. You get the feel of the whole service. (Ordonez, 2002)

We must consider however the possibility that physical memorialisation is superior to the online, because of the proximity of the memorial to the deceased. That is, online memorials may not seem 'real' to the bereaved, who may believe that their loved one is where the physical remains are located. Though, just as graves and static memorials can evoke memory through limited content and proximity to the deceased, I find the interactive nature of online memorials require less and less memory and imagination of the living. Consequently, photos, text, video, and sights and sounds make for an emotion-charging experience for the bereaved, and indeed any visitor to an online memorial, allowing the memories to be created for them, and perhaps mitigating the issues surrounding lack of proximity to the deceased.

Timeliness, cost, accessibility and creativity are not the only advantages of online memorialisation however. The web is also a favourable medium for preserving existing physical memorials from degradation and desecration. Physical cemeteries are fast becoming areas of disrepair, and preservationists are working to transfer the information in these places to electronic repositories – such as databases and virtual cemeteries thus preserving historical memory.

Finally, although I have been considering the web as an additional or alternate space to memorialise the dead, are physical and online memorialisation distinct and disparate rituals? Or are they utilised in collaboration to enhance memorialisation practice? In fact, physical space and cyberspace work in symbiosis on many occasions. Concisely, cyberspace, and specifically the web, provides numerous advantages to traditional (physical) memorialisation practice, in terms of timeliness, cost, accessibility, and a broader spectrum of creativity.

Conclusion

While millions of people die per year and a majority of those in the past were lost to anonymity, Internet technology is ensuring that every one of them and their descendants roaming the Earth today have the opportunity to be immortalised in some form. Their life can be commemorated online, on the event of their death in the physical world, and remembered by the general public via online memorials. In a society that is increasingly fragmented and where families and friends, often separated by significant distances, cannot actively participate in physical memorialisation, cyberspace is an available and effective space for memorialising the deceased.

Notes

1   Search terms used were: memorial, memorialisation, memorialising, tribute, 'In Loving Memory Of', 'To The Memory Of'.
2   This assertion assumes, of course, the management and financial responsibilities of the online resource are covered and continued for the life of the online memorial.

References

Alstatt, Amanda Joy (15 March, 1981–5 June 1997).
http://virtual-memorials.com/servlet/ViewMemorials?memid=6142&pageno=4
Conaway-Cameron, Suzie (2 August 2003), www.hist.umn.edu/~lek/suzie.htm
Cosslett, Tess (2002) '"History from below": time-slip narratives and national identity', *The Lion and the Unicorn*, 26(2): 243–5.
Davies, Jon (1994) 'One hundred billion dead: a theology of death', in Jon Davies (ed.), Ritual and Rememberence: *Responses to Death in Human Societies*. Sheffield: Sheffield Academic Press.
Diggle, Robert Bernard (1914–1993) Perpetual Memorial Websites www.memorials.com/diggle/index.htm
Dube, Edward Herbert (13 March 2002), www.angelfire.com/vt/busylizzie/link6.html
Frangos, Alex (2004) 'Three years on: memorials give comfort'. *The Wall Street Journal Online*, http://homes.wsi.com/propertyreport/architecture/20040913-frangos.html
Friedman, Russell and James, John W. (2002) 'Conclusionary rituals: things you need to know about funerals and memorial services', www.grief-recovery.com/Articles/conclusionaryrituals.htm
Geser, Hans (1998) 'Yours virtually forever: death memorials and remembrance sites in the WWW', online publication, http://socio.ch/intcom/thgeser07.htm
Hallam, Elizebeth and Hockey, Jenny (2001) *Death, Memory & Material Culture* (Oxford: Berg Publishers).
In Loving Memory of DebraAnn (n.d.) http://griefnet.Org/memorials/2003b/apr22-0590724320.html
Johnson, Debbi Hood (n.d.) 'Memorial for Bob "BJ" Johnson (AIDS)', http://gbgm-umc.org/cam/memorials/johnsononbi.html
Kübler-Ross, Elizabeth (1969) *On Death and Dying*. New York: Macmillan.
Kuenning, Delores (1987) *Helping people through grief*. Bloomington: Bethany House.
Marshall, Lindsay (14 December 2000) 'Some shadow of eternity: the internet and memorials to the dead', www.cs.ncl.ac.uk/research/pubs/trs/papers/718.pdf
Metcalf, Peter and Huntington, Richard (1991) *Celebration of Death: The Anthropology of Mortuary Ritual*. Cambridge: Cambridge University Press.
Miller, Jessica (n.d.) 'Jordon 1', www.geocities.com/South Beach/Shores/7972/jordon1.html
The Officer Down Memorial Page Inc. 'Deputy Keeper James B. Lippincott', 13 October (2003), www.odmp.org/reflections.php?oid=16848

Ordonez, F. (17 April 2002) Taking the funeral to the mourners', www.im.columbia.edu/student work/cns/2002-04-17/378.asp

Ramsland, K. (2002) 'Be a stud after death: creative use of remains', www.funeralserviceprofessional. com/FuneralServiceNews32902.html

Ruby, Jay (1995) *Secure the Shadow: Death and Photography in America*. Cambridge, MA: Massachusetts Institute of Technology.

Ryle, Gerard (2002) 'Six feet down under: call for an inquiry into the high cost of dying', *Sydney Morning Herald*, 30 September, www.smh.com.au/articles/2002/09/29/1033283388485.html

Sade-Beck, Liav (2003) 'Mourning and memorial culture on the Internet: The Israeli case', http://burdacenter.bgu.ac.il/publications/proposals2002–2003/Sade-Beck.pdf

Searl, Ed (2000) 'Reclaiming death', *Conscious Choice* online publication, www.consciouschoice. com/issues/cc1310/reclaimingdeath1310.html

Smith, Robbie (n.d), http://robbiehsmith.com

Tracy, Alice (n.d.) 'D Tracy Memorial', www.geocities.com/prisonmurder/dtracymemorial.html

van Gennep, Arnold (1960) *The Rites of Passage*. Chicago: University of Chicago press.

Veale, Kylie J. (2003) 'A virtual adaptation of a physical cemetery for diverse researchers using information science methods', *Computers in Genealogy*, B(4): 136–58.

Von Eckartsberg, Rolf (1998) 'Social and electronic immortality 'Online publication'. www.earth portal Messenger/immortal.html

Wertheim, Margaret (1999) *The Pearly Gates of Cyberspace: A History of Space from Dante to the Internet*. Sydney: Doubleday.

Woznick, connie (n.d.) 'Kenny, my son, taken too soon', www.webhealing.com/hon/conn.html.

Part V
Researching Death, Dying and Bereavement

Introduction

Sarah Earle

Research offers the potential to develop a sound evidence base which can underpin development in policy and practice. Practitioners, researchers, potential research participants, and their families and carers can all play a vital role in this process. The readings within this part of the book explore some of the dilemmas in research on death, dying and bereavement, offering insight into the ways in which these dilemmas can be overcome.

Part V begins by focusing on the key challenges in researching end-of-life issues. Reading 28, written by Marilyn Kendall and colleagues, starts by noting the limitations within the current literature, insofar as it lacks attention to the practicalities of carrying out research at the end of life. Drawing on a qualitative research study of researchers, patients and carers, Kendall and colleagues outline some of the barriers to conducting research in this area and offer suggestions for overcoming these. The authors argue that death and dying is surrounded by 'personal and social taboos' which can hinder research and, in particular, report that health professionals can act as 'overzealous gatekeepers' seeking to protect 'vulnerable', dying people. This reading challenges the notion of vulnerability and explores some of the issues relating to research design, methodology (the analysis of research methods) and ethical conduct in research at the end of life. The reading also highlights the difficulty of defining the 'end of life' and the impact of this for research.

Reading 29, by Margo J. Milne and Cathy E. Lloyd, examines the concept of respondent burden which they define as 'the sum of the physical, economic and/or psychological hardships associated with research participation'. Continuing to challenge the notion of vulnerability at the end of life, Milne and Lloyd explore the issue of researching 'sensitive' topics and ask the question: 'is death and dying a sensitive issue?' The authors review the literature in this area and conclude that participation in research at the end of life may not be as distressing as might be imagined and, in fact, that the personal costs may be outweighed by the benefits of participating in such research. In this reading Milne and Lloyd explore some of the ways in which researchers can seek to minimise the respondent burden. They also highlight the need to think about the costs to researchers working in the field.

Following on from this, the next reading focuses specifically on the role of the researcher in loss and grief research. Reading 30, by Louise Rowling, argues that while considerable attention is given to the needs of participants, little attention is paid to researchers' needs and experiences. Drawing on a qualitative research study of loss and grief in school communities in New South Wales, Australia, this reading focuses, in particular, on the role of empathy in research and the management of emotions. The author discusses the difficulty for researchers in managing their own feelings when respondents disclose personal and intimate stories of grief. And, as noted in the reading by Milne and Lloyd, Rowling suggests that participants can often benefit greatly from participating in research which involves 'telling their stories'.

In Reading 31, Judith Dorrell and colleagues draw on a qualitative study of young people living with HIV carried out in the UK. Drawing on interview data, the authors explore the importance of death, dying and bereavement in a study designed to focus on the affect of HIV on daily life, relationships, schooling and work, rather than on the issues of primary concern within this book. Focusing on two specific themes, Dorrell and colleagues explore the concepts of 'living with dying' and 'living with loss' discussing how these affect young people's lives. The reading concludes by highlighting that while living with HIV might only be one aspect of a person's life, it can serve to heighten young people's sense of mortality.

In the first reading in this part of the book Marilyn Kendall and colleagues suggest that the taboo of death and dying plays a significant role in research at the end of life. Whether this is generally true, or not, Reading 32 explores this issue further by focusing on the absence of death and dying in intellectual disability research. Stuart Todd begins his reading by arguing that the way in which society deals with death can tell us much about the nature of that society and, furthermore, that the social characteristics of people who are dying may well influence their care at the end of life. Exploring the concept of social death, Todd asks whether the neglect of death and dying in relation to people with intellectual disabilities (and their families and carers) reflects the symbolic and social death which hovers over their lives already. Todd concludes by arguing that the deaths of people with intellectual disabilities are not taboo, but devalued, and urges for the end of a 'death-free zone' when researching and caring for people with intellectual disabilities.

In Reading 33 Gayle Letherby focuses on the social and emotional experiences of reproductive loss, offering reflections on her auto/biographical work in this area as well as a critique of some of the literature in this field. The reading explores a wide range of issues including the difficulty of definition, a concern also identified by the authors of Reading 28, and the relationship between method and methodology; highlighting the importance of choosing methods which fit the needs of research, rather than the other way around. Letherby also discusses the importance of bringing men 'back in' to research on reproductive loss, which is often only defined as an experience which affects women. Concluding her reading, Letherby strongly urges researchers to 'make research count' in policy and practice settings, as well as in academic ones.

The final reading further examines the relationship between research and practice. Focusing specifically on bereavement research, Reading 34 by the Bridging Work Group notes that many practitioners regard research as irrelevant to their work and that many researchers believe that practice bears little relevance to the scholarly study of bereavement. However, the Bridging Work Group suggests that researchers and practitioners have much to learn from each other. In particular, they suggest that practitioners should expose themselves to research which has the potential to change and improve practice, as well as equip themselves – through learning, training and education – to critically evaluate the findings of such research studies. Similarly, they recommend that researchers should expose themselves to the experiences of practitioners working at the end of life, designing research that is relevant to the needs of practitioners and other stakeholders.

28

Key Challenges and Ways Forward in Researching the 'Good Death'

Marilyn Kendall, Fiona Harris, Kirsty Boyd, Aziz Sheikh, Scott A. Murray, Duncan Brown, Ian Mallinson, Nora Kearney and Allison Worth

Introduction

When an editorial in the *BMJ* posed the question, 'What is a good death?'[1] contributors concluded that we cannot answer this as we lack the necessary evidence from research, especially from the perspective of patients and carers.[2] Achieving a comfortable and dignified death requires research that supports the development of end of life care as an evidence based specialty.[1,3] It was in direct response to the *BMJ* good death theme issue that Macmillan Cancer Relief commissioned us to explore the reasons behind this lack of research evidence in end of life care.

Practical, ethical, methodological, and emotional difficulties are experienced by those conducting research into the end of life.[4-9] Clark called for more qualitative research with patients and families, cross cultural research, longitudinal studies that can identify the changing needs of patients and families, and the use of innovative methods that examine the difficulties of research in palliative care settings.[1] With some notable exceptions, however, few researchers have written specifically about the challenges involved with conducting end of life research.[6,8-10] This was confirmed by a systematic literature review in which we identified only small numbers of publications related to the practicalities of conducting such research.[11]

Methods

Methodological approach

We used qualitative methods to learn about the experiences, perceptions, and practice of relevant researchers and the views of people approaching the end of life and their carers. We defined end of life broadly as the months before the death of patients with advanced illness, whether or not they were receiving palliative care. We explored issues relating to research conducted with people in the last months to the last days of life and in bereavement.

Sampling and data generation

We identified a purposive sample of 34 researchers and completed interviews with 32 (Table 28.1). One person declined for personal reasons, and another was unavailable during the period of the study. Initially the researchers were identified from our systematic literature review,[11] which aimed to determine what methods are being used in cancer studies and how best to include the views of patients in the development of services. We included papers on research methods published in 1980–2004 that sought the views of people affected by cancer about end of life issues. This enabled us to identify researchers from a range of disciplines who were using diverse approaches to conducting end of life research. Some were researchers of international standing, who were asked to reflect on their own research experience and give an overview as managers of many projects; others were comparatively junior researchers with more current 'hands-on' experience. Many had also worked on non-cancer research. To follow up themes emerging from early interviews and to include more non-cancer work, we interviewed two transcribers and researchers with experience of working in specialties such as HIV/AIDS, dementia, and education, thus enabling us to learn from research methods in other sensitive subjects.

To complement the researchers' perspectives and to include the experience of patients and carers we held four focus groups that explored a range of users' views of the best ways to conduct research. Day hospice staff recruited a group of four patients with advanced cancer. They met on two occasions, firstly to discuss ways of conducting research and then to validate the researcher's interpretation of the discussion. The second group, of three patients specifically interested in research, was recruited from a cancer network database. The third group, consisting of four carers, was recruited through a community palliative care team.

FH conducted the interviews by telephone or face to face and also facilitated the service user focus groups. […]

Data analysis

The interviews with researchers and the focus group discussions were recorded, fully transcribed with accompanying field notes, and entered into NVivo version 2. We integrated, coded, and thematically analysed both datasets using an interpretive approach and a coding scheme derived both from the research questions and from issues that emerged during data generation and early analysis.[12] An anthropologist (FH) led the analysis with the ongoing involvement and input of two members of the research team with backgrounds in sociology and nursing and extensive experience of end of life research (MK and AW). We all regularly discussed emerging themes to include multidisciplinary perspectives (including patients, palliative medicine, and primary care) and further strengthen and develop the analysis. We agreed on four major themes.

Table 28.1   Main research methods used, disciplinary backgrounds, and locations of researchers interviewed in end of life research

Methods	No of participants
Interviews/focus groups	11
Participant observation	4
Arts/drama	4
Quality of life tools/surveys	3
Storytelling	2
Narratives/diaries	2
Mixed methods	6
Not specified	6
Discipline:	
Psychology/psycho-oncology	9
Nursing/medicine	7
Medical sociology	5
Social work	3
Medical anthropology	2
Creative arts	1
Not specified	5
Location:	
United Kingdom	25
Canada	3
United States	1
Sweden	1
Netherlands	1
Australia	1

Results

Most researchers with experience in both end of life and other research specialties thought end of life research should not be seen as a special case as the challenges were equally relevant in other topics of biomedical and social research. They cited the need for sensitivity, caution, and respect for the physical and emotional wellbeing of participants in any research.

The interviews with researchers and the discussions in user groups highlighted these issues for consideration in conducting end of life research: the design of end of life studies, recruiting participants, ethical conduct, and the emotional challenges faced by participants, researchers, and transcribers.

Designing end of life studies

Defining end of life

All the researchers discussed the ambiguities around the concept of end of life, which one health professional might define as the last 48 hours but others might use to refer to the last six months or even longer. In addition, the uncertainty surrounding any individual patient's prognosis and the fact that he or she may be unaware of their status as 'terminally ill' or receiving 'palliative care' render it difficult to identify and recruit patients who clearly have a limited life expectancy. Problems with defining and standardising the research numerator and denominator of people facing death has led many researchers to gather proxy views after death from informal and professional carers.

Methodological options

End of life researchers were using a range of established social science methods, each with its own strengths and weaknesses. Most researchers thought that a range of approaches and methods was needed, given the variety of issues and groups to be investigated. We found considerable interest in the combining of methods and approaches:

> 'Well at the moment the project we are doing … we are using a mixture of quantitative and qualitative methods to get at different issues and that actually seems to be working really well because it gives us a sort of broad overview of the experiences of lots of different people' (researcher 29).

While some discussed the importance of 'innovative methods' such as arts based research involving drama or poetry or using story boards, few had ventured beyond the mainstream methods. One senior researcher said that lack of support from funding bodies was a barrier to using more innovative research techniques. Several researchers suggested that approaches and methods from other sensitive issues, such as long term disability or domestic abuse, could be useful in end of life research.

Most participants in the focus groups expressed a preference for qualitative methods. Providing that the research is conducted sensitively, these methods allow people to raise and contextualise issues important to them:

> 'Let the patient introduce the subject, rather than the researcher asking questions that might not be to their liking' (participant in focus group 1).

Recruitment of participants

Gatekeepers

Researchers recognised the need to recruit sensitively, and most sought advice from health professionals on the suitability of participants. Some, however, reported that health professionals acted as overzealous gatekeepers, blocking recruitment or introducing a selection bias. This problem, they suggested, could be ameliorated by careful wording of patients' participation letters and by establishing good relationships with health professionals and keeping them fully informed.

All researchers agreed that research should be scrutinised and conducted ethically but also found the bureaucracy and time involved in submissions to ethics and research committees increasingly burdensome. Many spoke of the paternalism of ethics committees, which added to the access barrier imposed by clinicians acting as gatekeepers for perceived 'vulnerable' patients, rather than seeing them as individuals capable of making their own decisions:

'I think patients and family members are people, human beings in their own rights, citizens of the world and they can make decisions whether or not they want to take part in research' (researcher 14).

Inclusive approaches

Difficulties in including people from various ethnic communities were repeatedly highlighted, these recruitment problems reflecting demographic and language barriers and the fact that few people from minority groups access specialist palliative care. Given the recruitment difficulties within the majority population, it is not surprising that many studies fail to engage with people from these small populations. Many researchers, however, thought that greater efforts should be made to include these perspectives to ensure that culturally appropriate care is developed. Successful recruitment strategies included exploring what could be offered in return for participation (for example, information sessions about a particular issue, a social event, or art based activities); gaining the approval of community leaders; and considering issues from the perspective of service users to ensure the study design, research materials, and methods of dissemination are culturally appropriate.

Other hard to reach groups identified included people with physical, sensory, and cognitive impairment; those from socially deprived areas; children and young people; and all those with non-malignant conditions. Many researchers and members of the user focus groups suggested that there is a need for more inclusive approaches and methods and a greater commitment to recruiting from these groups:

'We are all largely middle class, middle aged, you know. We are not representative. We are people who are articulate and can speak out' (participant in focus group 2).

Do people facing the end of life want to participate in research?

Participants in the user focus groups confirmed the researchers' views that many people with advanced illness still want to participate in research. They thought that the perspectives of patients and carers must be included in research to develop suitable and effective services and support. The researchers reported that many people see their participation as an opportunity to 'give something back' in return for the care they, or their loved ones, have received or as an opportunity to try to improve services and support for people in the future. Participants in two of the focus groups spoke at length about the personal benefit of taking part in research:

'When I spoke to [researchers's name] it really helped me. Because I felt that it was somebody listening, and I know it helped me' (participant in focus group 2).

Some participants in focus groups raised concerns about the real value of participating in research, feeling that the efforts made were sometimes a token gesture as no feedback was received and no change resulted:

'We are speaking, we are saying our piece, and we go away feeling better, but years down the line you think, 'Well, did it make any differences?'' (participants in focus group 2).

Researchers also pointed out that research may not result in changes to patient services, and that participants should be made aware of this.

Maintaining ethical conduct

Talking about death

As some potential participants may not understand, or wish to be confronted with, their prognosis, researchers advised proceeding as if people do not know they are dying, unless there is an explicit acknowledgment to the contrary. Many researchers emphasised that this should be borne in mind in the design of information sheets and questionnaires for patients, as well as during interviews – for example, not using the phrase 'end of life' in information sheets:

'It's very difficult as a researcher, you are trying to ask questions and ascertain what this person knows about their illness and how they feel about it before you go a step further' (researcher 3).

Researchers emphasized the need to respond to cues given by people about their willingness to discuss end of life issues and cautioned against asking direct questions about death and dying. These ethical concerns overlaid by more general societal taboos surrounding death and dying, sometimes leading to a lack of confidence in researchers in approaching such discussions.

Researchers reported difficulties in giving feedback, such as copies of project reports, to participants without confronting them with information about end of life issues that some might prefer to avoid:

'How do you identify people who actually are dying and how do you write it up so that you don't upset some people because they still think they're going to get better?' (researcher 25).

Informed consent

Researching end of life issues necessarily means engaging with people (both patients and their families) who may be in extremely poor health and experiencing exhaustion, depression, or high levels of stress and anxiety. For this reason, researchers emphasised the importance of distinguishing between informed and valid consent. While it is good practice to ensure that research participants are fully informed about their role in a study (balanced with the need to ensure that they are not presented with information that may upset them), researchers underlined the importance of ensuring that, particularly in longitudinal research, once consent is given, its validity is regularly reconfirmed. Participants should be given several opportunities to withdraw, up until, and even during, interviews or focus groups.

Emotional challenges for participants, researchers, and transcribers

Some researchers, many of whom had also worked on non-cancer studies, considered the emotional challenges of conducting end of life research to be no greater than those in research with other groups such as people with long term disabilities or threatened with domestic violence or child abuse:

'I started off doing research with stroke patients and I couldn't have continued with that type of work because that was, you know, just some of the things that those people were going through, living with disability, wasn't going to get any better, it was going to get worse and the stress on their carers. Whereas dying is something that is going to happen to all of us and so in that sense it's not a problem for me' (researcher 7).

Some senior researchers thought it important to recruit experienced researchers for these studies, emphasising that often the most important factors are the skills and personal qualities of the researcher:

'Much of it comes down to the skills and the personality of the people who are collecting the data, that you really do need people who are skilled, who are able and who make it a positive interaction for the people concerned' (researcher 18).

Research managers often expressed concerns that end of life research placed heavy demands on junior researchers, who should be offered formal counselling sessions as well as informal debriefing and peer support. They also identified a lack of career structure, which made it difficult to retain skilled researchers.

Many researchers identified end of life research as demanding, but most also spoke of satisfaction gained. Witnessing enduring relationships restored faith in the human capacity to receive and give love and support. It inspired researchers to re-evaluate their own lives in more positive ways and, in some cases, face their own morality:

'It is, I think, a terrifically important field. It's important that we do begin to talk more about end of life care … so the reward for me is knowing that perhaps one is contributing in a small way to changing social attitudes and culture around end of life care' (researcher 13).

We questioned staff who transcribed end of life interviews because researchers had raised concerns about the emotional demands placed on them. The transcribers explained that events in their own lives could affect their reactions:

'A very close friend of ours died just about this time last year with cancer and for a while whenever I was typing I couldn't stop thinking about him and it made you look at it very differently' (transcriber 1).

Several researchers warned of the harm that can be caused by not paying attention to the emotional state of interviewees. They indicated the importance of knowing how to bring the interview to an end in a manner that left the interviewee in a safe emotional state and of ensuring access support if needed.

Discussion

The evidence from our study indicates that some people with advanced illness may want to take part in research. Researchers with experience in the specialty consider that end of life research is not essentially different from other types of research and not too difficult to conduct. Nevertheless, there is a dearth of research on the views of patients and carers on the good death. Some barriers are practical and methodological: uncertainty about defining end of life, patients lacking awareness of their prognosis, and overly protective gatekeepers hindering recruitment. Although they may be necessary, imaginative and inclusive methods are rarely used, reflecting the challenges in attracting funding for these approaches. More insidious barriers may lie in the societal taboos surrounding death and dying that affect such research.

[...]

Main finding in the context of the existing literature

Gatekeeping by health professionals and ethics committees has previously been identified as a barrier to end of life.[3,4,13,14] From our study, however, it is clear that many people at the end of their life would welcome the opportunity to participate in research. Many researchers suggested broadening and deepening our understanding of end of life research by developing innovative approaches and methods able to capture the perspectives of a wider range of people, conditions, and settings.[13-17]

Researchers were articulate about the professional and personal challenges faced, as revealed in previous literature,[4,6,8,17-19] but many, especially those who had worked in other types of research, challenged the idea that end of life research is a special case, more difficult or sensitive than many other areas of social research.[20,21] We summarise the barriers to researching end of life care and possible solutions in Table 28.2.

The personal and societal taboos surrounding death and dying present a major challenge, and funding bodies, ethics committees, and researchers are also affected by them. The concept of social death is well established in the literature: people can suffer a social death before their physical death as society turns away from the dying.[22] Some people's desire to participate in research at the end of life may itself be an example of resistance to social death, an opportunity to be an active and participating citizen again rather than an invalid or patient.

[...]

Table 28. 2   Barriers to researching end of life care and possible solutions

Barriers	
Difficulties in designing studies	Possible solutions
Lack of agreed definitions of palliative care, and end of life	Researchers to provide definitions to recruiters as part of study documentation
Difficulties of specifying/determining prognosis (or difficulty recognizing/defining end of life)	Use specific instruments or prognostic guides, or recruit at a stage in illness trajectory not at defined prognosis
Variable levels of awareness of diagnosis and prognosis in patients and carers	Explore participants' understanding and language they use to describe the illness, and talk with them at that level
Uncertainty about suitable methods	Match methods to research aims, resources, and local context. Consider mixed methods and innovative approaches from other specialties
Funding bodies tend to support only tried and tested methods	Encourage researchers from other specialities/ methods who have published successfully to participate in palliative care research groups. Researchers should argue case for innovative methods to examine problems associated with traditional research approaches, particularly in relation to hard to reach groups
Ethical issues	
Staff gatekeeping/ethics committee procedures and attitudes	Work closely with staff and keep them well informed. Clarify that issues around living with illness wil be discussed, and sensitive issues will be examined only if patient gives cues. Involve clinical staff in research steering groups
Maintaining informed consent in longitudinal studies	Regularly check willingness to maintain consent
Doubts among clinicians, ethics committees, and carers about willingness of people at end of life to participate in research	Provide evidence that people want to participate and can do so without harm. Include users in research development and project management
Challenges in recruiting participants	
Difficulties in recruiting representative range of people at end of life	Use range of recruitment techniques – for example, local media and community groups, health professionals, and innovative methods
High attention rates	Factor in attrition rates of 30–50% for longitudinal studies
Emotional challenges	
Researchers	Employ experienced researchers; offer training in advanced communication, palliative care induction. Plan interview workload (three a week). Provide debriefing and peer support sessions. Budget for external support and supervision
Transcribers	Include debriefing and support sessions as required.

Notes

1   Clark J. Patient centred death. *BMJ* 2003;327:174–5.
2   Bowling A. Research on dying is scant. *BMJ* 2000;320:1205.
3   Riley J, Ross JR. Research into care at the end of life. *Lancet* 2005;365:735–7.
4   Addington-Hall J. Research sensitivities to palliative care patients. *Eur J Cancer Care* 2002;11:220–4.
5   Entwistle V, Tritter J, Calnan M. Researching experiences of cancer: the importance of methodology. *Eur J Cancer Care* 2002;11:232–7.
6   Lawton J. Gaining and maintaining consent ethical concerns raised in a study of dying patients. *Qual Health Res* 2001;11:693–705.
7   Rowling L. Being in, being out, being with: affect and the qualitative researcher in loss and grief research. *Mortality* 1999;14:167–81.
8   Seymour J, Skilbeck J. Ethical considerations in researching user views. *Eur J Cancer Care* 2002;11:215–9.
9   Beaver K, Luker K, Woods S. Conducting research with the terminally ill: challenges and considerations. *Int J Palliat Nurs* 1999;5:13–17.
10 Seymour J, Ingleton C. Ethical issues in qualitative research at the end of life. *Int J Palliat Nurs* 2005;11:138–46.
11 Harris F, Kendall M, Murray SA, Worth A, Boyd K, Brown D, et al. *What are the best ways to seek the views of people affected by cancer about end of life issues?* London: Macmillan Cancer Relief, 2005.
12 Rose K, Webb C. Analyzing data: maintaining rigor in a qualitative study. *Qual Health Res* 1998;8:556–62.
13 Cook AM, Finlay AG, Butler-Keating RJ. Recruiting into palliative care trials: lessons learnt from a feasibility study. *Palliat Med* 2002;16:163–5.
14 Krishnasamy M. Perceptions of health care need in lung cancer. Can prospective surveys provide nationally representative data? *Palliat Med* 2000;14:410–8.
15 Gray R, Sinding C, Ivonoffski V, Fitch M, Hampson A, Greenberg M. The use of research-based theatre in a project related to metastatic breast cancer. *Health Expect* 2000; 3:137–44.
16 Gray RE. Performing on and off the stage: the place(s) of performance in arts-based approaches to qualitative inquiry. *Qual Inq* 2003;9:254.
17 Lee RM. Doing research on sensitive topics. London: Sage, 1993.
18 Seamark DA, Gilbert J, Williams S. Are postbereavement research interviews distressing to carers? Lessons learned from palliative care research. *Palliat Med* 2000;14:55–6.
19 Woods S, Beaver K, Luker K. Users' views on palliative care services: ethical implications. *Nurs Ethics* 2000;7:314–26.
20 British Sociological Associastion. Statement of ethical practice. www.britsoc.co.uk/equality/63.htm.
21 Association of Social Anthropologists. Ethical guidelines for good research practice. www.theasa.org/ethics/ethics_guidelines.htm.
22 Seale C. *Constructing death: the sociology of dying and bereavement.* Cambridge: Cambridge University Press, 1998.

29

Keeping the Personal Costs Down: Minimising Distress When Researching Sensitive Issues

Margo J. Milne and Cathy E. Lloyd

Whenever we ask people to participate in our research, we ask them, at the most basic level, to give up their time. There may be other costs as well however, and for our participants to give truly informed consent we need to know what these costs are likely to be. The total of these costs is the respondent burden. All research participation could be argued to involve some cost, if only in terms of time and inconvenience. However, the potential costs of participating in research into sensitive topics may go well beyond this (Lee, 1993).

This reading considers the nature of the respondent burden in research about sensitive issues. We discuss the nature of 'sensitive issues', reviewing some of the literature regarding whether participation in research about death and dying in particular is burdensome, and examine some ways that have been suggested of reducing any distress caused by such research.

Respondent burden

Bradburn (1977) defined respondent burden as the sum of the physical, economic and/or psychological hardships associated with research participation. He stressed, however, that the research interview is a social encounter, influenced by the norms prevailing when people voluntarily participate in social events. Factors motivating the individual to participate and provide information in that situation are therefore balanced against more burdensome factors. Tailoring Bradburn's definition to clinical and health care research, Ulrich et al. argue that respondent burden may vary in intensity and degree, depending on the risk level of the research, any procedures it entails, and the individual participant's condition, prognosis, mental state and support systems. They suggest that an individual with significant pain and other symptoms and/or a poor prognosis may be particularly burdened by being asked to commit their limited energy to research participation (Ulrich et al., 2005).

Researchers therefore have particular obligations to vulnerable populations, including dying patients as well as acutely ill persons, older people and people with cognitive impairments.

However, we currently lack a detailed understanding of the risks and burdens faced by dying patients and their families who participate in research, or how those risks can accurately be assessed (Daly and Rosenfeld, 2003).

Certain groups, for example those who attend a particular hospital out-patient department or who are on a register (for example, the UK National Childhood Tumour Registry), may be more frequently sought out as research subjects, owing to their availability in settings where research is conducted. One early report, The Belmont Report (1979) argued that such groups should be protected against being involved in research solely for administrative convenience. No matter how well each individual study is designed, participants in multiple studies may become physically exhausted and psychologically distressed (Ulrich et al., 2005).

What is a sensitive topic?

Lee and Renzetti (1990) defined a sensitive research topic as one potentially posing a substantial threat to those involved. They identified four categories of sensitive research:

- Research that intrudes into a deeply personal experience.
- Research that is concerned with deviance and social control.
- Research that impinges on the vested interests of powerful persons.
- Research that involves things sacred to those being studied.

Researchers assume that end-of-life issues must be sensitive because they are deeply personal. The emotionally charged nature of death and dying may make participants unsure of their ability to maintain an appropriate demeanour in their interaction with the researcher, a much prized characteristic (Goffman, 1971). The danger is that once an issue is identified as sensitive, other untested assumptions may follow. For instance, researchers may assume that people do not respond to sensitive questions because those questions cause them pain, whereas there may be other, equally valid explanations (Lloyd, 1996). There may be cultural, gender or age-related factors influencing the researcher–participant dyad – or quite simply, the participant may not like the researcher and not want to respond to his or her questions!

Participants in different types of research are likely to have very different experiences: for example, some researchers suggest that a participant in a qualitative research interview retains considerable control over the process. They argue that to assume automatically that interviews are potentially harmful risks being overprotective and potentially denying participants agency and control over what is said and how (Corbin and Morse, 2003).

Being overly concerned about potential risks also implies that the distress aroused by talking to a researcher is greater than that experienced when talking to a family member or friend (Corbin and Morse, 2003). It could be argued that recounting personal details to a stranger who has just come into one's life is indeed likely to be more distressing than recounting them to a friend or confidant. On the other hand, many of us have fallen into conversation with a stranger on a train or plane and disclosed personal information, safe in the knowledge that we will almost certainly never see our fellow traveller again. As psychiatrist Linda Austin said in *USA Today*, 'If you reveal something about yourself to a stranger, so what?' (Schmit, 1993, p. 1B). A research interview, however, is not the same as a casual conversation. Would all participants feel sufficiently confident and empowered to divert a line of questioning they perceived as distressing or overly intrusive, or would the inherent power structure of the interview make the expectation of answering too strong to resist?

Sometimes the sensitivity of a topic becomes apparent only once research is under-way, but the reverse can also be true: a researcher may approach a topic with caution only to find that his or her initial fears about 'sensitivity' were misplaced. The nature of research as a social encounter also means that a topic which one group finds sensitive may be found totally innocuous by another (Lee, 1993). Sensitivity can be seen as situated and constructed within the context of the cultural norms and taboos of the specific group with which an individual is identifying at that moment in time (Farquhar and Das, 1999).

In some situations, distress may be unavoidable. It may be the situation being researched rather than the research process itself that is causing the distress, and therefore unlikely that any strategies adopted by researchers can alleviate these feelings. Oster (2003) asks whether these feelings should in fact be avoided at all: perhaps participants want or need to feel and express them. Additionally, participants may feel obliged not to appear distressed when they see researchers' attempts to mitigate their feelings.

Is participating in end-of-life research burdensome?

Potential participants in research into end-of-life issues are often people who are already seriously ill. It can be argued that such individuals' participation may come at a signifi-cantly increased cost, given their vulnerability and compromised health status (Ulrich et al., 2005).

Casarett and Karlawish (2000), expanding on the topic of whether people receiving pal-liative care are 'vulnerable', suggest that subjects may be vulnerable because of dimin-ished decision-making capability. They are concerned that decision-making capacity may be impaired in patients near the end of life, making informed consent more difficult and sometimes impossible. While this may be the case, it is not a situation unique to palliative care research and, argue Casarett and Karlawish, does not provide grounds for special guidelines or restrictions. Investigators in fields such as dementia, psychiatric illness and intensive care have all developed strategies for assessing whether and how decision-making capacity should be assessed before patients are recruited into research (Casarett and Karlawish, 2000).

In some situations patients may feel under pressure to participate in research into end-of-life care, particularly if they depend on a particular institution or physician for their care. Again, it is reasonable to assume that these influences exist, but not that they are nec-essarily any more influential than in other forms of research (Casarett and Karlawish, 2000). There will always be people who are too emotionally fragile to talk about certain topics. It can be argued that those individuals will usually not volunteer to be interviewed.

As long as the request to participate is made in such a manner that potential participants are explicitly allowed to say 'no' without consequences for their treatment or care, those who are uncomfortable or distrustful of the interview process are free to refuse to participate (Corbin and Morse, 2003).

There may be particular characteristics associated with the experience of distress during research participation. For example, a recent study demonstrated that the probability of distress appeared to be lower in older family members, family members of older patients, and family members of patients who died of non-cancer illnesses. There was a higher incidence of distress among women (Takesaka, Crowley and Casarett, 2004). Overall however, this study found that only a minority of respondents reported any distress, and that such distress was typically reported as mild or moderate. Takesaka and her colleagues argue that such studies may therefore be much less distressing to participants than previously suspected (Takesaka, Crawley and Casarett, 2004).

The type of study being conducted may also impact on levels of distress. In the same study, Takesaka and her colleagues observed that a postal survey appeared to cause higher distress levels than a face-to-face interview research study. They hypothesised that postal surveys allow more time to reflect and therefore may be more likely to cause distress. It is also possible, they argued, that respondents were more comfortable with admitting distress anonymously, whereas those participating in interviews may have underreported their distress to avoid appearing critical of the interviewer. Finally, it is possible that the interviewer's presence was therapeutic and ameliorated the distress caused by the questions in the face-to-face studies (Takesaka, Crawley and Casarett, 2004).

Several studies have suggested that participants may welcome the chance to share their opinions about sensitive topics. Lee (1993), for instance, commented that research on sensitive topics often reveals a desire for catharsis rather than sanctuary among participants. Kalish and Reynolds found that very few respondents in their survey about attitudes to death and dying had negative responses to taking part, and around 44 per cent had positive responses, mentioning the value of the research interview as a learning experience or as an interesting and thought-provoking experience. The opportunity to express oneself to a concerned outsider on a topic usually considered taboo commonly results in expressions of relief and gratitude (Kalish and Reynolds, 1981).

Even if some distress is experienced, individuals may still find their overall experience of participation positive. In one study Davis et al. (1996), researching the effects of terminal illness on patients and their carers, described participants who wept throughout their interviews but nonetheless wanted to continue, while 90 per cent of participants in Michelson et al.'s (2006) recent study about end-of-life decision making with parents of children in neonatal intensive care units described the experience as 'good' or 'neutral'. Many participants described the interview process as relieving, even therapeutic, even when they had expressed intense emotion through tears. Other potential benefits described included increased awareness of end-of-life issues, clarification and/or affirmation of previous ideas, and positive impacts on future decision making by prompting advance care planning (Michelson et al., 2006).

Although there remains lack of agreement as to the extent of distress caused by research into end-of-life issues, it is almost universally acknowledged that some risk is involved. As ethical researchers we must make every attempt to reduce this risk wherever possible.

Qualitative research interviews

Qualitative interviews are widely used in research into death and dying, from programme evaluation to intimate portrayals of the dying process. There is, however, a lack of consensus on their suitability for use in researching sensitive topics.

On the one hand, as Michelson et al. (2006) argue, qualitative in-depth interviewing is well suited as a data collection method for sensitive issues because it explores subjects' experiences and emotions. Koenig, Back and Crawley suggest that qualitative research can address three types of issues in death and dying: 'basic' questions such as the nature of decision-making processes; 'applied' clinical issues such as how physicians respond to requests for hastened death; and quality improvements in clinical practice such as identifying institutional barriers to the delivery of effective pain control (Koenig, and Back and Crawley, 2003).

On the other hand, qualitative methodology has been identified as carrying particular risks for participants in research into sensitive topics. Themes of power differential between researcher and participant (Lee, 1993) and the uncertainty of the qualitative research process (Munhall, 1988) have been identified. Kavanaugh and Ayres (1998) argue that neither respondents nor interviewer are able to predict everything that will emerge during a qualitative interview. Situations may arise that necessitate abandoning further investigation of areas that are too painful for the participant to discuss. It is clearly unacceptable for investigators to advance their research agenda at the psychological expense of participants.

Potential participants may perceive focus-group discussions as a less threatening environment for discussing sensitive topics than one-to-one interviews (Farquhar and Das, 1999), but there is a risk that one participant may voice an opinion that is distressing to others in the group. Kitzinger and Barbour, for example, quote a suggestion made in one focus group that incest survivors should be sterilised as 'unfit parents' (Kitzinger and Barbour, 1999).

How can the burden of participation be reduced?

Various ways of reducing the burden of research participation and any potential distress have been suggested. For example, at the recruitment stage of their study of people with terminal illnesses and their carers, Davis et al. (1996) were concerned not to cause distress by the usual methods of increasing response rates such as 'cold-calling' or repeated reminders. Following an introductory letter with a suggested appointment time, they therefore made only one further attempt to contact the person.

Casarett and Karlawish (2000) have suggested various strategies for ensuring that participation is truly voluntary. They argue that it should be emphasised in the informed consent process that participation is truly voluntary, and future medical treatment is not contingent on participation. Indeed, this is now an integral part of the recommended patient information sheet for participants in NHS-based research in the UK (NHS, 2007).

Where the researchers are clinicians, it can be useful to recruit participants through a third party who is not associated with the patient's care. This helps to emphasise the distinction between research and clinical care, and helps makes it clear to patients that they can decline to participate in the research without compromising their clinical care (Casarett and Karlawish, 2000).

Consent should be periodically revisited to ensure that each individual's unique experience as a participant is being supported (Ulrich et al., 2005). In the specific context of the qualitative research interview, Munhall recommends the use of 'process consent', defined as the immediate renegotiation of consent as circumstances change or unexpected events occur during the interview (Munhall, 1988).

Where the research design includes more than one contact with each participant, the nature of the research relationship inevitably changes over time. Researchers need therefore to be aware of all behaviours relating to the study, not just during the interview itself, including such information as cancelled appointments and late attendance. These behaviours can be examined with the aim of identifying additional strategies that will reduce the potential for harm to participants (Kavanaugh and Ayres, 1998).

People with progressive disease have, by definition, needs that change over time. Longitudinal qualitative research can not only reflect these changes, but also allow participants time to disclose information at their own pace, and allow trust, empathy and a deeper understanding to emerge. Murray and Sheikh (2006) found that people with advanced cancer and chronic illness discussed deeply personal issues like dying more openly in subsequent rounds of interviews than in initial interviews. Repeat interviews also allow the researcher to access and make sense of patients' competing and often contradictory accounts of trying to remain positive while facing the real possibility of dying.

A flexible approach to interviewing has been recommended by some researchers as a more positive way of conducting research into sensitive topics. For example, Cowles (1998) directed the interview in and out of sensitive areas, offered rest breaks, and provided immediate therapeutic intervention when needed. Kavanaugh and Ayres (1988) suggest adapting the structure of the interview as necessary according to the individual's need for pacing, for instance, by taking breaks or postponing all or parts of interviews.

Similar sensitivity should be shown in focus groups on sensitive topics: for instance, the session could start with warm-up activities, move from less to more sensitive topics, and end with an opportunity for participants to clarify any possible confusions or misconceptions (Hoppe et al., 1995). Allowing participants to set their own ground rules can help them to feel safe in the group, by participating in the creation of safety (Farquhar and Das, 1999). To reduce the risk of distress during qualitative research, for example, during face-to-face interviews or focus-group discussions, and as a way of deflecting the issues away from the individual participant, some researchers have used vignettes, or case studies. Vignettes consist of text, images or other stimuli to which participants are asked to respond (Hughes and Huby, 2002). Unlike attitude statements on surveys, vignettes present participants with concrete, detailed situations that do not involve them personally. It therefore becomes possible to discuss norms and beliefs in a situated way which accepts the complexities normally surrounding them (Lee, 1993). Kalish and Reynolds (1981) found that it was necessary to ground questions in some sort of concrete context before respondents could answer meaningfully. For example, exploring attitudes to whether someone with cancer should be told that he or she was going to die, they asked respondents to imagine that a friend of theirs had been given this diagnosis, and whether they should be told. Because the situations presented to participants are hypothetical, there is a distancing effect. As a result, the vignettes are less personally threatening than direct questions would be, allowing sensitive topics to be discussed in a relatively neutral way (Lee, 1993).

Inevitably, vignettes offer only a partial representation of real life, but this can be harnessed by varying the factual information included in different vignettes and comparing the responses to them (Hughes and Huby, 2002). Some researchers have noticed, however, that participants' responses to vignettes tend to be simple, not reflecting the complexity of real-life decisions (Denk et al., 1997). By being asked to assume the role of a vignette character, respondents may be distanced from the necessity to give 'socially desirable' patterns of responding (Constant, Kiesler and Spraull, 1994). In a similar way, practitioners, commenting on hypothetical situations rather than the reality of their own practice, may also experience more freedom in their responses (Wilks, 2004).

Various ways of reducing the burden of participation in clinical research have been suggested. For example, Ulrich et al. suggest that where several studies are taking place at the same time, they should be integrated into one. They also suggest that a central registry of studies should be established and reviewed to avoid unnecessary duplication. Additionally, research participant advocates could be used to help potential participants better understand the studies being offered to them, monitor the amount of burden individual participants are experiencing, and help participants negotiate decision making (Ulrich et al., 2005). Researchers must also be aware of their own responsibilities as participant advocates, and research institutions should provide training in this important skill.

The costs of research on sensitive topics may also include costs to the researcher (Lee, 1993). For example, as Koenig, Back and Crawley (2003) suggest, the intense, personal nature of qualitative data gathering may require the development of empathic or caring relationships with research subjects. Where participants in end-of-life research subsequently die, this may be particularly distressing to the researcher. It is essential that the researcher has an appropriate support network in place, to help him or her deal with his or her own feelings about the research and its participants.

Conclusion

The evidence reviewed here suggests that participating in research on sensitive topics may not be as distressing as we sometimes fear – or if it is, that distress can be counterbalanced by benefits gained. More research is needed though: we need to find out, for instance, how individuals with different characteristics react to research on sensitive topics, to help us minimise the risk of causing distress. We also need to establish how individuals react to the burdens placed upon them by their individual circumstances and the demands placed upon them by participation in research, as well as the benefits they derive from participation.

Further research is also needed on how cultural, ethnic and gender influences impact on the relationship between researcher and participant, and specifically how they could influence the researcher's ability to recognise distress in participants. Through methodological research such as this, we can do our best to ensure that our work as researchers is ethically sound, and does not inflict unreasonable costs on our participants.

References

Austin, L. (2003) quoted in Schmit, J. (1993) 'Deep secrets told among passengers', *USA Today*: 1B–2B.

The Belmont Report (1979) Ethical Principles and Guidelines for the Protection of Human Subjects of Research. The National Commission for the Protection of Human Subjects of Biomedical and Behavioral Research: Department of Health, Education and Welfare.

Bradburn, N. (1977) 'Respondent burden', in L. Reeder (ed.) *Health Survey Research Method: Second Biennial Conference*. Williamsburg, VA: US Government Printing Office. pp. 49–53.

Casarett, D.J. and Karlawish, J.H.T. (2000) 'Are special ethical guidelines needed for palliative care research?', *Journal of Pain and Symptom Management*, 20: 130.

Constant, D., Kiesler, S. and Sproull, L. (1994) 'What's mine is ours, or is it? A study of attitudes about information sharing', *Information Systems Research*, 5: 400.

Corbin, J. and Morse, J.M. (2003) 'The unstructured interactive interview: issues of reciprocity and risks when dealing with sensitive topics', *Qualitative Inquiry*, 9: 335–54.

Cowles, K. (1988) 'Issues in qualitative research on sensitive topics', *Western Journal of Nursing Research*, 10: 163–79.

Daly, B.J. and Rosenfeld, K. (2003) 'Maximizing benefits and minimizing risks in health services research near the end of life', *Journal of Pain and Symptom Management*, 25: S33.

Davis, B.D., Cowley, S.A. and Ryland, R.K. (1996) 'The effects of terminal illness on patients and their carers', *Journal of Advanced Nursing*, 23: 512–20.

Denk, C.E., Benson, J.M., Fletcher, J.C. and Reigel, T.M. (1997) 'How do Americans want to die? A factorial vignette survey of public attitudes about end-of-life medical decision-making', *Social Science Research*, 26: 95.

Farquhar, C. and Das, R. (1999) 'Are focus groups suitable for "sensitive" topics?' in R. Barbour and J. Kitzinger (eds) *Developing Focus Group Research: Politics, Theory and Practice*. London: Sage. pp. 47–63.

Goffman, E. (1971) *Relations in Public: Microstudies of the Public Order*. Harmondsworth: Penguin.

Hoppe, M., Wells, E., Morrison, D., Gillmore, M. and Wilsdon, A. (1995) 'Using focus groups to discuss sensitive topics with children', *Evaluation Review*, 19: 102–14.

Hughes, R. and Huby, M. (2002) 'The application of vignettes in social and nursing research', *Journal of Advanced Nursing*, 37: 382–6.

Kalish, R. and Reynolds, D. (1981) *Death and Ethnicity: A Psychocultural Study*. Farmingdale, NY: Baywood Publishing.

Kavanaugh, K. and Ayres, L. (1998) '"Not as bad as it could have been": assessing and mitigating harm during research interviews on sensitive topics', *Research in Nursing & Health*, 21: 91–7.

Kitzinger, J. and Barbour, R. (1999) 'The challenge and promise of focus groups', in R. Barbour and J. Kitzinger (eds) *Developing Focus Group Research: Politics, Theory and Practice*. London: Sage. pp. 1–20.

Koenig, B.A., Back, A.L. and Crawley, L.M. (2003) 'Qualitative methods in end-of-life research: recommendations to enhance the protection of human subjects', *Journal of Pain and Symptom Management*, 25: S43.

Lee, R. (1993) *Doing Research on Sensitive Topics*. London: Sage.

Lee, R. and Renzetti, C. (1990) 'The problems of researching sensitive topics: an overview and introduction', *American Behavioral Scientist*, 33: 510–28.

Lloyd, M. (1996) 'Condemned to be meaningful: non-response in studies of men and infertility', *Sociology of Health & Illness*, 18: 433–54.

Michelson, K.N., Koogler, T.K., Skipton, K., Sullivan, C. and Frader, J. (2006) 'Parents' reactions to participating in interviews about end-of-life decision making', *Journal of Palliative Medicine,* 9: 1329.

Munhall, P. (1988) 'Ethical considerations in qualitative research', *Western Journal of Nursing Research,* 10: 150–62.

Murray, S.A. and Sheikh, A. (2006) 'Serial interviews for patients with progressive diseases', *The Lancet,* 368: 901–2.

NHS (National Health Service) (2007) *Information Sheets and Consent Forms: Guidance for Researchers and Reviewers.* Version 3.2. National Patient Safety Agency.

Oster, C. (2003) 'Harm minimisation as technologies of the self: some experiences of interviewing people with genital herpes', *Nursing Inquiry,* 10: 201–3.

Schmit, J. (1993) 'Deep secrets told among passengers', *USA Today,* 1B–2B.

Takesaka, J., Crowley, R. and Casarett, D. (2004) 'What is the risk of distress in palliative care survey research?', *Journal of Pain and Symptom Management,* 28: 593.

Ulrich, C., Wallen, G., Fiester, A. and Grady, C. (2005) 'Respondent burden in clinical research: when are we asking too much of subjects?', *IRB: Ethics & Human Research,* 27: 17–20.

Wilks, T. (2004) 'The use of vignettes in qualitative research into social work values', *Qualitative Social Work,* 3: 78–87.

30
The Role of the Qualitative Researcher in Loss and Grief Research

Louise Rowling

Qualitative methods such as repeated in-depth interviews are frequently used in research on sensitive issues such as HIV/AIDS, loss and grief and child abuse. The research process can be highly emotional, both for the participants and the researcher. While the ethical dilemmas that this poses for participants have been elaborated, little attention has been given to researchers' experiences and their needs.

[...]

Using examples from two years of fieldwork in a study of loss and grief in school communities, this article will explore the dilemmas encountered using 'self as instrument' in the research process. These dilemmas include: the clash of the ontological beliefs brought to the research; identifying, monitoring and managing the emotional impact of spontaneous, intimate self-disclosure in participants' stories. [...]

The study

The research process reported here involved an institutional case study design using qualitative methods of in-depth repeated intensive interviewing (Lofland & Lofland, 1984), participant observation and document analysis over two years of fieldwork in 1992–93. School sites for the case studies were chosen that optimized the potential for explicating the substantive topic of concern – loss and grief in school communities (Ely, 1991; Stake, 1994). One of the schools, Kair High School (pseudonym) is a large multicultural comprehensive high school in the Sydney metropolitan area of New South Wales, Australia. There are some 120 teaching staff and about 1350 students, 75% of whom speak a language other than English at home. The other school, Midway High School (pseudonym) is

Excerpts from 'Being in, being out, being with: affect and the role of the qualitative researcher in loss and grief research' by Louise Rowling, *Mortality*, 4(2): 167–81, 1999, Taylor & Francis Ltd, reprinted by kind permission of the publisher and author (Taylor & Francis Ltd., www.informaworld.com).

a semi-rural school about 300 kilometers from Sydney. There are about 90 staff and roughly 700 students attending the school, drawn from the town and from the surrounding countryside. While the students' background and the physical size and location of the schools differed, significantly different research findings (reported elsewhere – Rowling, 1995, 1996a, b) did not emerge.

[...]

In this reading, verbatim quotes of the participants will be used to exemplify particular issues. They were obtained from the transcribed tape recordings of interviews. Excerpts from my research journal [R/J] (Holly, 1989) kept throughout the field work will be used to exemplify my role as the chief 'data collection' instrument. [...]

Dilemmas encountered

Clash of ontological beliefs

The intent to establish a collaborative non-exploitative approach in a constructivist paradigm (Punch, 1994) to the study of this particular research topic, created a major dilemma for me. The collaborative relationship with the research participants that I had originally envisioned was based on my desire for equality and sharing in the creation of the research findings. This was my concept of being fully 'in' the research, based on my previous action research experiences. Yet this being 'in' was problematic.

Emotions were a key component of the research. This involved, for the participants, the resurgence of emotions in the retelling of experiences in interviews and the re-experiencing of emotions triggered as interview transcripts were read. For me, as the researcher, it involved my immediate non-verbal emotional responses to interviewees' stories (such as tears coming to my eyes); and the emotional responses that occurred as participants described events that resonated with my life experiences. Advice in textbooks (e.g. Bailey, 1987) emphasizes the importance of maintaining interviewer/interviewee distance in conducting research. Distance could imply detachment – indifference and coldness to emotional responses of participants. Yet participants' emotions were the data I wanted, to help understand their experiences. I believed that being detached would not elicit this data. I had wanted to be fully immersed in the research interview but found I had to manage my emotional reactions – to 'create some distance' in terms of my overt emotional response and involvement, to allow interviews to progress. I also had to develop skills and management techniques to monitor the possible entanglement of my life experiences in the 'hearing' of participants' stories. There was a clash between my beliefs about my role in such a collaborative research approach, the need to focus on the participants' construction and interpretation of their experiences, not mine; and the emotionality of the research topic – loss and grief.

My concern about not being 'in' the research and appearing cold and indifferent, presented me with the practical dilemma of how to build rapport, trust and acceptance with participants in order to explore deeply personal issues, without the emotional connections I believed needed to be a part of such relationships. It was my view that, in this research design, empathy would be an essential facilitating factor. While researchers who interview participants once or twice might effectively establish a productive research relationship by being sympathetic, I believed that this would not sustain a long-term project of personal exchanges at a heightened emotional level. For me, being accepted by participants dictated social obligations (Punch, 1994), but I was also aware that I was not an ongoing part of their social world. My research journal recorded my feelings about this some 12 months into the fieldwork:

> The problem is, I have developed trust with these people, who are sharing personal concerns and experiences of loss. Now they treat me as a friend, a confidante. Natural social reciprocity in social relations would have me talking about everyday things about myself. But I dare not do this. (R/J, 12/92)

I eventually accepted the apparent paradox of this 'empathic distance' as a part of the researcher's role in this type of study with grief as the topic.

While maintaining 'empathic distance' had been of great concern to me in terms of social obligations, it was not experienced as dissonant for at least one of the participants. To explore the participants' perception of my role in the research, I asked them in the final interview how they perceived that role. Harry (pseudonym) explained:

> I must admit I hadn't thought about your role in the research. It is an interesting point, because it would be difficult to step out of what you are doing. I guess in a sense I have seen what your role has been as very comfortable, it seems pretty natural, as well as being able to achieve your professional goal. We've talked about a lot of things of a fairly personal nature, in one sense, certainly from what I have talked to you about …
> You have been able to keep that at professional level. Yet I think that for what I have been talking about there must have been some personal connection with your own experiences. You haven't shared any of that except when you said you had to come to terms with your mother's death. I thought you were human then! […] (Harry, 11 years' teaching experience)

The parts of myself I presented in the interview were perceived by Harry as my professional role, with a touch of 'being human'.

With hindsight, I might have been too restrictive in maintaining 'empathic distance' but the fact that this research was for a dissertation and the paradigm I was working in was a new one for me, prompted me to err on the side of caution. This stance is one that researchers need to work out themselves, but all participants both male and female reported that my gender lessened the 'distance'. This is an issue that space does not permit elaboration on here. But feminist researchers (Oakley, 1981; Stanley & Wise, 1991) would support the influence of gender of the researcher in research.

Clash between the 'researcher I' and the 'counsellor I'

Another dilemma faced in this research related to a past career as a counsellor and my current role as a researcher. […] In the beginning, the research process had been slow. […] I failed to probe too deeply early in the research about loss and grief, first, because the precise role I should adopt was not clear in my mind: 'How much distance should I maintain from my participants to keep my research role?'; and second: 'How could I care for my respondents?' This I now understand to be a clash between what Peshkin (1988) refers to as the various 'Is' we bring to the research process. In this case it was a clash between my 'Research I' and my 'Counsellor I'. In my research journal, after I had interviewed a teacher about his experience of telling a class about the death of the parent of one of their classmates, I recorded:

> The territory I was charting hit me … a teacher revealed the impact of recent personal loss experiences on his role as a teacher. This was the heart of what my research was about, but I had been unprepared for it. I came away from that interview feeling disturbed and uneasy. I had let someone down – that 'I' as a researcher had opened up some issues – but the 'Counsellor I' had, mindful of my research role, not reached out to help. The bell had rung, we had not made a contract that if what we talked about raised difficult issues, that I would provide a safety net. The realisation of the dilemma between the two roles haunted me for days. It resulted in the resolution, to preface future interviews where I was specifically going to focus on loss and grief, with the proviso/contract that if anything did arise that they felt they needed to talk more about, that I could supply them with names of people who could help. I also resolved to tell them that they could stop the interview at any stage and to ask them at the end, if they were okay to return to class (R/J, 9/92).

[…]

Coyle & Wright (1996) make suggestions about the use of counselling skills in in-depth interviews. They advocate the use of basic counselling techniques that allow the interviewer to 'create conditions in which the interviewee can derive therapeutic benefit' (p. 434). For them, the purpose of utilizing counselling skills is to perform clarifying, account forming and cathartic functions (Coyle & Wright, 1996). Rosenblatt (1995) further elucidates these therapy/research aspects, maintaining that the boundaries are not useful. He offers the concept of 'therapeutic experiences' (Nadeau, cited in Rosenblatt, 1995: 151), that is, interviews that are 'transformative or growth – producing moments, but [not] … focused on growth or healing'.

[…]

One of the things that encouraged participants in this study to be open was that it was 'research'. The intent of discovery of the issues on my part and for teachers, students, parents and other school community members, and the possibility of others benefiting from the participants' involvement in the research, motivated their participation. It appeared that being involved in research facilitated disclosure, disclosure some may not feel comfortable with in a counselling session where they perceive themselves as 'needing help'. It is my belief that in the research interaction they were 'powerful', they were offering their experience so that it might help others. […]

Despite it being an emotional experience, participants did not refuse being repeatedly interviewed. Each interview transcript was returned to the participant and usually formed the basis for the next interview. This facilitated their reflection and helped develop rapport. In this instance someone 'doing research' gave permission for people to talk about what for many is still a taboo topic and/or an experience of powerlessness. The research process provided the conditions for the participants to feel powerful about an experience that, for many, was disempowering. In this research the valuing of participants' perspectives was one factor that facilitated their feelings of 'power' – power that was created through the form the research process took. Regaining a sense of control in one's life might also be achieved through bereavement counselling. In this instance it might be that the research process acted as an intervention. Other researchers have also reported the positive impact for participants of 'telling their story' (Kellehear, 1989; Rosenblatt, 1995).

[...]

The emotional impact

The emotional impact of the research was another dilemma I encountered. The nature of sensitive issues, created by emotional responses of individuals and the meaning of the experiences (Rowling, 1996b) meant that subjectivity was important in researching them, not only the subjective experiences of the participants, but also the researcher's subjectivity. In my case this meant my existing knowledge of the field of loss and grief, my comfort level with people's sadness, and my experience as a teacher, counsellor, academic and researcher. In other words, the knowledge I wanted to construct was from particular experiences and expressions of human beings in a particular context. I, as the researcher, also brought knowledge, beliefs and experiences to the research process. Subjectivity, rather than being a hindrance, was vitally important to begin to develop an understanding of grief experiences in the context of school communities. This orientation to research has been emphasized by many feminist researchers (Oakley, 1981; Stanley & Wise, 1991). It is a key element in researching sensitive issues: 'personal involvement is more than dangerous bias – it is the condition under which people come to know each other and to admit others into their lives' (Oakley, 1981: 58). Researching sensitive issues needs an empathic involvement because of the intimate nature of the research topics and consequent subjective experiences in the research process.

   The study included in-depth repeated intensive interviews. This resulted in a highly interactive research process. Some of the stories that were told to me were of great sadness and pain. I was aware that doing research using qualitative methods, using myself as the main instrument, would involve emotional experiences. I knew the topic itself was highly emotional, but the spontaneous sharing by participants of their life experiences sometimes caught me unaware and left me feeling humbled and with a deep respect for the resilience of human beings. It also meant that there were times when the events and reactions that were being described resonated with my own life experiences. This always presented a dilemma for me: should I say 'I too have experienced that' in an attempt to link their experience to my own and thereby facilitate connection in the interview relationship, knowing I ran the risk of the interview being diverted to me? Or should I maintain my research distance and document my response in my research journal? It was the latter response that

I chose, for in the back of my mind was the message from grief counselling that people's experiences are unique and that likening their experience to yours is not helpful. [...]

Nothing that I read in planning this study prepared me for the emotionality of the research process. I read recommendations about how I should address confidentiality, harm, deception and privacy, but there was not much written on such things as the impact on the researcher of listening to people talk about their grief, their fears and anxieties, sometimes being expressed for the first time and in times of crisis. Participants told me of events in their lives that had great emotional impact on them: at the time they occurred, and in their retelling. These accounts had an emotional impact on me as I heard them. Kellehear (1989) refers to this as the 'trauma' in the research context.

[...] During the research I continually experienced emotional reactions to interviews. I was unprepared for the intimacy and spontaneity of revelations and the prolonged impact of two years of fieldwork on this topic. Interviews were affected by feelings of anxiety 'heightened by the anticipation of interacting with vulnerable subjects involved in sensitive situations' (Cowles, 1988: 173). I experienced anxiety in making contact with people who, because of their traumatic experience, became the focus of my interest. I experienced anxiety when I knew I was going into an interview where I would be probing someone to tell me about their feelings about current events – their own impending death, the death of a spouse or the death of a parent. Thoughts that ran through my head included, 'What will this parent who has cancer look like?' 'Do I have a right to question someone about a recent deeply personal loss?' 'How can I provide some sort of protection for them after I leave?' I had to console myself with the fact that the interviews were voluntary, people could tell me as much or as little as they wanted.

[...]

On reflection I realized I had brought to the research process 'feeling rules' (Young & Lee, 1996) about how a researcher should act. Most recommendations about the qualities of a researcher using qualitative methods relate to technical skills. Guidance is not offered about management of one's own emotional reactions, yet the 'researcher cannot isolate himself from the feelings of loss and anxiety in others and himself [sic]' (Koocher, 1974: 20). [...]

References

Bailey, R.D. (1987). *Methods of social research*. New York: Free Press.

Coyle, A. and Wright, C. (1996). Using the counselling interview to collect research data on sensitive topics. *Journal of Health Psychology, 1*, 431–440.

Cowles, K.V. (1988). Issues in qualitative research on sensitive topics. *Western Journal of Nursing Research, 10*, 163–179.

Ely, M. (ed.) (1991). *Doing qualitative research: circles within circles*. London: Falmer Press.

Holly, M.L. (1989). *Writing to grow. Keeping a personal-professional journal*. Portsmouth, New Haven: Heinemann.

Kellehear, A. (1989). Ethics and social research. In J. Perry (ed.), *Doing fieldwork* (pp. 61–72). Geelong, Deakin University Press.

Kellehear, A. (1996). Unobtrusive methods in delicate situations. In J. Daly, *Ethical intersections: health research, methods and researcher responsibilities*. St Leonards: Allen and Unwin.

Koocher, G.P. (1974). Conversations with children about death – ethical considerations in research. *Journal of Child Psychology, 3*, 19–21.

Lofland, J. and Lofland, L.H. (1984). *Analyzing social settings*. New York: McGraw Hill.

Nadeau, J.W. (1998). *Families making sense of death*. Thousand Oaks, CA: Sage.

Oakley, A. (1981). Interviewing women: a contradiction in terms. In H. Roberts (ed.), *Doing feminist research* (pp. 30–61). London: Routledge.

Peshkin, A. (1988). In search of subjectivity – one's own. *Educational Researcher, 17*, 17–22.

Punch, M. (1994). Politics and ethics in qualitative research. In N.K. Denzin & Y.S. Lincoln (eds), *Handbook of Qualitative Research* (pp. 83–98). Thousand Oaks, CA: Sage.

Rosenblatt, P. (1995). Ethics of qualitative interviewing with grieving families. *Death Studies, 19*, 139–156.

Rowling, L. (1995). Disenfranchised grief of teachers. *Omega. International Journal of Death and Dying, 31*, 317–329.

Rowling, L. (1996a). Learning about life: teaching about loss. In R. Best (ed.), *Education Spirituality and the Whole Child*. London: Cassell.

Rowling, L. (1996b). A comprehensive approach to handling sensitive issues in schools with special reference to loss and grief. *Pastoral Care in Education, 4*, 17–21.

Stake, R.E. (1994). Case studies. In N.K. Denzin & Y.S. Lincoln (eds), *Handbook of Qualitative Research* (pp. 236–248). Thousand Oaks, CA: Sage.

Stanley, L. and Wise, S. (1991). Method, methodology and epistemology in feminist research processes. In L. Stanley (ed.), *Feminist Praxis* (pp. 20–59). London: Routledge.

Young, E.H. and Lee, R. (1996). Fieldworker feelings as data: 'emotion work' and 'feeling rules' in first person accounts of sociological fieldwork. In V. James and J. Gabe (eds), *Health and the sociology of emotions* (pp. 97–113). Oxford: Blackwell.

31

Growing up with HIV: The Experiences of Young People Living with HIV Since Birth in the UK

Judith Dorrell, Sarah Earle, Jeanne Katz and Shirley Reveley

Introduction

As treatment for HIV has improved, children with the infection are living longer and healthier lives, and with mortality rates declining and survival rates improving, this has become a medical success story (Sharland, Gibb and Tudor-Williams, 2002; Gibb et al., 2003; Foster and Lyall, 2005). For many people, the introduction of effective treatment has transformed HIV from an acute terminal illness into a chronic condition and, as a result, there are increasing numbers of older children and young people growing up with HIV. One of the greatest achievements has also been the dramatic reduction in children becoming infected at birth (mother to child transmission). However, in the UK there is a small, but significant number of children and young people who live with HIV, most of them having been infected at birth, before such effective treatment became available (Brown and Lourie, 2000; Gibb et al., 2003). These children and young people face a range of complex issues, and although they are not large in number, they are an important and sometimes forgotten part of the AIDS epidemic. HIV services and care historically have tended to focus on adults, with children and young people's issues becoming marginalised. This has been in part due to their small numbers, but also the dominance of adult services and care in this field. The development of paediatric treatment and medical management of paediatric HIV has tended to lag behind that of adults (McKinney and Cunningham, 2004). Despite the improved treatment, young people still live with an uncertain future and there is still no cure for HIV. Many live with medical crises and some will need to come to terms with the idea of dying prematurely. These young people may also experience multiple losses in their families because of HIV; some may have lost their mother, father or both parents; others may have lost siblings or members of their extended family (Brown and Lourie, 2000).

While there have been several clinical studies on young people and HIV (Gibb et al., 2003; Walker et al., 2004), and some studies which examine service provision in the UK (Lewis 2001; Conway 2006), there is limited research on the social and psychological impact of living with HIV infection for young people (Thorne et al., 2002; Green and

Smith, 2004). This reading draws on research carried out as part of a doctoral study exploring the lives of young people infected with HIV. The next section offers a brief background to the research, followed by a discussion on research methods. The final section of the reading explores how young people articulate their fears of dying and their experiences and feelings about living with loss.

Background to the research

In the UK, the numbers of children and young people infected with HIV is small, in 2006, there were less than 1200 under 19 years of age known to be infected living in the UK – 50 per cent of these being over the age of 10 (Conway 2006; National Study of HIV, 2006). Most of these young people have been infected perinatally (at birth or shortly after). As the young people with HIV in the UK come from diverse ethnic backgrounds, they are not a homogenous group (Lewis, 2001; Green and Smith, 2004; Miah, 2004; Conway, 2006; NAT, 2006; NCB, 2006). In a study of the development of transitional care in a large London HIV clinic, researchers found that 85 per cent of the parents of perinatally infected children originate from countries outside the UK, predominantly from African countries, although most of the children and young people were either born or lived in the UK for many years (Dodge and Melvin, 2003).

Researching young people living with HIV

This reading draws on ongoing qualitative research which aims to document the experiences of young people with perinatally acquired HIV so as to further understanding of how HIV affects young people's lives. Ethical approval for the study was granted by the Open University Human and Participants Material Ethics Committee and the Local NHS Ethics Committee and Research Governance Committee of the hospital. An enhanced Criminal Records Bureau check was also required in order to interview the young people.

Participants who fulfilled the selection criteria were recruited to the study. The selection criteria included children/young people:

- perinatally infected with HIV (having HIV since birth)
- between the ages of 13 and 24 years
- aware of HIV status for at least one year and feel sufficiently comfortable to talk about HIV
- who have been in the hospital service for at least 6 months.

The research adopted a purposive sampling method and participants were recruited from a specialist adolescent clinic in a large London hospital. The study was piloted with two young people and, at the time of writing, 20 young people have been interviewed. The study used semi-structured in-depth interviews with young people aged between 13 and 24 years. The interviews focused on topics such as how HIV affects daily life; relationships with family and friends; intimate relationships; school/work; and the future. It was important that the young people felt enabled to talk openly about HIV and had known about their status for some time in order to minimise any potential distress. Also it was important for them to be familiar with the clinic before being approached to participate in the study. The young people were interviewed alone in a private room in the clinic without their parent/carer or guardian present. As talking about HIV is not easy because it involves talking about personal and sensitive issues (Miah 2004; Melvin 2007; Wiener and Battles, 2006; Weiner et al., 2007), and there is always the potential risk of distress, it was important to ensure there was good support and care in place. Following the interviews, the young people were given details of support organisations and there was easy access to a psychologist or clinical nurse specialist to speak to should they be upset.

The interviews lasted between one and three hours; they were audio-taped and transcribed verbatim. Many themes emerged from the data, but the concepts of 'living with dying' and 'living with loss' were prominent. It is these themes which are now considered.

Living with dying

The fear of dying looms large in the lives of the young people interviewed for this study. Many talked about 'living in the shadow of HIV'. For example, Rebecca aged 18 said:

> HIV is always in my head, it is always there whatever I do, whenever I sleep, when I wake HIV is there, it never goes away that fear of dying.

Some young people have lived with the expectation of death around them for many years, having been diagnosed at a time when there was limited treatment available for children, as Paul (24 years old) – one of the respondents – commented:

> At that time, we were just not expected to live, we were meant to die, I was surprised when I just kept on living.

Most of young people interviewed live in families where one or more family members have HIV or have died from HIV, and therefore some will have observed the illness trajectory at first hand. Although there is now much more effective treatment available, the progress of HIV remains unpredictable and the fear of illness is reflected in what the young people said, for example:

> Living with HIV is sometimes like living with dying, I am always waiting to become ill, waiting to deteriorate, waiting for my time. (Liam, 17 years old)

> When I fall ill, I get sad cos I think the worst, and I think I am not going to make it this time, I have been ill quite a lot. (Carmel, 18 years old)

The fear of death was one of the common reactions reported by the young people when they were told about having HIV. They reported feeling frightened, feeling a fear of dying and fearing they would die soon. Some young people expressed feeling a need to condense their living into fewer years because they were unsure as to how long they had left to live.

They expressed needing to live for now and not to look too far into the future. Another respondent, Emily (18 years old), expresses this as follows:

> I feel as if I have to do it all quickly because I don't know how long I will stay well, I haven't got time to waste.

The young people interviewed clearly identified living with the fear of dying as an issue and felt that living with HIV resulted in a heightened sense of their mortality. For these young people, this is further reinforced by their experiences of multiple losses in the family.

Living with loss

Although treatment has changed the course of this disease for many, most of these young people will have experienced the long-term illness and loss of a parent, sibling or other family member from HIV. When parents/carers die it can lead to family disruption, separation and relationship breakdown (Lewis, 2001; Rotherham-Borus et al., 2005; Lyon and D'Angelo, 2006; Weiner and Battles, 2006). Such breakdown may result in young people being cared for by foster carers, grandparents or other family members (Lewis, 2001; Miah, 2004; Conway, 2006). When there is a death from HIV, it is often difficult for families (and the young person) to be open about the cause of death due to the fear of discrimination and stigma. When a family member dies from HIV young people spoke about having to lie about what their parent or sibling had died from, and they found this very distressing, and they found it equally hard to share their grief with anyone, because they could not tell the truth. For example:

> I didn't tell people what my brother died of, when they asked I just lied, well it was partly the truth, he did die from a lung infection, but it was caused by HIV. (Paul, 24 years old)

> I just told them he died of cancer, what else could I say? (Emily, 18 years old)

Living with HIV involves keeping many secrets, often these are family secrets which can create barriers in young people's social relationships. Living with an illness that you cannot discuss with people you meet every day presents difficulties for young people and problems from keeping secrets have been reported by other researchers (Lewis 2001; Battles and Weiner 2002; Bond, Dorrell and Honigsbaum, 2000; Brown and Lourie, 2000). HIV remains a stigmatised condition and as a sexually transmitted infection brings a complex mix of issues for a young person to deal with. Young people may perceive that they have to keep the family secret, as in disclosing their own status to people they are also disclosing their mother's infection and this is a difficult issue for them. Talking about HIV in their families may risk raising issues that have not been addressed by parents in relation to how they became infected. The data suggest that a young person's HIV status is not always disclosed even within families that live together, for example, Charlotte (18 years old) says:

> I don't tell my sister because I wouldn't do that to my mum, it wouldn't be fair to her as she has told no one, not even my sister knows, only me as I have it too.

Young people express great loyalty to their parents and do not want to be the cause of their distress. They are mindful that disclosing their own status or talking openly about HIV may cause difficulties for their families. Young people seek to protect parents by keeping their status secret and not discussing it, as Luke and Emma comment:

> I can't talk about HIV to Mum and Dad as I know it upsets them so I don't feel able to talk to them, I don't think they want to talk about it. I just know I can't tell anyone. I think they want to protect me, but sometimes I think it would help to talk to them about it, it might make it a bit easier. (Luke, 16 years old)

> We never spoke about it, we all just pretended it wasn't there, but it was. (Emma, 17 years old)

In other studies young people report feeling sad, depressed, lonely and isolated from family and friends (Lewis, 2001; Miah, 2004; Lyon and D'Angelo, 2006). They fear other people finding out and find it difficult not being able to talk about HIV in their families. In some families not everybody is told about HIV, in others all the family may be aware, but it may never be spoken about. Young people, such as Luke and Emma, are aware that talking about HIV for some of parents may be upsetting, so they learn to keep silent (Bond, Dorrell and Honigsbaum, 2000; Lewis, 2001; Melvin, 2003; in press). Some of the other respondents in this study talked about the need to keep their HIV status a secret from friends:

> The bit I hate is lying to my friends, but if I did tell them how could I explain why I didn't trust them enough to tell them before? (Carmel, 18 years old)

Young people observe how HIV is viewed differently from other illnesses, such as cancer and they comment on how it feels impossible to be open about living and dying from HIV, because of the fear of the stigma and discrimination. Sarah (18 years old) – another respondent – makes this point:

> You know if he had died from cancer I would have got loads of sympathy and people would be kind, but with HIV, you can't even tell people the truth, all the sadness has to stay inside for ever.

The loss of a brother or sister is also common for this group and these losses reinforce the reality to the young people that they may be the next one to die. A brother or sister is part of the peer group for young people and a death of someone close in age has profound effects.

> When my brother died, it was a case of when was it my turn, you know that was definitely it, I thought well Mum's gone, my brother's gone, so next in line is me, so it's me next. (Paul, 24 years old)

Outside the small number of people that may know in their family, most young people do not talk about HIV with friends and therefore when a brother or sister dies, most say they have no one to talk to about their loss. At the same time as experiencing this loss they are reminded of and fear their own death. Evidence suggests that many of these young people have limited and somewhat fragile support networks, and little emotional support (Nostlinger et al. 2004, 2006; Rotherham-Borus, 2005). This is emphasised by the comment made by Paul below:

> I think when my brother died I felt the pain of my mum dying and there was pain in that place, I was 13 years old. When he died, I just felt that I basically took it upon me and all of my brother's goals he had and I put them on my shoulders and I did all of them for him. (Paul, 24 years old)

The young people interviewed in this study emphasised that they want their lives to be meaningful and want to leave their mark on their world, like any other young person, but this becomes more important when living with a condition that may limit your lifespan. This is reflected in what they say, for example:

> I have to make my life count, or what does it all mean? I will have gone through all this for nothing. (Emma, 17 years old)

> No one can cure you, the tablets won't make you better so all the time you just live day by day, not planning too much, but whatever you do, make sure you really live, make it worthwhile. (Ben, 17 years old)

Most of the young people interviewed had experienced the loss of a close family member from HIV, and while they tried to make sense of these losses, young people are reminded of the stigma of HIV, as they do not feel able to talk openly. They carry the additional burden of secrecy and fear of disclosure of their condition. While they know there is no cure for HIV, they see their lives of value and worth, and most try to find a way to focus on living positively.

Conclusion

Living with HIV is difficult for young people but new treatment has made a significant difference by extending their lives. The social stigma of HIV remains and the difficulties of not being able to talk openly to friends and family about HIV means that many of these young people feel isolated and lonely. Unlike adults, these young people have grown up in the presence of HIV which has been an integral part of their narrative and as such the virus is always part of their identity. For example, Paul (24 years old) says:

> I have two worlds, my normal one and then my HIV one, I am alone in my HIV world, but that's ok.

While it is not possible to predict how these young people's health and lives may develop and how HIV will affect their future, many are living fulfilling lives. Some have become parents, most are either working or studying and many see HIV as just one part of their lives, in spite of the fears they have about dying and their experiences of loss. As one young person said:

> I am more than just HIV, I am a young person who just happens to have HIV, so what, I am still here and I am going to live the life I want for as long as I can. (Matt, 18 years old)

References

Bond, K., Dorrell, J. and Honigsbaum, N. (2000) *What Do The Children Tell Us?* Project Report. European Forum on HIV/AIDS Children and Families.

Battles, H.B. and Weiner, L.S. (2002) 'From adolescence through young adulthood: psychosocial adjustment associated with long term survival of HIV', *Journal of Adolescent Health*, 30 (3): 161–81.

Brown, L.K., Lourie, K.J. and Pao, M. (2000) 'Children and adolescents living with HIV and AIDS: a review', *Journal of Child Psychology and Psychiatry*, 41 (1): 81–96.

Conway, M. (2006) *Developing Support Services for Children, Young People and Families Living with HIV: A Handbook for Service Providers*. London: National Children's Bureau.

Dodge, J. and Melvin, D. (2003) 'From family clinic to adolescent services: 12 years of a specialist HIV service for children and families', *HIV Medicine*, 5(1): 4–46 and also at www.blackwell-synergy.com/doi/abs

Foster, C. and Lyall, E.G.H. (2005) 'Children with HIV: improved mortality and morbidity with combined antiretroviral therapy', *Current Opinion Infectious Diseases*, 18 (3): 253–9.

Gibb, D.M., Duong, T., Tookey, P.A., Sharland, M., Tudor-Williams, G., Novelli, K., Butler, K, Riordan, A., Farrelly, L., Masters, J., Peckham, C.S. and Dunn, D.T. (2003) 'Decline in mortality, AIDS, and hospital admissions in perinatally HIV-1 infected children in the United Kingdom and Ireland', *British Medical Journal*, 327: 1019–23.

Green, G. and Smith, R. (2004) 'The psychosocial and health needs of HIV-positive people in the United Kingdom: a review', *HIV Medicine*, 5 (1): 5–46.

Lewis, E. (2001) *Afraid to Say: The Needs and Views of Young People Living with HIV/AIDS*. London: National Children's Bureau.

Lyon, M.E. and D'Angelo, L.J. (eds) (2006) *Teenagers, HIV, and AIDS: Insights from Youths Living with the Virus*. Westport, Connecticut: Praeger.

McKinney, R.E. and Cunningham, C.K. (2004) 'Newer treatments for HIV in children: infectious diseases and immunization', *Current Opinion in Pediatrics*, 16 (1): 76–9.

Melvin, D. (2003) 'Children living with HIV: psychological concerns', *HIV Nursing*, 3: 5–7.

Melvin, D. (in press) *Psychosexual Development in Adolescents Growing up with HIV Infection in London*.

Miah, J. (ed.) (2004) *Talking with Young People and Families about Chronic Illness and Living with HIV*. London: National Children's Bureau.

NAT (National AIDS Trust) (2006) *Dispersal of Asylum Seekers Living with HIV*. London: NAT.

NCB (National Children's Bureau) (2006) *Children and Young people living with HIV/AIDS*. Amanda El No. 228. London: National Children's Bureau.

NSHPC (2006) *National Study of HIV in Pregnancy and Childhood Quarterly Update*. No. 66, April. London: NSHPC.

Nostlinger, C., Jonckheer, T., De Belder, E., Van Wijngaerden, E., Wylock, C., Pelgrom, J. and Colebunders, R. (2004) 'Families affected by HIV: parents' and children's characteristics and disclosure to the children', *AIDS Care*, 16 (5): 641–8.

Nostlinger, C., Bartoli, G., Gordillo, V., Roberfroid, D. and Colebunders, R. (2006) 'Children and adolescents living with HIV positive parents: emotional and behavioural problems', *Vulnerable Children and Youth Studies*, 1 (1): 29–43.

Rotherham-Borus, M.J., Flannery, D., Rice, E. and Lester, P. (2005) 'Families living with HIV', *AIDS Care*, 17 (8): 978–87.

Sharland, M., Gibb, D.M. and Tudor-Williams, G. (2002) 'Advances in the prevention of paediatric HIV in the United Kingdom', *Archives of Disease in Childhood*, 87: 178–80.

Thorne, C., Newell, M.L., Botet, F.A., Bohlin, A.B., Ferrazin, A., Giaquinto, C., de Jose Gomez, I., Mok, J.Y.Q., Mur, A. and Peltier, A. (2002) 'Older children and adolescents surviving with vertically acquired HIV infection', *Journal of Acquired Immune Deficiency Syndromes*, 29: 396–401.

Walker, S.A., Doerholf, K.A., Sharland, M.B. and Gibb, D.M. (2004) 'Response to highly active anti-retroviral therapy varies with age: the UK and Ireland Collaborative HIV Study', *AIDS*, 18 (14): 1915–24.

Weiner, L.S. and Battles, H.B. (2006) 'Untangling the web: a close look at diagnosis disclosure among HIV infected adolescents', *Journal of Adolescent Health*, 38: 307–9.

Weiner, L., Mellins, C.A., Marhefka, S. and Battles, H.B. (2007) 'Disclosure of an HIV diagnosis to children: history, current research, and future directions', *Journal of Developmental and Behavioural Pediatrics*, 28 (2): 155–66.

32

The Absence of Death and Dying in Intellectual Disability Research

Stuart Todd

If there is any certainty concerning the meaning and impact of living with intellectual disability, it is simply this: people so identified will, as we all must, die. A fundamental argument of this paper is that while death is inevitable, the experience of death and dying may not be universal. Intellectual disability may thoroughly exert its influence in death as it will have done in life. It may remain a significant feature governing the nature of individuals' death and their remembrance just as it will surely have done during those fateful moments when the identity was initially suspected, the label applied (Booth, 1978), and, thereafter, at significant turning points in their life-careers (See for example, May, 1988). There exists considerable evidence that the social characteristics of dying individuals can dramatically influence the type of care they receive (Sudnow, 1967; Lawton, 2000) in much the same ways as they influence the care of individuals more generally (Becker, 1952; Jeffrey, 1979; Kelly, 1982). Yet, despite the distinct possibility that intellectual disability will shape the way these final stages of life are managed and understood, death and dying appear to be excluded or, at least, overlooked as substantive research topics in their own right. Beyond the issue of mortality, researchers have been oddly reticent to consider the social and emotional contexts of the deaths of people with intellectual disabilities or of the experiences of and demands placed upon their carers. As a consequence, death and dying remain largely neglected issues, screened off from wider appreciation in a private and impenetrable zone of experience. The costs stemming from such privatization can only be imagined.

The aim of this [reading] is to argue that, sociologically at least, the social issues of death warrant focused attention and that researchers should deal with this inevitable and most enigmatic aspect of human existence. In so doing, important discussions can be conducted concerning the difficulty that people with intellectual disabilities and their relatives, friends and care staff undoubtedly, if all too silently, encounter in the times before and after death. Furthermore, as well as examining some of the troubles and dilemmas that dying poses, an understanding of the nature of the times before and after death will provide deep insight into the social and cultural phenomenon which give shape to living with intellectual disability. A study of how any society deals with death can be highly informative about the nature of that society itself (Frankenberg, 1987; Seale, 1998).

From 'Death does not become us: The absence of death and dying in intellectual disability research' by Stuart Todd, *Gerontological Social Work*, 38: 225–40, 2002, Taylor & Francis, reprinted by kind permission of the publisher and author (Taylor & Francis, www.informaworld.com).

This [reading] does not outline with any adequate comprehensiveness or precision what a sociological perspective offers to the understanding of dying and death. [...] It is concerned more with death as a social phenomenon rather than with biological survival, although there are important issues to be resolved around the latter (Eyman & Borthwick-Duffy, 1994). The concerns here related to issues of the quality of care to dying people – managing death awareness. [...]

The trouble with death: it's not life!

[...] The relative absence of studies of death and dying within the study of intellectual disability might be readily understood as just another expression of the generalized tabooed treatment of death in our society. Put simply, the dearth of research work can be attributed to more widespread social and cultural practices of dealing with death and dying by locating them within forbidden and dangerous zones of interest. Death, thus handled, can be securely entombed (Ariès, 1974: Elias, 1985: Gorer, 1965).

Yet any such argument sits uneasily with an increasingly accepted view that death and dying have, over the past three decades, become areas of intensive scholarly and lay discourse (for example, Armstrong, 1987; Field, 1989; Glaser and Strauss, 1965; Gorer, 1965; Kellehear, 1984; Kübler-Ross, 1969; Mellor and Schilling, 1993; Sudnow, 1967; Walter, 1994). Walter (1994: 1–2), for example, comments on the 'revival of death' as a pervasive feature of late modern societies, writing that the plethora of works on these issues generally:

... sounds like a society obsessed with death, not one that denies it.

Such curiosity has yet to extend to the area of intellectual disabilities. General textbooks on intellectual disability, and research on a range of relevant concerns, for example, residential care, aging and health, do not seem typically to include death or dying as areas of particular concerns beyond that of mortality. The personal, emotional and social dimensions of dying and death for individuals, carers and professionals seem to be beyond the realm of our concerns. Death appears to be a side-stepped issue which may be viewed as an illegitimate and unwelcome intruder, detracting from our more typical dealings with the lifestyles of people with intellectual disabilities. Blacher (1998: 412), for example, in a commentary upon studies of mortality across types of residential settings urges:

In my opinion, mortality is the wrong question to consider. The question to consider involves life not death in the community.

Without wishing to take too much from a single comment, it does seem to demonstrate a striking sentiment which would probably find resonance across the field of intellectual disabilities more generally. That is, in the choice between life and death, life must win. The choice no doubt alludes to the efforts which have taken place over recent years to establish and advance the social bond of people with intellectual disabilities within their communities. Death may pose a disruptive threat to such ambitions given its capacity for reminding us of the ultimate power of nature over culture (Giddens, 1991). Furthermore, side-stepping death may be interpreted as confronting and defying the symbolic and social deaths which have hovered over their lives in the past. That is to say that, in life, people with intellectual disabilities have been too eagerly treated as without culture and, therefore, already dead. We have been, perhaps, 'fighting death tooth and nail' (Bauman, 1993) in all its symbolic forms and, in the process, have overlooked the fact that death comes in physical form with social and emotional implications. Biological and social deaths are far from identical and the latter acknowledges that the social existence of an individual may be diminished or removed before they are biologically dead (Sudnow, 1967). The potential for the pre-mortem disintegration of personhood and the acute withdrawal from social interaction which dying poses can be seen as essential dimensions of the lives of people with intellectual disability some years before their deaths. As Mulkay (1993: 42) writes, it is:

possible for extended social death sequences to stretch deeply back into people's existence as living organisms.

This tendency is surely recognized in the lives of people with learning disabilities who have been unduly and eagerly removed from their communities to die symbolically within institutions, settings which could be characterized as the descendants of society's initial practices of social exclusion: namely cemeteries (Baudrillard, 1993). Goffman (1961), for example, wrote of the processes of 'mortification' whereby individuals were taken out of symbolic, as well as physical circulation and disciplined to the imperatives of institutional life. The metaphor of death is repeated in forceful fashion in Blatt and Kaplan's (1966) 'A Christmas in purgatory'. Residential services for people with intellectual disabilities have been easily viewed as social cemeteries, places to which parents were once asked to send their offspring and to think of them as having died. Death has also been used as a metaphor to understand the reactions of parents to the discovery that a son or daughter has a learning disability. Parents are defined as undergoing a form of 'bereavement' en-route to their successful adjustment (Bicknell, 1988) Yet, while we may reject the appropriation of death metaphors to capture life, when physical death occurs. Oswin's (1984: 226) poignant account of the silence of human services is matched, it seems, only by research blindness. She describes how one set of bereaved foster parents of a child with intellectual disabilities were:

… dreadfully upset that the professionals, who had encouraged the affectionate relationship to develop between them and the little boy, did not seem to appreciate the extent of their bereavement. 'It has never been mentioned, how upset we felt about him dying. It should have been told to us in the beginning that some children could die, but nothing was ever said … and nobody wants to talk about it now either'. They attended monthly meetings of special foster parents organized by social workers, but the death of the little foster boy had not been referred to at any of the meetings. They could not explain what sort of help they would have liked for their grief, but they just knew that they felt very bereft and were hurt because it did not seem that any of the professionals understood or cared that they were sad and needed an opportunity to talk about what had happened. … a few weeks after he had died they were approached by a social worker who, knowing they had a vacancy, hoped to fill his dates with a new child. They had been very upset by this. The last thing they wanted was a social worker immediately trying to fill the dead child's place with a new child.

Oswin's account of these grieving foster parents underlines that, in discounting death, life is simply devalued. If the lives of people with intellectual disabilities are to count as significant, then surely their deaths must also have some consequence. We can reject the death metaphors in our field but not embodied dying and death and their very real social impact. The choice of research focus between issues of life and death is surely superfluous. Death can only not count for those who have never lived or for those we wish to be lost from memory in unmarked graves (Lovell, 1997). To tackle issues of death and dying as they impinge upon the lives of people with intellectual disabilities avows rather than denies their social bond since, as Berger (1973), for example, writes:

Every human society is, in the last resort, men (sic) banded together in the face of death.

Handling bad news: death awareness

There can be no dying, from a sociological and personal point of view, without an awareness of dying. Therefore, an important starting point for research activity concerns the question of awareness of dying and the beliefs people with intellectual disabilities bring with them to the dying process. Williams (1990) has argued that awareness of impending death is an important feature which reflects dimensions of control over the dying process between medical professionals, carers, relatives and the dying individual him/herself. However, there is also a need to determine and describe what people with intellectual disabilities understand about the nature of death itself. Lipe-Goodson and Goebel (1983) argued that many people with intellectual disabilities understand the concept of death, although their level of understanding will be a function of severity of impairment, age and experience. Indeed it does appear that death and dying are treated as taboo areas in discourses amongst family members, professionals and people with intellectual disabilities (French and Kuczaj, 1985; Hollins and Esterhuyzen, 1997; Seltzer and Luchterhan, 1994). A critical point for study is the nature of the beliefs people with intellectual disabilities hold about dying and death and how these are shaped through social relationships.

The extent to which professionals and relatives may conceal death as a typical and inevitable part of life becomes of critical importance when an individual is deemed to have entered the dying process. At this point, people's views of death and dying take on a more palpable form. Glaser and Strauss (1965) described four main forms of awareness contexts which were distinguished in terms of the different levels of knowledge over the dying individual's condition held by individuals, their families and medical staff. The contexts ranged from closed awareness where the diagonosis and prognosis were kept secret from individuals to open awareness where the knowledge was shared openly by all parties. This work was conducted in a period when an increasing proportion of deaths were occurring in hospitals, settings associated with the invisibility of the dying process, the sequestration of the dying, the increasing medicalization of dying and death and a tendency for closed awareness contexts to predominate (Ariès, 1981; Sudnow, 1967). Over the past two decades, there has been a definite shift in health professionals' views regarding the communication of terminal prognosis (Armstrong, 1987; Seale, 1991) and this is, in itself seen as an indication of a more enlightened regime of care for people who are dying. However, we know very little about how such matters are handled for people with intellectual disabilities who are dying and who is deemed the most suitable person for delivering such news.

The task of managing disclosure may well fall to relatives or direct care staff who may not see it as their responsibility and may find little encouragement and support to adopt it as their own. The analytic usefulness of the now famous four-point typology of death awareness has been used to study the information control practices that parents and staff employ in handling information concerning the status and meanings of intellectual disability as an aspect of self-identity (Todd and Shearn, 1997; Todd, 2000). They argue that here closed awareness contexts predominate and make links between such practices wider social control mechanisms, highlighting the implications they may have for effective participation in decision-making fora. Does a similar conspiracy of silence exist over dying and to what extent is the individual at the center of a potentially dramatic set of events? Awareness contexts may also have important emotional implications for those who care for people with intellectual disabilities. Dealing with dying through closed awareness contexts can be emotionally demanding for staff and relatives since they may not be able to show their concern and have to manage situations for their potential leakage of information (Field, 1989). As a result of such difficulties, individuals may prefer to restrict the time they spend with dying individuals, thereby hastening their social deaths. The role of care staff in supporting individuals who are dying has been considered to be demanding and requiring much support (May, 1995; Field, 1989).

[…]

Summary

This [reading] has suggested that the social issues of death, dying and bereavement represent important but neglected research areas, and has had the simple objective of bringing such issues to the awareness of researchers as ones both for practical reform and for deciphering what living with intellectual disability entails. […] While the problems of daily living will continue to provide a focus for research, we must remember that life does not go on forever. […] For sure, many investigators are committed to research which seeks to provide insight into the characteristics of a good and eventful life but to remove people from the collective drama of death is to potentially undermine such ambitions. The deaths of people with intellectual disabilities are not so much taboo, rather, they are forbidden metaphorically and perhaps devalued experientially. If intellectual disability is to be a death-free zone it can only be so because it is seen as offering an impoverished life.

References

Ariès, P. (1974) *Western Attitudes Towards Death*. London: Marion Boyars.
Armstrong, D. (1987) 'Silence and truth in death and dying', *Social Science & Medicine,* 24: 651–8.

Baudrillard, J. (1993) *Symbolic Exchange and Death*. London: Sage.

Baumann, Z. (1993) *Mortality, Immortality and other Life Strategies*. Oxford: Polity Press.

Becker, H.S. (1952) 'Social class variations in the teacher–pupil relationship', *Journal of Educational Society*, 25(April): 451–65.

Berger, P. (1973) *The Social Reality of Religion*. Harmondsworth: Penguin.

Blacher, J. (1998) 'Much ado about mortality: debating the wrong question', *Mental Retardation*, 36: 412–15.

Blatt, B. and Kaplan, F. (1966) *Christmas in Purgatory: A Photographic Essay in Mental Retardation*. Newton: Allyn and Bacon.

Booth, T. (1978) 'From normal baby to handicapped child: unravelling the ideas of subnormality in families of mentally handicapped children', *Sociology*, 12: 203–22.

Elias, N. (1985) *The Loneliness of the Dying*. Oxford: Basil Blackwell.

Eyman, R.K. and Borthwick-Duffy, S.A. (1994) 'Trends in mortality rates and predictors of mortality', in M.M. Seltzer, M.W. Krauss and M. Janciki (eds), *Life Course Perspectives on Adulthood and Old Age*. Washington. DC: AAMR.

Field, D. (1989) *Nursing the Dying*. London: Tavistock/Routledge.

Frankenberg, R. (1987) 'Life: cycle, trajectory or pilgrimage? A social production approach to Marxism, metaphor and mortality', in A. Bryman, B. Bytheway., P. Allat and T. Keil (eds), *Rethinking the Life Cycle*. London: Macmillan.

French, J. and Kuczaj, D. (1985) 'Working through loss and change with people with learning disabilities', *Mental Handicap*, 20: 108–10.

Giddens, A. (1991) *Modernity and Self-Identity*. Cambridge: Polity Press.

Glaser, B.G. and Strauss, A.L. (1964) 'Awareness contexts and social interaction', *American Sociological Review*, 29: 669–79.

Goffman, E. (1961) *Asylums*. Harmondsworth: Penguin.

Gorer, G. (1965) *Death, Grief and Mourning*. London: Cresset Press.

Hollins, S. and Esterhuyzen, A. (1997) 'Bereavement and grief in adults with learning disabilities', *British Journal of Psychiatry*, 170: 497–501.

Jeffrey, R. (1979) 'Normal rubbish: deviant patients in casualty departments', *Sociology of Health and Illness*, 1(1): 90–107.

Kellehear, A. (1984) 'Are we a death denying society? A sociological review', *Social Science & Medicine*, 18: 713–23.

Kelly, M. (1982) 'Good and bad patients': a review of the literature and theoretical critique', *Journal of Advanced Nursing*. 7: 147–56.

Kübler-Ross, E. (1969) *On Death and Dying*. New York: Macmillan.

Lawton, J. (2000) *The Dying Process: Patients' Experiences of Palliative Care*. London: Routledge.

Lovell, A. (1997) 'Death at the beginning of life', in D. Field, J. Hockey and N. Small (eds), *Death, Gender and Ethnicity*. London: Routledge.

Lipe-Goodson, P.S. and Goebel, B.L. (1983) 'Perception of age and death in mentally retarded adults', *Mental Retardation*, 21: 68–75.

May, C. (1995) To call it work somehow demeans it: the social construction of talk in the care of terminally ill people. *Journal of Advanced Nursing*, 22: 556–61.

May, D. (1988) *Living with Mental Handicap: Transitions in the Lives of People with Mental Handicap*. London: Jessica Kingsley.

Mellor, P.A. and Shilling, C. (1993) 'Modernity, self-identity & the sequestration of death', *Sociology*, 27: 411–31.

Mulkay, M. (1993) 'Social death in Britain', in D. Clark (ed.), *The Sociology of Death*. Oxford: Blackwell.

Oswin, M. (1984) *They Keep Going Away*. London: King Edward's Hospital Fund for London.

Seale, C. (1998) *Constructing Death: The Sociology of Dying and Bereavement*. Cambridge: Cambridge University Press.

Seltzer, G.B. and Luchterhan, C. (1994) 'Health and well-being of older persons with developmental disabilities', in M.M. Seltzer, M.W. Krauss and M. Janciki (eds), *Life Course Perspectives on Adulthood and Old Age*. Washington. DC: AAMR.

Sudnow, D. (1967) *Passing On: The Social Organization of Dying*. Englewood Cliffs, NJ: Prentice Hall.

Todd, S. (2000) 'Working in the public and private domains: staff management of community activities for and identities of people with intellectual disability', *Journal of Intellectual Disability Research*, 66: 600–20.

Todd, S. and Shearn, J. (1997) 'Family dilemmas and secrets', *Disability & Society*, 12: 341–66.

Walter, T. (1991) Modern death: taboo or not taboo? *Sociology,* 25: 293–310.

Walter, T. (1994) *The Revival of Death*. London: Routledge.

Williams, R. (1990) *A Protestant Legacy*. Oxford: Clarendon Press.

33

Researching Reproductive Loss

Gayle Letherby

First thoughts

> ... conception is one of the few events that changes the course of an individual's life
> for ever. That course can be modified after the event but it cannot be undone. (Price,
> 1988: 148)

Reproductive loss is of interest to different types of researchers. Medical research is
likely to focus on the causes of reproductive loss and the possibilities of reducing it,
demographers will be interested in the impact of such events to populations and demographic trends. In a recent article in the *International Journal of Andrology* (the branch
of medicine concerned with men's health, particularly male infertility and sexual dys-
function), Brady E. Hamilton and Stephanie J. Ventura (2006), drawing on published
reports of the US government's Centres for Disease Control and Prevention National
Centre for Health Statistics, provide a detailed descriptive overview of trends in the
United States with reference to birth, fertility and abortion data. Social scientists are also
concerned with rates and trends and the implications of this for current and future populations. But they are also concerned with the social and emotional experiences of reproductive loss and the experience of researching this issue. It is specifically these concerns
that I focus on in this reading.

Early concerns and related issues

In 2003 I published a book focusing on the relationship between the feminist research
process and feminist knowledge production. In it I began by reflecting on my own first
experience of solo research which happened to be an auto/biographical (see below for further explanation of auto/biography) study of the experience of miscarriage:

> From the first day of [my undergraduate degree] I knew that I wanted mine to be
> based on an empirical study of the experience of miscarriage. ... I felt that the expe-
> rience was misunderstood and under-researched, yet I was apprehensive about the
> project. ... Would I find enough people to speak to? Would we both feel comfortable

during the interview situation? Would I ask the 'right' questions? Would I do justice to their experiences in the writing-up stage? I was also … worried that I might cause the people to whom I spoke distress by reminding them of things they would rather forget …

Acutely sensitive to all of my 'fears' … I embarked on the fieldwork. I interviewed ten women and corresponded with two women and one man. … All of the women I approached were happy to talk to me (the two I corresponded with rather than talked to, lived a long way away and both sent me a taped account of their experiences) … some even contacted me and asked if I would like to interview them. Prior to, or at the beginning of each interview I told each respondent that I had also had a miscarriage. From then on, each interview was peppered with my experiences, questions on what I knew of support groups, statistics etc. and sometimes sentences ended with 'Isn't it?; 'Don't you think?' etc. …

Committed to representing the experience of all, I had planned to talk to five men about their experience; but they were more difficult to contact. I asked several of my female respondents if their partners would be willing to talk to me. All refused except one, who wrote down a brief description of how he felt. Eventually, I stopped asking women if their partners would speak to me and although I also knew a man who I considered asking, after so many rejections I was too nervous to do so …

Although we only met the once, all the women to whom I spoke or with whom I corresponded told me very personal and intimate details about their lives. There was often reference to very negative emotions: grief, anger, pain, jealousy … (Letherby, 2003: 11–13 reproduced from research diary 1989/90, and see Letherby, 1993).

All of the issues raised in my first research diary are relevant to a more general consideration of researching reproductive loss and in the main body of this reading I pick up on several of the issues highlighted above. Thus, my concern is with:

- defining reproductive loss
- methods, methodologies and dilemmas, and researching reproductive loss
- bringing women and men 'back into' research on reproductive loss
- politics and praxis when researching reproductive loss.

Defining reproductive loss

The adoption of a lifecourse approach is useful to understanding reproductive loss. Traditionally the lifecycle approach was considered to be the most appropriate way to understand individual lives but this implies a rigid set of transitions and implies an 'ideal' life within which death and birth should occur only at the 'right time'. This approach does not account for factors such as premarital pregnancy, infertility, stillbirth nor other issues, such as divorce or premature terminal illness (Cotterill, 1994). Given this, the lifecourse approach which 'encompasses social and demographic changes which affect all our lives, as well as the personal biographical events in each individual's lifecourse' (Cotterill, 1994: 112) would seem to be more appropriate for many people's lives.

A lifecourse approach then allows us to consider reproductive loss as a disruption to individual and family lifecourses (Exley and Letherby, 2001), what Julia Frost et al., (2007) – writing specifically about miscarriage although applicable to all reproductive loss – call the 'loss of possibility'. Furthermore, it is necessary to identify just what we mean by reproductive loss. Perinatal loss is often associated – in medical and lay discourse – with miscarriage, neonatal death, stillbirth and therapeutic abortion. But what of 'infertility' (medically defined as the inability to get pregnant after 12 months of trying or the inability to carry a baby to term), elective abortion, adoption or mothers and fathers who have their baby/ies taken away from them, which all also result in a loss or losses for individuals and families? This question provides us with an indication of the importance and power of language in this instance. Loss may be defined differently by different people and as researchers we need to consider who defines as well as who experiences 'loss'. In addition this is one (among many) areas where medical language can hinder rather than help for whereas women and men who have experienced loss may prefer to speak of babies, death and goodbyes health care professionals may refer to foetuses, termination and disposal (see. Lovell, 1983, Letherby, 1993; de Crespigny and McCullough, 1999).

Methods, methodologies and dilemmas, and researching reproductive loss

When undertaking any research careful reflection about issues of method (the tools for data gathering, for example, questionnaires, interviews, conversational analysis) and of methodology (the analysis of the methods used) are essential. Liz Kelly, Sheila Burton and Linda Regan (1994) argue that appropriate methods should be chosen to suit research areas rather than research areas being chosen to 'fit' favourite techniques. In addition, Ann Oakley suggests that the 'most important criteria for choosing a particular research method is not its relationship to academic arguments about methods, but its fit with the question being asked in the research' (2004: 191). Given that reproductive loss is, as noted above, an experience about which it is important to be sensitive, it might seem that the qualitative interview, which not only enables respondents to 'tell it how it is' from their own perspective but also gives them some influence on the direction of the research process, may be the best method to use. However, this is a simplistic assumption as some respondents may prefer to complete a questionnaire or write a letter rather than talk, and our understanding of medical experience prior to and following reproductive loss may be better understood via a large-scale survey, observation or documentary analysis. As with many other research areas flexibility is necessary (see Reinharz, 1992; Stanley and Wise, 1993; Letherby and Zdrodowski, 1995 for further discussion).

Any research project involving patients, patient records and/or health care professionals now needs external ethical approval from a local medical ethics committee. For those working in the academy it may also be necessary to obtain similar approval from the university ethics committee. In addition, many professional associations provide guidelines on ethical practice in research to their members (for example, British Sociological Association, www.britsoc.org.uk; British Psychological Society, www.bps.org.uk). If a research project has ethical approval, this protects both the researched and the researchers but it is important to be aware of the limitations of ethical guidelines and committees. As Truman (2003) notes, it is impossible to be sure that the concerns of those approving a project will be the concerns of those being researched and as a project progresses it is likely that new issues will arise that no one has predicted.

Another early concern for the researcher is access to and recruitment of respondents. Different dilemmas will be encountered when focusing on an already established/identifiable group (such as hospital outpatients' group, counsellors at a pregnancy advisory service or a perinatal bereavement group) or when recruiting respondents via self-selection methods (such as through adverts in the media, at hospitals and doctors' surgeries). It may be necessary to access the first type of respondent via gatekeepers and the respondents themselves may worry about the effect being involved (or not being involved) in the research might have on their treatment. However, self-selecting respondent populations may have their own agendas and this may affect the data in terms of an overfocus on problems and negative experiences (Letherby, 2003).

Reproductive loss can be an emotive issue both for researchers and respondents and displays of emotion can be difficult and even dangerous for both the researcher and the researched. Angela McRobbie argues that the researcher may feel that they are 'holidaying on people's misery' and then leaving the respondent to deal with the consequences alone while they leave with what they came for (1982: 5). And as Janet Finch (1984) adds, giving people a chance to focus on an experience which is often 'taboo' can bring forward vulnerable people who may 'give away' more (both substantively and emotionally) than they later feel comfortable with. Barbara Katz-Rothman (1986), on the other hand, writes about how her research on reproductive loss made her feel:

> My next book is going to be on flower arranging. That seems safe enough – the sociology of flower arranging. That's the ticket. Something pleasant, lovely, no tears, no anguish. I need a rest.
>
> My last book ... was no joy. It was a book on women's experiences with amniocentesis for prenatal diagnosis ...
>
> It was like lifting the proverbial rock and having it all crawl out – ugliness, pain, grief, horror, anger, anguish, fear, sadness. Women in their fifth month of pregnancy afraid to feel their babies move – because they may not be babies at all, but genetic mistakes, eventual abortuses. Women having abortions but using the language of infanticide, because these are not 'accidental' pregnancies, but wanted babies. It was a nightmare. (Katz-Rothman, 1986: 48)

Despite this, others have argued that it is morally indefensible to distract someone from focusing on something that they feel the need to talk/write about, and being able to reflect on and re-evaluate experiences as part of the research can be therapeutic and/or help the respondent to re-evaluate their position (see Cotterill, 1992; Opie, 1992; Letherby, 2002). Geraldine Lee-Treweek and Stephanie Linkogle (2000) argue that it is possible to intellectualise away emotion by focusing upon other aspects of data, but they suggest that by using and analysing our emotional experiences we can add to our understandings of respondents' lives.

Bringing women and men 'back into' research on reproductive loss

Traditionally, social science was concerned with the public domain – the marketplace, the state, the workplace – 'the sphere where history is made' (Smith, 1974: 6). The personal and the private were of less interest and consequently many of the issues of particular concern to women where at best marginalised, at worst ignored. In 1987 Sandra Harding argued that while studying women was not new, studying them from the perspective of their own experiences so that women could understand themselves and their social world had 'virtually no history at all'. In the last 20 years things have improved, not least because of feminist influence in the social sciences. Women's lives are indeed more visible now and it is possible to argue that in some areas – family, health and reproduction included – more research is needed on male experience. David Morgan (1981; 1992) argues that if we are to 'take gender seriously', we must bring men back in. He adds that in accepting that 'man' is not the norm and 'woman' the deviation, we need to consider the social construction of both femininity and masculinity and focus our research on women's and men's experience.

Thinking specifically about reproduction, it is commonly assumed that this area of life is 'women's business'. However, most women do not make reproductive choices in isolation from men, and men, both as medics and as partners, have significant influence on women's experience (Annandale and Clark, 1996; Earle and Letherby, 2003; Abbott, Wallace and Tyler, 2005). Of course women are never just women and it is also important to consider how gender interacts with other differences such as ethnicity, age, sexuality and so on (Maynard, 1994; Doyal, 1995). Stereotypical assumptions about masculine behaviour may make it harder for men to express emotions such as grief and distress (Hochschild, 1983; James, 1989) which may result in male experience of reproductive loss being neglected, not least because of the problems in finding men willing to be involved in research (Letherby, 1993; Murphy, 1998). It is also likely that expectations of men to be 'strong' in such situations confirm the view that men suffer less, which in turn affects researchers', research funders' and ethics committees' views and deliberations when considering researching men's experience of reproductive loss.

Ironically, given the historical research focus on men and male experience, female researchers have traditionally been portrayed as 'more accessible and less threatening than men' which coupled with their 'superior' communicative abilities has thought to make the interactions of fieldwork generally easier (Warren, 1988: 45). This is not only sexist but denies the hard work that women and men do in the field. While there are suggestions that men may find it easier to talk to women if the topic is socially defined as 'female' (McKee and O'Brien, 1983), others argue that there needs to be more consideration of the significance of same and cross-gender researcher–respondent relationships (Padfield and Procter, 1996).

Politics and praxis when researching reproductive loss

As C. Wright Mills suggests:

> The social scientist is not some autonomous being standing outside society, the question is where he [*sic*] stands within it. (1959: 204)

Further, he encourages us:

> learn to use your life experience in your intellectual work: continually to examine it and interpret it. In this sense craftsmanship [*sic*] is the centre of yourself and you are personally involved in every intellectual product which you work. (ibid.: 216)

Nearly 50 years on it has now become commonplace for the researcher to locate her/himself within the research process and produce 'first person' accounts. This involves a recognition that, as researchers, we need to realise that our research activities tell us things about ourselves as well as about those we are researching (Steier, 1991). Further, there is recognition among social scientists that we need to consider how the researcher as author is positioned in relation to the research process: this includes reference to motivations and values and how the research process affects the research product in relation to choice and design of the project, fieldwork experience and analysis, editorship and presentation (Iles, 1992; Sparkes, 1998; Letherby, 2003).

It is recognised that many researchers are connected in some way to the issues that they research (Katz-Rothman, 1996) in terms of their own experience or that of someone close to them. This may be particularly the case in such an emotive issue as reproductive loss and clearly I am – as a biologically childless woman who has undertaken research on (among other things) miscarriage and 'infertility' and 'involuntary' childlessness[1] – an example of this. Yet, I suggest that research is always auto/biographical in that when reflecting on and writing our own autobiographies we reflect on our relationship with the biographies of others and when writing the biographies of others we inevitably refer to and reflect on our own autobiographies (Letherby, 2000). However, this does not mean that researchers should always do research on people like themselves (Wilkinson and Kitzinger, 1996). Research is not better or worse because we are closely connected to it by experience, but our connection does make a difference and we need to acknowledge this in our analysis and presentation of the data. Also, although not all researchers will be as affected as Katz-Rothman (1986, see above), research often promotes personal as well as intellectual growth and change for researchers.

Those who work for an emancipatory model of social research argue that in order to be ethically sound and non-exploitative, research should be 'for' rather than 'of' those that are studied (Oakley, 1981; 1999). From this perspective it is important to 'make research count' in policy and practice settings as well as in academic ones. But in order to do this researchers may need to find alternative ways – beyond the academy – to promote their work (Burawoy, 2005; Letherby and Bywaters, 2007). This may involve working closely with research stakeholders (including respondents and sometimes funders) and/or with the media.

Reflections

Since completing my first experience of research on reproductive loss I have conducted two other related studies. For my doctoral research I was concerned with exploring the social and emotional experience of 'infertility' and 'involuntary' childlessness (completed in 1997), and more recently, as part of a series of projects the experience of teenage pregnancy and young parenthood, a project focusing on the experiences of support prior to and following termination and miscarriage. Both of these projects have led me to reflect further on the issues considered here. Another researcher, with different personal concerns and research interests would likely to have written this short reading differently; yet another example of the significance of auto/biography. Nevertheless, just as research accounts are likely to have significance for others in similar situations, hopefully my research reflections resonate with other researchers' experiences.

Note

1   I write 'infertility' and 'involuntary' childlessness in single quotation marks to highlight the problems of definition.

References

Abbott, P. Wallace, C. and Tyler, M. (2005) *An Introduction to Sociology: Feminist Perspectives.* Third edition. London: Routledge

Annandale, E. and Clark, J. (1996) 'What is gender? Feminist theory and the sociology of human reproduction', *Sociology of Health and Illness*, 18 (1): 17–44.

Burawoy, M. (2005) 'For public sociology', *American Sociological Review* 70: 4–28.

Cotterill, P. (1992) 'Interviewing women: issues of friendship, vulnerability and power', *Women's Studies International Forum*, 15 (5/6): 593–606.

Cotterill, P. (1994) *Friendly Relations? Mothers and Their Daughters-In-Law.* London: Taylor and Francis.

de Crespigny, L. C. and McCullough, F. L. (1999) 'Mothers and babies, pregnant women and fetuses', *BJOG: An International Journal of Obstetrics and Gynaecology*, 106 (12): 1235–37.

Doyal, L. (1995) *What Makes Women Sick? Gender and the Political Economy of Health.* Basingstoke: Macmillan.

Earle, S. and Letherby, G. (eds) (2003) *Gender, Identity and Reproduction: Social Perspectives.* Basingstoke: Palgrave.

Exley, C. and Letherby, G. (2001) 'Managing a disrupted lifecourse: issues of identity and emotion work', *Health*, 5(1): 112–32.

Finch, J. (1984) '"It's great to have someone to talk to": the ethics and politics of interviewing women', in C. Bell. and H. Roberts (eds), *Social Researching: Politics, Problems, Practice.* London: Routledge and Kegan Paul. pp. 70–87.

Frost, J., Bradley, H., Levitas, R., Smith, L. and Garcia, J. (2007) 'The loss of possibility: scientisation of death and the special case of early miscarriage', *Sociology of Health and Illness*, 29 (7): 1003–22.

Harding, S. (1987) *Feminism and Methodology*. Milton Keynes: Open University Press.

Hamilton, B. E. and Ventura, S. J. (2006) 'Fertility and abortion rates in the United States, 1960–2002', *International Journal of Andrology*, 29 (1): 34–45.

Hochschild, A. R. (1983) *The Managed Heart: The Commercialisation of Human Feelings*. London: University of California.

Iles, T. (ed.) (1992) *All Sides of the Subject: Women and Biography*. New York: Teacher's College Press.

James, N. (1989) 'Emotional labour: skills and work in the social regulation of feelings', *Sociological Review*, 37 (1): 5–152.

Katz-Rothman, B. (1986) 'Reflections: on hard work', *Qualitative Sociology*, 9 (1): 48–53.

Katz-Rothman, B. (1996) 'Bearing witness: representing women's experiences of prenatal diagnosis', in S. Wilkinson and C. Kitzinger (eds), *Representing the Other: A Feminism and Psychology Reader*. London: Sage. pp. 50–2.

Kelly, L., Burton, S. and Regan, L. (1994) 'Researching women's lives or studying women's oppression? Reflections on what constitutes feminist research', in M. Maynard and J. Purvis (eds), *Researching Women's Lives From a Feminist Perspective*. London: Taylor and Francis. pp.27–48.

Lee-Treweek, G. and Linkogle, S. (eds) (2000) *Danger in the Field: Risk and Ethics in Social Research*. London: Routledge.

Letherby, G. (1993) 'The meanings of miscarriage', *Women's Studies International Forum*, 16 (2): 165–180.

Letherby, G. (2000) 'Dangerous liaisons: auto/biography in research and research writing', in G. Lee-Treweek and S. Linkogle (eds), *Danger in the Field: Risk and Ethics in Social Research*. London: Routledge. pp. 91–113.

Letherby, G. (2002) 'Challenging dominant discourses: identity and change and the experience of "infertility" and "involuntary childlessness"', *Journal of Gender Studies*, 11: (3): 277–88.

Letherby, G. (2003) *Feminist Research in Theory and Practice*. Buckingham: Open University Press.

Letherby, G. and Zdrokowski, D. (1995) 'Dear researcher: the use of correspondence as a method within feminist qualitative research', *Gender and Society*, 9(5): 576–93.

Letherby, G. and Bywaters, P. (2007) *Extending Social Research: Application, Implementation, Presentation*. Buckingham: Open University Press.

Lovell, A. (1983). 'Some questions of identity: late miscarriage, stillbirth and perinatal loss', *Social Science and Medicine*, 17 (11): 755–61.

Maynard, M. (1994) '"Race", gender and the concept of "difference" in feminist thought', in H. Asfar and M. Maynard (eds), *The Dynamics of 'Race' and Gender: Some Feminist Interventions*. London: Taylor and Francis. pp. 9–25.

McKee, L. and O'Brien, M. (1983) 'Interviewing men: taking gender seriously', in E. Gamarnikow, D. Morgan, J. Purvis and D. Taylorson (eds), *The Public and the Private: Social Patterns of Gender Relation*. London: Heinemann.

McRobbie, A. (1982) 'The politics of feminist research: between talk, text and action', *Feminist Review*, 12: 26–57.

Mills, C. W. (1959) *The Sociological Imagination*. London: Penguin.

Morgan, D. (1981) 'Men, masculinity and the process of sociological inquiry', in H. Roberts, (ed.), *Doing Feminist Research*. London: Routledge and Kegan Paul. pp. 83–113.

Morgan, D. (1992) *Discovering Men*. London: Routledge.

Murphy, F. A. (1998) 'The experience of early miscarriage from a male perspective', *Journal of Clinical Nursing*, 7(4): 325 32.

Oakley, A. (1981) 'Interviewing women: a contradiction in terms?', in H. Roberts (ed.), *Doing Feminist Research*. London: Routledge. pp. 30–61.

Oakley, A. (1999) 'People's ways of knowing: gender and methodology', in S. Hood, B. Mayall and S. Oliver (eds), *Critical Issues in Social Research*. Buckingham: Open University Press. pp. 154–70.

Oakley, A. (2004) 'Response to "Quoting and counting: an autobiographical response to Oakley"', *Sociology,* 38 (1): 191–2.

Opie, A. (1992) 'Qualitative research, appropriation of the "other" and empowerment', *Feminist Review*, 40: 52–69.

Padfield, M. and Proctor, L. (1996) 'The effect of interviewer's gender on the interviewing process: a comparative enquiry', *Sociology,* 30 (2): 355–66.

Price, J. (1988) *Motherhood: What it Does to Your Mind.* London: Pandora Press.

Reinharz, S. (1992) *Feminist Methods in Social Research.* Oxford: Oxford University Press.

Smith, D. (1974) 'Women, the family and corporate capitalism', in M.L. Stephenson (ed.), *Women in Canada.* Toronto: New Press.

Sparkes, A. (1998) 'Reciprocity in critical research? Some unsettling thoughts', in G. Shacklock and J. Smyth (eds), *Being Reflexive in Critical and Social Educational Research.* London: Falmer. pp. 67–82.

Stanley, L. and Wise, S. (1993) *Breaking Out Again: Feminist Ontology and Epistemology.* London: Routledge.

Steier, F. (1991) *Research and Reflexivity.* London: Sage.

Truman, C. (2003) 'Ethics and the ruling relations of research', *Sociological Research Online,* 8(1) www.socresonline.org.uk/8/1/truman.

Warren, C. (1988) *Gender Issues in Field Research.* Newbury Park, CA: Sage.

Wilkinson, S. and Kitzinger, C. (eds) (1996) *Representing the Other.* London: Sage.

34

Bridging the Gap between Research and Practice in Bereavement

Bridging Work Group[1]

The existence of a gap between research and practice in the area of bereavement is part of a larger problem that plagues many fields […]. Many practitioners regard research as holding little relevance for their work, and many researchers believe that clinical practice has little to contribute to the scientific study of bereavement. Consider the conclusions of the editor of the respected peer-reviewed journal *Family Process*:

> Many clinicians tell me that they neither read nor value the research data being produced, and that they basically fail to see any relationship it has to the realities of their practice. … While clinicians ignore research, many investigators dismiss clinical knowledge and skills. Many admit that they do not seek to integrate the clinical wisdom of therapists and teachers, and do not believe such an integration would improve the quality and relevance of the research they conduct. (Anderson, 2003, p. 323–324).

In the view of some scholars, diametrically opposed values maintain the gap and obstruct efforts to bridge it. Many clinicians find only such ideas as self-actualization and human potential personally meaningful and consider only qualitative, in-depth descriptive studies capable of capturing the complexity of human intentionality. In contrast, many researchers spurn these humanistic concepts as lacking empirical foundation and prefer concepts that can be reliably measured and tested using quantitative methods (Sheldon et al., 2003).

Connecting practitioners and researchers in bereavement

Some efforts have occurred in the past several years to address the gap between research and practice of those working in the areas of death, dying, and bereavement. […]

Excerpts from 'Bridging the gap between research and practice in bereavement' by Bridging Work Group, *Death Studies*, 29: 93–122, 2005, Taylor & Francis, reprinted by kind permission of the publisher and Irwin Sandler (Taylor & Francis, www.informaworld.com).

The current article reports on the work of the group on bridging the gap between research and practice (which will be referred to as the *Bridging Group*) including our conceptual framework [...] and recommendations for activities to bridge the gap between bereavement research and practice.

Orienting conceptual framework

Three basic assumptions provided the orienting framework for The Bridging Group: (a) Researchers and practitioners have much to learn from each other. (b) The bridge between researchers and practitioners is bi-directional, so that information needs to flow both ways in order to improve research and practice. (c) Recommendations for directions to bridge the gap must be based on an understanding of the current nature of the gap between research and practice.

The Bridging Group conceptualized the gap as a problem of cross-cultural communication. [...] Dramatically differing values, rewards, work settings and approaches to work separate the cultures of grief researchers and of practitioners (Jordan, 2000a; Silverman, 2000). To begin, let us consider the culture of practitioners.

One group of practitioners is hospice caregivers. Hospice caregivers provide a variety of services to terminally ill persons, and what counts ultimately is relieving the manifold forms of pain (physical, interpersonal, emotional, spiritual) so that hospice patients die a good death. Decision making in hospice is time-limited and situation-bound, namely, what will help this dying person at this time. Promotion and salary merit increases are linked to quality work as part of an interdisciplinary team. The work life of the hospice worker is dominated by the crush of demands to meet pressing (and emotionally demanding) needs of patients' and the practical requirements to complete necessary paperwork. Administrators in non-profit practice settings are under continuous pressure to secure adequate funding so that caregivers can meet the daily needs of their clients/patients. In an environment driven by these daily pressures, low priority is given to reading research papers on interesting but somewhat esoteric issues that do not speak to the immediate pressures of the job.

Now let us consider the culture of grief researchers. Many grief researchers work as faculty in university environments that value and expect contributions to prestigious peer-reviewed journals that often give priority to findings of theoretical rather than practical significance. Promotion, prestige, and salary merit increases depend heavily on success as a researcher, which is assessed by record of publications, citations by other scholars in the field, and obtaining external funding for research. Although teaching and public service are valued, they are secondary to success in scholarship and research. Questions driving researchers often have high general theoretical significance to their discipline, but seldom focus on practical issues that are relevant to the everyday realities of practitioners' needs. While there are growing expectations from major funding sources that researchers will work as part of interdisciplinary teams, the focus of this work is often on theoretical issues that cut across disciplines rather than on solving practical problems of society. Research universities structure faculty time so that they have time to devote to thinking about issues of theoretical and long-term interest to the discipline rather than be distracted by short-term problems of the organization, which are often the domain of a subgroup of faculty who specialize in university administration.

Bridging the gap separating the two cultures of research and practice requires understanding of and appreciation for the different values, rewards, work settings, and approaches to work that separate these two cultures (Jordan, 2000a; Neimeyer, 2000). Collaboration, under-standing, and mutual appreciation will produce practitioners and researchers informed by the different issues important to the diverse stakeholders in the health care and research systems, by the need for respectful translation of what practitioners and researchers do, and by orga-nizational assessments that identify institutional beliefs, practices, and rewards.

The connections between research and practice in the bereavement field are especially complex because both researchers and practitioners are engaged in work encompassing the tripartite continuum: treatment, problem prevention, and health promotion. These points on the continuum each ask specific questions using distinctive and often overlapping the-oretical models and research methods. Training in both research and practice occurs within specific academic disciplines, and licensed practitioners remain accountable for regulation of practice to their disciplines. For these reasons, the gaps between research and practice in bereavement have multiple locations and dimensions. [...]

Steps toward bridging the gap

We recognized that developing a bridging plan would need to occur in steps and would involve both conceptualizing the issues and making initial recommendations and mobiliz-ing key organizations to focus on the agenda of bridging the gap between research and practice. As a first step in conceptualizing the issues, we identified three actions salient to bridging the research-practice gap. These actions are (a) promoting, teaching, and engag-ing in evidence-based practice; (b) using multi-systemic approaches to generate and dis-seminate research and practice innovations; and (c) identifying and evaluating common and divergent conceptual frame-works and assumptions that guide research and practice.

Promoting evidence-based practice

In health care disciplines, the most widely accepted definitions of evidence-based practice are adapted from Sackett and associates (2000; see Institue of Medicine, 2001) who empha-size integrating clinical expertise with preeminent research evidence and patient values. While it was not the job of the Working Group to resolve the differences of opinion in the field, we recognized that valuable evidence can emerge from quantitative studies (e.g., ran-domized controlled trials of interventions), qualitative studies and clinical practice and that each type of evidence has critical strengths and limitations. For example, properly con-ducted randomized experimental trials provide the most convincing evidence concerning the effects of an intervention program to affect specified outcomes. The evaluation of ran-domized trials has progressed to address increasingly complex and interesting questions such as What are the processes that mediate the effects of interventions? How do the effects differ across sub-groups of the population? and What are the long-term effects of interven-tions over time? (Flay, 1986). However, these trials often are conducted under conditions that do not match the settings in which practice is usually conducted or the types of clients typically seen in practice settings, limiting their direct applicability to practice (Flay, 1986). Also, these trials are very expensive and are relatively rare in the bereavement area.

Qualitative methods offer some distinct advantages when studying complex processes or at an exploratory phase of research (Denzin & Lincoln, 2000). Qualitative methods are especially useful for intensively examining little-known complex social phenomena. Examples are Myra Bluebond-Langner's (1978) study of terminally ill children, Dennis Klass's (1988; 1999) studies of bereaved parents, Glaser and Strauss's (1965, 1968) studies of how dying is managed in a hospital, and Janice Nadeau's (1998) study of family meaning-making. Qualitative methods help bring to life people, problems, and situations, and give a human face to research. These methods enable researchers to learn people's perceptions and motives in depth. At the same time, however, for an increase of understanding, qualitative researchers sacrifice the precision of measurement offered by quantitative research (Stake, 2000). Qualitative research typically is limited to examining a few cases and cannot produce generalizable results. While qualitative research can test nomothetic causal hypotheses (e.g., see Chambliss, 1996; Van DerWal, 2001), it cannot rule out extraneous influences and alternative explanations and therefore provides a limited methodology for testing hypotheses (Chambliss & Schutt, 2003). Some researchers propose using mixed-methods research, in which both quantitative and qualitative methods are used to explore appropriate questions in complementary ways (Neimeyer & Hogan, 2001; Tashakkori & Teddli, 2003).

Most of the research evidence on practice currently available has been generated in academic settings under conditions and with populations that do not translate well into diverse practice contexts. In response, practitioners and funders have intensified support for practice-based research, in which clinicians in diverse settings collaborate with each other and with academic centers on the design, implementation, and evaluation of interventions (Hayes, Barlow, & Nelson-Gray, 1999; Nutting, Beasley, & Werner, 1999). Fundamentally, practice-based research studies compare patient outcomes or rates of change for a group receiving a particular intervention as compared with a group that did not receive the care. Participants in the intervention and comparison groups are matched as closely as possible for characteristics like age that might contribute to those outcomes. Practitioners in a number of disciplines, including primary care family physicians, nurses, and clinical psychologists, have created practice-based research networks in which participants decide together on tools for implementing and evaluating an intervention (Brokevec, Echementia, Ragusea, & Ruiz, 2001). Networking practice-based research makes it possible to increase sample size and share dissemination and implementation of findings.

[…]

Using multi-systemic approaches to generate and disseminate research and practice innovations

Disseminating new information requires identifying the multiple stakeholders who have an impact on the flow and synthesis of information and/or who are gatekeepers of the implementation of research findings. Although interventions in any sphere may improve the process of bridging the research-practice gap, we assert that attending to the complexity in these multiple systems and appreciating institutional constraints on dissemination and implementation will most effectively span the divide. Stakeholders include, among others, service providers from different disciplines and in different settings, health care systems, funders of bereavement services and research, the public that uses bereavement services, students in many social science and human service fields, and researchers in the area of bereavement. Each category of stakeholder brings its own perspective on the issues involved in developing evidence-based practice and needs to be involved in developing approaches in bridging the gap between research and practice (Kellam & Langevin, 2003). Furthermore, different stakeholders may rely on different mechanisms to obtain knowledge of new innovations and emerging findings, and different sources of information may have different credibility for different groups. For example, practitioners and researchers may rely on different sources of information and may have different standards for what they consider as credible and valuable information. One step toward bridging the gap between research and practice is to better understand the sources of information that are used and valued by these groups.

Identifying and evaluating conceptual frameworks that guide research and practice

Over the past decade many of the preeminent conceptual frameworks in bereavement have been challenged. For instance, attention has been called to the importance of unmasking myths about loss and grief (Wortman & Silver, 1989, 2001), of extending coping with loss beyond the grief work hypothesis (Stroebe & Schut, 1999, 2001), of questioning the effectiveness of interventions that are simply assumed to be helpful for all mourners (Jordan & Neimeyer, 2003), and of understanding the implications of approaches that might pathologize cultural differences or individual variation in grief responses (Shapiro, 1996; Dennis Klass, personal communication, March 1, 2004; Walter, 1999). Questions about the dominant conceptual frameworks provide challenges for both research and practice. Research needs to develop and test theoretical models that may be derived from different conceptual perspectives, and may require new measures and new methodologies. Practitioners need to reconsider the outcomes of their work, and how they can resolve their practice with emerging empirical evidence concerning who needs and benefits from services. We maintain that the challenges to both research and practice should serve as an impetus for greater collaboration between the two endeavors.

[…]

Recommendations for bridging the gap between research and practice

The Bridging Group found both areas of divergence and potential pathways for connection between researchers and practitioners, and that bridging the gap between these two cultures will require change in both research and practice. There are important findings from research that should now be integrated into practice and there remains a critical need for more research on the effectiveness of services currently being offered. Recent literature reviews have suggested that there is a disturbing lack of demonstrated efficacy for many bereavement interventions (Jordan & Neimeyer, 2003). We are concerned about the apparent lack of time, knowledge, and willingness among bereavement caregivers to keep current with research in grief studies that might improve their practice. We are also concerned that on the part of researchers, there appears to be a frequent failure to design, implement and disseminate studies that will have a direct benefit to caregivers and the bereaved. However, ensuring that high-quality research is synthesized and used in practice settings requires closer collaboration and respectful two-way communication between researchers and practitioners.

We offer three principles to help build a bridge between researchers and practitioners. These principles apply equally to those interested in improving services to the bereaved, including researchers, practitioners, administrators, curriculum writers, students, and funding agencies. In addition, we offer specific recommendations for researchers, practitioners, and professional organizations and training programs.

Principle 1: Recognize that researchers and practitioners live in very different cultures, with different norms, values, priorities and ways of construing bereavement and the professional world in which they must function (Silverman, 2000). Therefore, both researchers and practitioners should educate themselves about the worldview, working environments, resources, strengths and constraints of the settings in which the other functions.

Principle 2: Recognize that communication between researchers and practitioners is a reciprocal process. The responsibility for fostering communication between the two cultures lies with professionals engaged in each activity. Efforts to bridge the gap will require efforts on the part of all concerned to communicate with those from the other culture.

Principle 3: Foster dialogue and collaboration between researchers and practitioners. This includes use of print and electronic media, professional meetings, training programs, continuing education seminars and actual participation in each other's professional activities. Extend the dialogue to also include other stakeholders in bereavement care, including consumers of bereavement services, managed care and insurance companies, students in training to be either researchers or practitioners and the large number of lay and paraprofessional caregivers who also deliver assistance to the bereaved (funeral directors, support group facilitators and emergency personnel). In order to translate these principles into practice we make the following recommendations.

Recommendations for practitioners

Practitioners and encouraged to:

1   Expose themselves to research that has implications for improving the delivery of services. Do this "ongoing learning" regularly through reading of books and journals, attendance at research oriented workshops and conferences, and through Web-based resources.
2   Base interactions with clients on clearly articulated theory that has been supported by empirical research. Be appropriately cautious about new models and techniques that lack empirical support. Practitioners should investigate whether there are empirical data to support the efficacy of new models and interventions they employ.
3   Be willing to reconsider and revise theoretical models, care delivery programs, and clinical practices based on new information emerging from research.
4   Obtain knowledge and skills that enable them to critically evaluate both qualitative and quantitative studies in bereavement care. This knowledge acquisition

includes gaining a basic understanding of the requirements and constraints of the scientific method needed to produce meaningful and valid information.

5   Incorporate relevant research findings into the content of their educational and training efforts, whether to professionals or the public (see *Recommendations* for educational organizations and training programs below).

6   Look for opportunities to participate in the design, implementation, write-up dissemination, and evaluation of research that is relevant to their practice. When this participation is not possible, cultivate person-to-person relationships with researchers in the field whose work they find relevant.

7   Integrate research findings and research practices into the regular work of their setting or agencies. Encourage program administrators to include time for the review of research in the job descriptions of their staff. Share findings from new studies in staff meetings and case presentations. Ask staff who have attended conferences, participated in Internet discussions or read about research findings in books and articles to summarize those findings for other staff on regular occasions. Encourage the development of ongoing evaluation of clinical services delivered in their setting.

Recommendations for researchers

Researchers are encouraged to:

1   Expose themselves to the loss experiences that are central to the work of bereavement caregivers. For example, consider participation in the delivery of services to dying and bereaved persons. This participation could include obtaining supervised clinical training, either paid or volunteered. Researchers should also make explicit the foundations of their research, including the theoretical models and personal loss experiences that have shaped their choice of research questions, methods and conclusions.

2   Design research that will be of relevance to practitioners and consumers of bereavement care. Focus on investigations that take into account the complexity, flexibility, and adaptation required to provide services in actual practice settings. Use multiple methods of research design, including qualitative methodology, for identification and exploration of bereavement phenomena. Also use practice-based effectiveness studies of clinical services as they are actually delivered to obtain information on the usefulness of new and existing interventions.

3   Pay particular attention to the validity and reliability of measurement methods as they apply to the experience of loss. For example, the use of standard measures of psychiatric symptoms as outcome measures alone may be inadequate to assess many grief-related phenomena.

4   Develop collaborative teams of practitioners, consumers, and researchers who will be involved in the conceptualization, design, implementation, analysis, dissemination, and evaluation of studies that may have a bearing on the delivery of services to the dying and bereaved. Conduct studies that pay particular attention to research problems that are identified "in the field" as important problems for practitioners. Enhance this process by developing personal relationships with

bereavement practitioners. Seek feedback from recipients of bereavement care regarding the design of measures and studies.

5   Include in the dissemination of their research studies more thorough discussions of the clinical implications of their findings for practitioners and consumers of services. Pay attention to the specific changes in clinical models and techniques that may be implied by the findings of studies. Keep in mind that many people who deliver bereavement care may have little or no professional training in bereavement care (such as lay facilitators of bereavement support groups, funeral directors, etc.). Make the report of findings simple, clear, and understandable for all potential audiences.

6   Include relevant clinical material such as case studies, audio and videotapes of clinical work, and discussions with providers and recipients of end-of-life and bereavement care services when providing training in research methods.

7   Seek multiple modalities for disseminating the results of their research to practitioners and consumers. These dissemination sources include books, professional journals, the Internet, professional and lay conferences, academic course content, print and electronic media, and independent organizations.

Recommendations for educational organizations and training programs

Recognizing that professional organizations and training programs have a key role to play in bridging the gap, we encourage such groups to:

1   Encourage instructors for courses, seminars, symposia, conferences, and workshops to include updates on research that is relevant to practitioners.

2   Provide opportunities for instruction in the methods and utilization of research for new and experienced practitioners as part of their training.

3   Encourage researchers in their programs to participate in the direct delivery of services as part of their training.

4   Create multiple venues for interaction and dialogue between researchers and practitioners. These venues could include pre-meeting institutes and symposia at conferences, organization newsletters, Internet web sites, and other settings where researchers could learn from one another.

Conclusion

[…] We see this report as one step to advance an ongoing process that will need to include active efforts of researchers, practitioners, as well as major organizations that are involved in the field to build a bridge between science and service, and thereby strengthen our understanding of bereavement and care for the bereaved.

Note

1. The Bridging Work Group consisted of Irwin Sandler, Chair, and (in alphabetical order) David Balk, John Jordan, Cara Kennedy, Janice Nadeau, Ester Shapiro. The manuscript is a revision of a report developed for the Center for the Advancement of Health, which provided support for the development of the project. Special appreciation is expressed to Tracy Kolian and Janice Genevro who managed the development of the report for the Center for the Advancement of Health.

References

Anderson, C.M. (2003). Cassandra notes on the state of the family research and practice union. *Family Process, 42,* 323–329.

Bluebond-Langner, M. (1978). *The private worlds of dying children.* Princeton, NJ: Princeton University Press.

Borkovec, T.D., Echemendia, R.J., Ragusea, S.A., and Ruiz, M. (2001). The Pennsylvania Practice Research Network and future possibilities for clinically meaningful and scientifically rigorous psychotherapy effectiveness research. *Clinical Psychology: Science and Practice, 8,* 155–167.

Chambliss, D.F. (1996). *Beyond caring: Hospitals, nurses, and the social organization of ethics.* Chicago: University of Chicago Press.

Chambliss, D.F and Schutt, R.K. (2003). *Making sense of the social world: Methods of investigation.* Thousand Oaks, CA: Pine Forge Press.

Denzin, N. and Lincon, Y. (2000). *Handbook of qualitative research* (2nd ed.). Thousand Oaks, CA: Sage.

Flay, B.R. (1986). Efficacy and effectiveness trials (and other phases or research) in the development of health promotion programs. *Preventive Medicine, 15,* 451–474.

Glaser, B. and Strauss, A. (1965). *Awareness of dying.* Chicago: Aldine.

Glaser, B. and Strauss, A. (1968). *Time for dying.* Chicago: Aldine.

Hayes, S.C., Barlow, D.H., and Nelson-Gray, R.O. (1999). *The scientist practitioner: Research and accountability in the age of managed care.* Boston: Allyn & Bacon.

Institute of Medicine. (2001). *Crossing the quality chasm: A new health system for the 21st century.* Washington, DC: The National Academies Press.

Jordan, J.R. (2000a). Research that matters: Bridging the gap between research and practice in thanatology. *Death Studies, 24,* 457–468.

Jordon, J.R. and Neimeyer, R.A. (2003). Does grief counseling work? *Death Studies, 27,* 765–786.

Kellam, S.G. and Langevin, D.J. (2003). A framework for understanding "evidence" in prevention research and programs. *Prevention Science, 4*(3), 137–153.

Klass, D. (1988). *Parental grief: Solace and resolution.* New York: Springer.

Klass, D. (1999). *The spiritual lives of bereaved parents.* Philadelphia: Brunner/Mazel.

Nadeau, J.W. (1998). *Families making sense of death.* Thousand Oaks, CA: Sage.

Neimeyer, R.A. (2000). Grief therapy and research as essential tensions: Prescriptions for a progressive partnership. *Death Studies, 24,* 603–610.

Neimeyer, R.A. and Hogan, N. (2001). Quantitative or qualitative? Measurement issues in the study of grief. In M.S. Stroebe and R.O. Hansson et al. (eds), *Handbook of bereavement research: Consequences, coping and care* (pp. 89–118). Washington, DC: American Psychological Association.

Nutting, P.A., Beasley, J.W., and Werner, J.J. (1999). Practice-based research networks answer primary care questions. *Journal of the American Medical Association, 37*, 1092–1104.

Sackett, D.L. Straus, S.E., Richardson, W.S., Rosenberg, W., and Haynes, R.B. (2000) *Evidence-based medicine: How to practice and teach EBM* (2nd ed.). New York: Churchill Livingstone.

Shapiro, E. (1996). Family bereavement and cultural diversity: A social developmental perspective. *Family Process, 35*, 313–332.

Sheldon, K.M., Joiner, T.E., Pettit, J.W., and Williams, G. (2003). Reconciling humanistic ideals and scientific clinical practice. *Clinical Psychology: Science & Practice 10*, 302–315.

Silverman, P.R. (2000). Research, clinical practice, and the human experience: Putting the pieces together. *Death Studies, 24*, 469–478.

Stake, R.E. (2000). Program evaluation particularly responsive evaluation. In D.L. Stufflebeam, G.F. Madaus, and T. Kellaghan (eds), *Evaluation models: Viewpoints on educational and human services evaluation* (pp. 343–362). Boston: Kluwer Academic Publishers.

Strobe, M.S. and Schut, H. (1999). The dual process model of coping with bereavement: Rationale and description. *Death Studies, 23*, 197–224.

Strobe, M.S. and Schut, H. (2001). Models of coping with bereavement: A review. In M.S. Stroebe, R.O. Hansson, W. Stroebe, and H. Schut (eds), *Handbook of bereavement research: Consequences, coping, and care* (pp. 375–403). Washington, DC: American Psychological Association.

Tashakkori, A. and Teddli, C. (2003). *Handbook of mixed-methods in social and behavioral research*. Thousand Oaks, CA: Sage.

Van Der Wal, D.M. (2001). *The maintenance of a caring concern by the care-giver*. Unpublished doctoral dissertation, University of South Africa.

Walter, T. (1999). *On bereavement: the culture of grief.* Buckingham, England: Open University Press.

Wortman, C.B. and Silver, R.C. (1989). The myths of coping with loss. *Journal of Consulting and Clinical Psychology, 57*, 349–357.

Wortman, C.B. and Silver R.C. (2001). The myths of coping with loss revisited. In M.S. Stroebe, R.O. Hansson, W. Stroebe and H. Schut (eds), *Handbook of bereavement research: Consequences, coping, and care* (pp. 405–429). Washington, DC: American Psychological Association.

Index